Head and Neck Surgery: Clinical Updates and Perspectives

Head and Neck Surgery: Clinical Updates and Perspectives

Editors

Luca Giovanni Locatello
Oreste Gallo

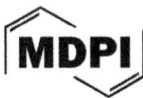

Basel • Beijing • Wuhan • Barcelona • Belgrade • Novi Sad • Cluj • Manchester

Editors
Luca Giovanni Locatello
Udine University Hospital
Udine, Italy

Oreste Gallo
Careggi University Hospital
Florence, Italy

Editorial Office
MDPI
St. Alban-Anlage 66
4052 Basel, Switzerland

This is a reprint of articles from the Special Issue published online in the open access journal *Journal of Clinical Medicine* (ISSN 2077-0383) (available at: https://www.mdpi.com/journal/jcm/special_issues/complications_head_neck_surgery).

For citation purposes, cite each article independently as indicated on the article page online and as indicated below:

Lastname, A.A.; Lastname, B.B. Article Title. *Journal Name* **Year**, *Volume Number*, Page Range.

ISBN 978-3-0365-9248-0 (Hbk)
ISBN 978-3-0365-9249-7 (PDF)
doi.org/10.3390/books978-3-0365-9249-7

© 2023 by the authors. Articles in this book are Open Access and distributed under the Creative Commons Attribution (CC BY) license. The book as a whole is distributed by MDPI under the terms and conditions of the Creative Commons Attribution-NonCommercial-NoDerivs (CC BY-NC-ND) license.

Contents

About the Editors . . . . **vii**

Luca Giovanni Locatello and Oreste Gallo
The Many Faces of Head and Neck Surgery in 2022 and Looking Ahead!
Reprinted from: *J. Clin. Med.* **2022**, *11*, 3174, doi:10.3390/jcm11113174 . . . . **1**

Luca Giovanni Locatello, Giuseppe Licci, Giandomenico Maggiore and Oreste Gallo
Non-Surgical Strategies for Assisting Closure of Pharyngocutaneous Fistula after Total Laryngectomy: A Systematic Review of the Literature
Reprinted from: *J. Clin. Med.* **2022**, *11*, 100, doi:10.3390/jcm11010100 . . . . **5**

Cheng-Hsun Chuang, Tzu-Yen Huang, Tzer-Zen Hwang, Che-Wei Wu, I-Cheng Lu, Pi-Ying Chang, et al.
Accumulation of Experience and Newly Developed Devices Can Improve the Safety and Voice Outcome of Total Thyroidectomy for Graves' Disease
Reprinted from: *J. Clin. Med.* **2022**, *11*, 1298, doi:10.3390/jcm11051298 . . . . **17**

Konstantinos Mantsopoulos, Michael Koch, Heinrich Iro and Jannis Constantinidis
Olfactory Neuroblastomas: What Actually Happens in the Long-Term?
Reprinted from: *J. Clin. Med.* **2022**, *11*, 2288, doi:10.3390/jcm11092288 . . . . **27**

Stéphane Hans, Grégoire Vialatte de Pemille, Robin Baudouin, Aude Julien-Laferriere, Florent Couineau, Lise Crevier-Buchman, et al.
Post-Laryngectomy Voice Prosthesis Changes by Speech-Language Pathologists: Preliminary Results
Reprinted from: *J. Clin. Med.* **2022**, *11*, 4113, doi:10.3390/jcm11144113 . . . . **41**

Giancarlo Pecorari, Giuseppe Riva, Andrea Albera, Ester Cravero, Elisabetta Fassone, Andrea Canale and Roberto Albera
Post-Operative Infections in Head and Neck Cancer Surgery: Risk Factors for Different Infection Sites
Reprinted from: *J. Clin. Med.* **2022**, *11*, 4969, doi:10.3390/jcm11174969 . . . . **45**

Stéphane Hans, Robin Baudouin, Marta P. Circiu, Florent Couineau, Quentin Lisan, Lise Crevier-Buchman and Jérôme R. Lechien
Open Partial Laryngectomies: History of Laryngeal Cancer Surgery
Reprinted from: *J. Clin. Med.* **2022**, *11*, 5352, doi:10.3390/jcm11185352 . . . . **55**

Mélanie Gigot, Antoine Digonnet, Alexandra Rodriguez and Jerome R. Lechien
Salvage Partial Laryngectomy after Failed Radiotherapy: Oncological and Functional Outcomes
Reprinted from: *J. Clin. Med.* **2022**, *11*, 5411, doi:10.3390/jcm11185411 . . . . **67**

Pierre Philouze, Olivier Malard, Sébastien Albert, Lionel Badet, Bertrand Baujat, Frédéric Faure, et al.
A New Animal Model of Laryngeal Transplantation
Reprinted from: *J. Clin. Med.* **2022**, *11*, 6427, doi:10.3390/jcm11216427 . . . . **77**

Peter Kántor, Lucia Staníková, Anna Švejdová, Karol Zeleník and Pavel Komínek
Narrative Review of Classification Systems Describing Laryngeal Vascularity Using Advanced Endoscopic Imaging
Reprinted from: *J. Clin. Med.* **2023**, *12*, 10, doi:10.3390/jcm12010010 . . . . **85**

Urszula Kacorzyk, Marek Kentnowski, Cezary Szymczyk, Ewa Chmielik, Barbara Bobek-Billewicz, Krzysztof Składowski and Tomasz Wojciech Rutkowski
Results of Primary Treatment and Salvage Treatment in the Management of Patients with Non-Squamous Cell Malignant Tumors of the Sinonasal Region: Single Institution Experience
Reprinted from: *J. Clin. Med.* **2023**, *12*, 1953, doi:10.3390/jcm12051953 . . . . **99**

Gabriele Molteni, Nicole Caiazza, Gianfranco Fulco, Andrea Sacchetto, Antonio Gulino and Daniele Marchioni
Functioning Endocrine Outcome after Endoscopic Endonasal Transsellar Approach for Pituitary Neuroendocrine Tumors
Reprinted from: *J. Clin. Med.* **2023**, *12*, 2986, doi:10.3390/jcm12082986 . . . . **115**

Marta Rogalska, Lukasz Antkowiak, Anna Kasperczuk, Wojciech Scierski and Maciej Misiolek
Transoral Robotic Surgery in the Management of Submandibular Gland Sialoliths: A Systematic Review
Reprinted from: *J. Clin. Med.* **2023**, *12*, 3007, doi:10.3390/jcm12083007 . . . . **127**

Angelo Eplite, Claudio Vicini, Giuseppe Meccariello, Giannicola Iannella, Antonino Maniaci, Angelo Cannavicci, et al.
Multi-Level 3D Surgery for Obstructive Sleep Apnea: Could It Be the Future?
Reprinted from: *J. Clin. Med.* **2023**, *12*, 4173, doi:10.3390/jcm12134173 . . . . **137**

Serena Jiang, Luca Giovanni Locatello, Giandomenico Maggiore and Oreste Gallo
Radiomics-Based Analysis in the Prediction of Occult Lymph Node Metastases in Patients with Oral Cancer: A Systematic Review
Reprinted from: *J. Clin. Med.* **2023**, *12*, 4958, doi:10.3390/jcm12154958 . . . . **143**

About the Editors

Luca Giovanni Locatello

Luca Giovanni Locatello, MD, is an Otorhinolaryngologist who is currently working at the Department of Otorhinolaryngology at the Academic Hospital, "Santa Maria della Misericordia", ASUFC, Udine, Italy. After graduating cum laude from the University of Udine, he completed a residency in Otorhinolaryngology at the University of Pisa and in Florence, Italy. He has authored over 70 scientific papers in peer-reviewed journals regarding many fields of the ear, nose, and throat.

Oreste Gallo

Oreste Gallo, MD, is a Full Professor and the Chief of the Department of Otorhinolaryngology at the Careggi University Hospital, University of Florence, Florence, Italy. He graduated from and completed his residency in Otorhinolaryngology at the University of Florence, Italy. He has performed thousands of ear, nose, and throat surgical procedures and has a particular interest in oncological head and neck surgery. He has published over 200 scientific articles, investigating a myriad of biological and surgical issues in this discipline.

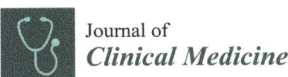

Editorial

The Many Faces of Head and Neck Surgery in 2022 and Looking Ahead!

Luca Giovanni Locatello [1],* and Oreste Gallo [2,3]

1. Department of Otorhinolaryngology, Sant'Antonio Abate Hospital, Azienda Sanitaria Universitaria Friuli Centrale, 33028 Tolmezzo, Italy
2. Department of Otorhinolaryngology, Careggi University Hospital, Largo Brambilla 3, 50134 Florence, Italy; oreste.gallo@unifi.it
3. Department of Clinical and Experimental Medicine, University of Florence, 50139 Firenze, Italy
* Correspondence: lucagiovanni.locatello@asufc.sanita.fvg.it; Tel.: +39-0433488679

Head and neck (HN) cancer, which mainly presents in the form of squamous cell carcinoma, was the seventh most common cancer worldwide in 2018, with approximately 890,000 new cases and 450,000 deaths [1]. Its incidence is rising in both less developed countries, due to the increased exposure to classical risk factors (tobacco smoking and alcohol), as well as in high-income nations, due to the spreading of high-risk serotypes of human papillomavirus (HPV-16 and HPV-18) [2]. Survival rates range from 70–80% at five years for early HN cancer (i.e., with neither nodal metastasis at presentation nor evidence of extra-organ extension) to an estimated overall survival of 30–40% at advanced stages [1,2]. Unfortunately, the latter is the most common clinical presentation, and a recent study from the USA showed that the age-adjusted incidence rates for stage IV HN cancer have significantly increased by 26.1% over the last two decades [3].

The first historical report of such a disfiguring disease dates back to the Ancient Egyptians and Greeks (with the first description of a case of oral cancer); it was in the Roman Empire, though, that *Aulus Cornelius Celsus* was credited to have performed the first HN operation in the form of a lip tumor excision [4,5]. Back to the present day, we know that the surgical removal of HN cancer remains a cornerstone of its management, along with chemo-radiation "organ-preserving" strategies [6]. More interestingly, the recent literature suggests that HN surgery must be performed shortly after a cancer diagnosis because time-to-surgery may represent an independent prognostic factor [7].

The field of head and neck surgery has been profoundly revolutionized, like many others, by the technological advances in recent decades, and open, microscopic, endoscopic, and robotic techniques have allowed us to achieve unprecedented results [8–10]. Many overlapping areas now exist in the HN surgery discipline, and otolaryngologists must work with (and learn from) plastic surgeons, neurosurgeons, and maxillofacial surgeons. For example, we are now capable of performing a totally endoscopic transnasal removal of sinonasal malignancies, even when invading the dural membrane; we can offer our patients "scarless" transaxillary or transoral thyroidectomy; or we can perform robotic transoral pharyngectomy and partial/total laryngectomies, or even endoscopic-assisted lateral skull base dissections [11–15].

As the boundaries of HN surgery expand, the chance of impairing or even permanently damaging critical structures (cranial nerves, major vessels, brain, etc.) and related physiological functions (swallowing, phonation, sense of smell and taste, etc.) increase [16]. The intratemporal and extratemporal facial nerves during otological and parotid surgery, and the superior and inferior laryngeal nerves during thyroid and parathyroid surgery, respectively, are well-known anatomical examples of this. The extensive demolition of oral, pharyngeal, and sinonasal structures instead requires a fine application of regional or free flaps in order to at least partially regain the functionality of the upper aerodigestive

Citation: Locatello, L.G.; Gallo, O. The Many Faces of Head and Neck Surgery in 2022 and Looking Ahead!. *J. Clin. Med.* **2022**, *11*, 3174. https://doi.org/10.3390/jcm11113174

Received: 29 May 2022
Accepted: 31 May 2022
Published: 2 June 2022

Publisher's Note: MDPI stays neutral with regard to jurisdictional claims in published maps and institutional affiliations.

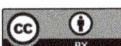

Copyright: © 2022 by the authors. Licensee MDPI, Basel, Switzerland. This article is an open access article distributed under the terms and conditions of the Creative Commons Attribution (CC BY) license (https:// creativecommons.org/licenses/by/ 4.0/).

tract. Sometimes, and despite all efforts, permanent tracheostomy and gastrostomy tube dependency rates are non-negligible (up to 64% in some series), a fact which is unavoidably associated with a poor quality of life [17,18]. There are some surgical complications that we must prevent and manage, sometimes by applying classical techniques: for instance, in transoral robotic surgery, bleeding is a very common event, and the transcervical ligation of the lingual artery has been shown to reduce the risk of fatal hemorrhage but not its incidence [19]. For skull base tumors, instead, the preoperative embolization of the internal carotid artery along with a deep knowledge of the microscopic and endoscopic landmarks now permit a safe dissection for previously considered unresectable tumors (e.g., endoscopic nasopharyngectomy operations for post-RT nasopharyngeal carcinoma) [20].

Many patient-related predictive factors of complications have been identified, such as age or the presence of comorbidities; on the other hand, because HN surgery is being more commonly performed as a salvage strategy, we tend to operate on previously irradiated patients who are, by definition, fragile [21]. Preoperative screening for patients who are most at risk and a rigorous surgical technique are the mainstay for reducing these complications, which can sometimes be managed in a conservative (medical) manner [22]. In conclusion, the prognosis of HN cancer has not improved by a large extent in the last century, and if we exclude oropharyngeal HPV-related cases, a little over half of the patients who are diagnosed with this disease will survive beyond 5 years. As we are continuously refining our diagnostic and therapeutic approaches to HN disorders, the aforementioned risks and complications are, and will always be, present. Optimistically, we believe that by following sound evidence-based clinical recommendations, and thanks to the diffusion of novel technologies, devices, and surgical expertise, the incidence of these adverse events will be brought nearly to zero. As Guest Editors of this Special Issue, we would like to conclude this Editorial by thanking the authors who have submitted their excellent papers so far, the reviewers for their punctual remarks, and all the staff of the *Journal of Clinical Medicine* for their constant support.

Author Contributions: Conceptualization, L.G.L. and O.G.; writing—original draft preparation, O.G.; writing—review and editing, L.G.L. and O.G. All authors have read and agreed to the published version of the manuscript.

Funding: This research received no external funding.

Conflicts of Interest: The authors declare no conflict of interest.

References

1. Chow, L.Q.M. Head and neck cancer. *New Engl. J. Med.* **2020**, *382*, 60–72. [CrossRef] [PubMed]
2. Hashim, D.; Genden, E.; Posner, M.; Hashibe, M.; Boffetta, P. Head and neck cancer prevention: From primary prevention to impact of clinicians on reducing burden. *Ann. Oncol.* **2019**, *30*, 744–756. [CrossRef] [PubMed]
3. Thompson-Harvey, A.; Yetukuri, M.; Hansen, A.R.; Simpson, M.C.; Adjei Boakye, E.; Varvares, M.A.; Osazuwa-Peters, N. Rising incidence of late-stage head and neck cancer in the United States. *Cancer* **2020**, *126*, 1090–1101. [CrossRef] [PubMed]
4. Goldstein, J.C.; Sisson, G.A. The history of head and neck surgery. *Otolaryngol. Head Neck Surg.* **1996**, *115*, 379–385.
5. Folz, B.J.; Silver, C.E.; Rinaldo, A.; Fagan, J.J.; Pratt, L.W.; Weir, N.; Seitz, D.; Ferlito, A. An outline of the history of head and neck oncology. *Oral Oncol.* **2008**, *44*, 2–9. [CrossRef] [PubMed]
6. Forastiere, A.A.; Ismaila, N.; Lewin, J.S.; Nathan, C.A.; Adelstein, D.J.; Eisbruch, A.; Wolf, G.T. Use of larynx-preservation strategies in the treatment of laryngeal cancer: American Society of Clinical Oncology clinical practice guideline update. *J. Clin. Oncol.* **2018**, *36*, 1143–1169. [CrossRef]
7. Rygalski, C.J.; Zhao, S.; Eskander, A.; Zhan, K.Y.; Mroz, E.A.; Brock, G.; Kang, S.Y. Time to surgery and survival in head and neck cancer. *Ann. Surg. Oncol.* **2021**, *28*, 877–885. [CrossRef]
8. Stammberger, H.; Posawetz, W. Functional endoscopic sinus surgery. *Eur. Arch. Oto-Rhino-Laryngol.* **1990**, *247*, 63–76. [CrossRef]
9. Urken, M.L.; Weinberg, H.; Buchbinder, D.; Moscoso, J.F.; Lawson, W.; Catalano, P.J.; Biller, H.F. Microvascular free flaps in head and neck reconstruction: Report of 200 cases and review of complications. *Arch. Otolaryngol. Head Neck Surg.* **1994**, *120*, 633–640. [CrossRef]
10. Fisch, U. Infratemporal fossa approach to tumours of the temporal bone and base of the skull. *J. Laryngol. Otol.* **1978**, *92*, 949–967. [CrossRef]
11. Tan, C.T.; Cheah, W.K.; Delbridge, L. "Scarless"(in the neck) endoscopic thyroidectomy (SET): An evidence-based review of published techniques. *World J. Surg.* **2008**, *32*, 1349–1357. [CrossRef] [PubMed]

12. Chuang, C.-H.; Huang, T.-Y.; Hwang, T.-Z.; Wu, C.-W.; Lu, I.-C.; Chang, P.-Y.; Lin, Y.-C.; Wang, L.-F.; Wang, C.-C.; Lien, C.-F.; et al. Accumulation of Experience and Newly Developed Devices Can Improve the Safety and Voice Outcome of Total Thyroidectomy for Graves' Disease. *J. Clin. Med.* **2022**, *11*, 1298. [CrossRef] [PubMed]
13. Mantsopoulos, K.; Koch, M.; Iro, H.; Constantinidis, J. Olfactory Neuroblastomas: What Actually Happens in the Long-Term? *J. Clin. Med.* **2022**, *11*, 2288. [CrossRef]
14. Isaacson, B.; Killeen, D.E.; Bianconi, L.; Marchioni, D. Endoscopic Assisted Lateral Skull Base Surgery. *Otolaryngol. Clin. North Am.* **2021**, *54*, 163–173. [CrossRef] [PubMed]
15. Weinstein, G.S.; O'Malley, B.W., Jr.; Desai, S.C.; Quon, H. Transoral robotic surgery: Does the ends justify the means? *Curr. Opin. Otolaryngol. Head Neck Surg.* **2009**, *17*, 126–131. [CrossRef] [PubMed]
16. Smith, J.D.; Correll, J.A.; Stucken, C.L.; Stucken, E.Z. Ear, Nose, and Throat Surgery: Postoperative Complications After Selected Head and Neck Operations. *Surg. Clin.* **2021**, *101*, 831–844.
17. Patel, S.N.; Cohen, M.A.; Givi, B.; Dixon, B.J.; Gilbert, R.W.; Gullane, P.J.; Goldstein, D.P. Salvage surgery for locally recurrent oropharyngeal cancer. *Head Neck* **2016**, *38*, E658–E664. [CrossRef]
18. Morton, R.P.; Crowder, V.L.; Mawdsley, R.; Ong, E.; Izzard, M. Elective gastrostomy, nutritional status and quality of life in advanced head and neck cancer patients receiving chemoradiotherapy. *ANZ J. Surg.* **2009**, *79*, 713–718. [CrossRef]
19. Stokes, W.; Ramadan, J.; Lawson, G.; Ferris, F.R.L.; Holsinger, F.C.; Turner, M.T. Bleeding Complications After Transoral Robotic Surgery: A Meta-Analysis and Systematic Review. *Laryngoscope* **2021**, *131*, 95–105. [CrossRef]
20. Wang, Z.Q.; Xie, Y.L.; Liu, Y.P.; Zou, X.; Chen, J.H.; Hua, Y.J.; Gu, Y.K.; Ouyang, Y.F.; Yu, Z.K.; Sun, R.; et al. Endoscopic Nasopharyngectomy Combined with Internal Carotid Artery Pretreatment for Recurrent Nasopharyngeal Carcinoma. *Otolaryngol. Head Neck Surg.* **2022**, *166*, 490–497. [CrossRef]
21. Locatello, L.G.; Mastronicola, R.; Cortese, S.; Beulque, E.; Salleron, J.; Gallo, O.; Dolivet, G. Estimating the risks and benefits before salvage surgery for recurrent head and neck squamous cell carcinoma. *Eur. J. Surg. Oncol.* **2021**, *47*, 1718–1726. [CrossRef] [PubMed]
22. Locatello, L.G.; Licci, G.; Maggiore, G.; Gallo, O. Non-Surgical Strategies for Assisting Closure of Pharyngocutaneous Fistula after Total Laryngectomy: A Systematic Review of the Literature. *J. Clin. Med.* **2022**, *11*, 100. [CrossRef] [PubMed]

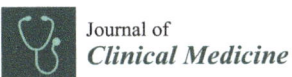

Review

Non-Surgical Strategies for Assisting Closure of Pharyngocutaneous Fistula after Total Laryngectomy: A Systematic Review of the Literature

Luca Giovanni Locatello [1,*,†], Giuseppe Licci [1,†], Giandomenico Maggiore [1] and Oreste Gallo [1,2]

1. Department of Otorhinolaryngology, Careggi University Hospital, Largo Brambilla, 3, 50134 Florence, Italy; giuseppe.licci@unifi.it (G.L.); maggiore2@virgilio.it (G.M.); oreste.gallo@unifi.it (O.G.)
2. Department of Experimental and Clinical Medicine, University of Florence, 50134 Florence, Italy
* Correspondence: locatello.lucagiovanni@gmail.com; Tel.: +39-055-7947989
† These authors contributed equally to this work.

Abstract: Background: Pharyngocutaneous fistula (PCF) is a frequent complication after total laryngectomy, with an incidence of up to 65%. Many conservative or invasive approaches are available and the choice among them is usually made on a case-by-case basis. The aim of the present review is to critically summarize the available evidence of the effectiveness of the non-surgical management of PCF. Methods: A systematic review and a meta-analysis of the literature were conducted, according to the PRISMA guidelines. Studies investigating botulinum toxin therapy, scopolamine transdermal patch, hyperbaric oxygen therapy (HBOT), and negative pressure wound therapy (NPWT) were assessed. Complete fistula closure after the initiation of non-surgical treatment was the main outcome. Results: After the application of selection criteria, a total of seven articles and 27 patients were included in the present review. All the eligible studies were descriptive case series, while only one article used a standard group as a comparison. The mean age was 63.3 and 14 patients (51.9%) had previously received RT. The reported comorbidities were diabetes, ischemic heart disease, hypertension, dyslipidemia, COPD, and atrial fibrillation. With a mean healing time of 25.0 days, the overall success rate was 92.6%. Conclusions: Non-surgical treatment of PCF is only based on the experience of small series. Although success rates seem promising, the absence of properly designed comparative studies does not allow us, at present, to identify ideal candidates for these non-invasive management strategies for PCF.

Keywords: head and neck; fistula; complications; non-surgical treatment; otorhinolaryngology

1. Introduction

Pharyngocutaneous fistula (PCF) is a frequent complication after total laryngectomy, with a reported incidence between 3% and 65% [1]. This event considerably increases the length of hospital stay and costs, may delay the start of postoperative radiotherapy (RT), and can heavily affect the patient's psychological status [2]. PCF is usually diagnosed 7 to 11 days after surgery [2], and while there is still no gold standard test (e.g., blue dye test, etc.) for an early diagnosis [3], fever in the early postoperative period represents an excellent predictor of its development [4].

Once PCF is diagnosed, standard wound treatment is usually implemented, in terms of compressive dressings, antibiotics coverage, and artificial nutrition. Closure can be expedited by invasive/surgical approaches (use of pedicled or free flaps, endoscopic repair) or by non-surgical strategies, such as the use of hyperbaric oxygen therapy, botulinum toxin injection, or negative pressure (or vacuum-assisted) therapy [1,5]. While excellent reviews have been published on the management of post-reconstructive head and neck salivary fistulas [5], or about the reduction strategies of salivary flow in head and neck cancer patients [6], no specific paper has ever focused on non-surgical treatment of PCF, which remains largely empirical and anecdotal. In the present review, we want to critically summarize the available evidence on the efficacy of the non-surgical treatments of PCF after total laryngectomy.

2. Materials and Methods

2.1. Literature Search

Following the preferred reporting items for systematic reviews and meta-analyses (PRISMA) guidelines [7], we conducted a literature search on articles published from January 1980 up to July 2021, using the PubMed database in order to identify all the studies reporting the outcomes of non-surgical strategies for the treatment of PCF.

The following keywords were used: "treatment AND pharyngocutaneous fistula" (596 results, 517 in English, 1 in Italian); "Management AND pharyngocutaneous fistula" (185 results, 167 in English, 0 in Italian); "Closing AND pharyngocutaneous fistula" (78 results, 67 in English, 1 in Italian); "Botulinum AND pharyngocutaneous fistula" (2 articles, 2 in English); "Botulinum AND salivary fistula" (47 articles, 40 in English, 0 in Italian); "Botulinum AND saliva" (172 articles, 149 in English, 0 in Italian); "Hyperbaric oxygen therapy AND pharyngocutaneous" (4 articles, 3 in English, 0 in Italian); "Oxygen AND pharyngocutaneous fistula" (4 articles, 3 in English, 0 in Italian); "HBOT AND pharyngocutaneous fistula" (1 article, 1 in English); "Vacuum Assisted Closure Therapy AND pharyngocutaneous fistula" (11 results, 9 in English, 0 in Italian); "Negative pressure wound therapy AND pharyngocutaneous fistula" (16 results, 13 in English, 0 in Italian); "Scopolamine AND pharyngocutaneous fistula" (0 results); "Scopolamine AND fistula" (13 results, 13 in English, 0 in Italian).

Only studies describing the clinical outcomes of patients presenting with a PCF and who were exclusively treated with non-surgical methods were selected. Articles were excluded based on the following criteria: studies describing other types of fistulas or wounds in the head and neck region (e.g., oro-cutaneous fistulas, post-parotidectomy fistulas, etc.); cases with the concurrent implementation of an invasive approach (for example, vacuum-assisted closure therapy/VAC and the associated need for returning to the operating room, or the need of general anesthesia); and articles written in languages other than Italian and English. In order to avoid unnecessary bias, cases reporting combined medical treatments for a single-treatment-resistant fistula were also excluded. Bibliographic research and the removal of duplicates were performed by the reference management software Mendeley Version 1.19.8 for macOS.

2.2. Data Collection

Titles and abstracts of the extracted papers were carefully evaluated according to the aforementioned criteria. Full texts were then analyzed in order to extract the following data: patients' age; sex; previous RT on head and neck region; the presence of medical comorbidities; TNM stage; type of head and neck surgery (total laryngectomy or pharyngo-laryngectomy) and the possible use of a free or pedicled flap for reinforcing the pharyngeal suture; time elapsed (expressed in days) from surgery to fistula presentation; time from fistula appearance to its closure; and other associated postoperative complications.

2.3. Definition of the Outcome and Statistical Methods

The aim of this study was to quantify the success rate, defined as complete fistula closure, after the initiation of a non-surgical strategy and in addition to standard wound therapy. Standard descriptive statistics were used to summarize the extracted data and Microsoft® Excel (Version 16.52, Redmond, WA, USA) was used to perform the calculations.

3. Results

After the application of selection criteria, a total of seven articles were included in the present review and the PRISMA flowchart is represented in Figure 1. Non-surgical strategies for PCF closure included botulinum toxin therapy (2 studies), HBOT (2 studies), and NPWT/VAC (3 studies) for a total of 27 patients. In all cases, these treatments were specifically added to the standard PCF care that included compressive dressings, systemic broad-spectrum antibiotics administration, and enteral artificial nutrition, usually by a nasogastric feeding tube.

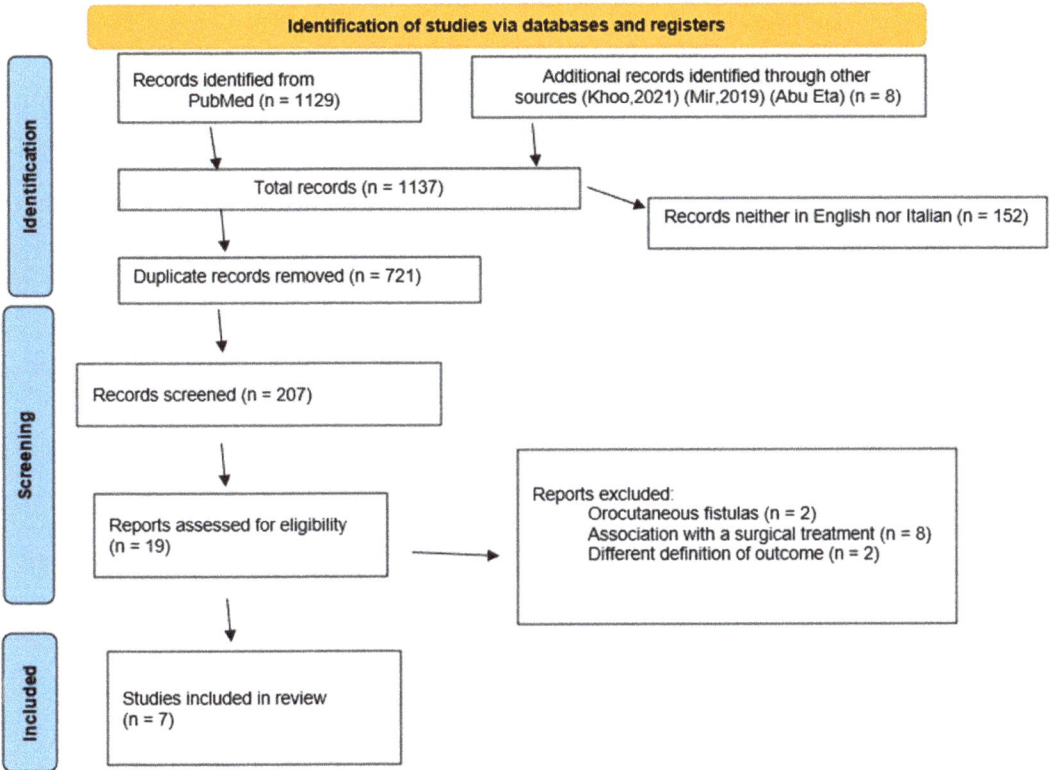

Figure 1. PRISMA flow diagram depicting the selection of the papers included in the present review.

In the whole cohort, there was only one female and the mean age was 63.3. Primary tumors' stages ranged from T2N0 to T4N2, and 14/27 patients (51.9%) had previously received RT. PCF was diagnosed a mean of 9.6 days after surgery and it healed about 25.0 days after its appearance. Comorbidities were seldom reported and only a few (3) studies have specifically investigated them: diabetes mellitus (2), ischemic heart disease (2), hypertension (2), dyslipidemia (3), COPD (1), and atrial fibrillation (1).

The detailed outcomes for the use of HBOT, NPWT, and botulinum toxin therapy are presented in Tables 1–3, respectively. The overall success rate was 92.6% but no formal comparison with a control group was ever made. In most cases, conservative treatments were used primarily, but in 11% of cases, they were also used after failed surgical treatment (2 pectoralis major flap, 1 radial forearm free flap). The reason for choosing one therapeutic process rather than another was never explicitly motivated. Finally, we have stratified patients according to previous RT status: those who have never been irradiated (13) had a mean healing time of 14.5 days versus 35.4 days in the RT group. Success rates were therefore 100% versus 85.7%, but the statistical comparison could not be performed due to missing data.

Table 1. Overview of the clinical outcomes of patients treated for PCF using hyperbaric oxygen therapy (HBOT). Acronyms: NA, not available; M, male; F, female; PMF, pectoralis major myocutaneous flap; DM, diabetes mellitus; HTN, hypertension; IHD, ischemic heart disease; PAF, paroxysmal atrial fibrillation.

Reference (Year, Country)	Study Type (Period)	N° of Cases (Sex)	Mean Age	Tumor Site	cTNM/pTNM	Type of Surgery	Previous RT (Number of Patients)	Previous Surgical Treatment for Fistula Healing	Comorbidities	Time for Fistula Presentation (Days after Surgery)	Mean Time for Fistula Healing (Days)	Success Rate (%)
Neovius et al. (1997, Sweden) [8]	Retrospective (1993–1995)	2 (2M/0F)	58.5	Laryngeal	T2-3 N0 M0	NA	2	NA	NA	NA	45	50%
R. Abu Eta et al. (2016, Israel) [9]	Retrospective (2008–2013)	8 (8M/0F)	63	Glottic-supraglottic	T3-4 N0-2b M0	8 total laryngectomy + 6 PMF	8	0	1 DMII 1 HNT 2 IHD 2 Dyslipidemia	12.75	41.5	87.5%

Table 2. Overview of the clinical outcomes of patients treated for PCF using negative pressure wound therapy (NPWT). Acronyms: NA, not available; M, male; F, female; PMF, pectoralis major myocutaneous flap; RFFF, radial forearm free flap; DM, diabetes mellitus; HTN, hypertension.

Reference (Year, Country)	Study Type (Period)	N° of Cases (Sex)	Mean Age	Tumor Site	cTNM/ pTNM	Type of Surgery	Previous RT (Number of Patients)	Previous Surgical Treatments for Fistula Healing	Comorbidities	Time for Fistula Presentation (Days after Surgery)	Mean Time for Fistula Healing (Days)	Success Rate (%)
Andrews et al. (2008, USA) [10]	Case series (NA)	1 (1M/0F)	75	larynx	T3-N0-M1	Salvage + radial forearm reconstruction	1	0	NA	NA (dehiscence soon after the surgery)	28	100%
Loaec et al. (France, 2014) [11]	Case series (2011–2013)	5 (5M/0F)	67.4	Larynx-oropharynx	T3-4 N0-2 M0	1 total laryngectomy; 1 total circular pharyngolaryngectomy + RFFF; 2 partial laryngectomies, 1 transmandibular oropharyngectomy	0	1 reoperation for Hematoma + debridement (NPWT for the recurrence of fistula) 1 RFFF	1 COPD	7.6	17.8	100%
Teixeira et al. (2017, Portugal) [12]	Case series (NA)	2 (1M, 1F)	64	Pyriform sinus	pT3N0M0	2 total laryngectomies (+1 RFFF)	1	1 PMF	1DMII+, HNT obesity, splenectomy nephrectomy in the context of polyarteritis nodosa	NA	22	100%

Table 3. Overview of the clinical outcomes of patients treated for PCF using botulinum toxin therapy. Acronyms: NA, not available; M, male; F, female; PMF, pectoralis major myocutaneous flap.

Reference (Year, Country)	Study Type (Period)	N° of Cases (Sex)	Mean Age	Tumor Site	cTNM/pTNM	Type of Surgery	Previous RT (Number of Patients)	Surgical Treatment for Fistula Healing	Comorbidities	Time for Fistula Presentation (Days after Surgery)	Mean Time for Fistula Healing (Days)	Success Rate (%)
Marchese et al. (2008, Italy) [13]	Case series (2004–2006)	6 (6M/0F)	62.5	Larynx-hypopharynx	NA	NA	1	0	NA	7	6.7	100%
Guntinas-Lichius et al. (2002, Germany) [14]	Case series (NA)	3 (3M/0F)	58	Larynx-oropharynx	rpT4 N2a-b M0	2 Laryngectomy + neck dissection; 1 Median mandibulotomy, tumor resection, radial forearm flap, neck dissection	1	1 PMF (failed)	NA	9.6	23.3	100%

4. Discussion

The optimal management of PCF begins preoperatively, with a proper assessment of the risk factors in each patient: poor nutritional status (measured by hypoalbuminemia), previous head and neck radiation therapy, or systemic chemotherapy can all increase the chance of PCF development [15]. These findings are probably due to the exacerbation of the obliterative endarteritis and fibrosis induced by the (chemo) radiation itself in local tissues [16]. While malnutrition should be aggressively corrected during the whole perioperative period [17], in the setting of a salvage laryngectomy/pharyngolaryngectomy the prophylactic use of a reinforcing flap has been shown to significantly decrease PCF risk [18]. In addition, while early oral feeding seems to increase PCF risk according to a recent meta-analysis [19], early oral hydration may actually reduce this probability (by a possible mechanical detersion of infected fluids and saliva on pharyngeal suture) [20].

Another point to remember is that preventing PCF development remains of the uttermost importance: a recent interesting experience has presented a "fistula-zero project" after total laryngectomy which is mainly based on a watertight horizontal pharyngeal closure, the reinforcing flap for post-RT patients, and the use of salivary bypass tubes [21]. Besides prevention, a key aspect is to make an early diagnosis of fistula. For instance, blue dye oral testing can help in intraoperative and early postoperative periods, with the advantage of being low in cost and easily administered [3]. Another early predictive test for PCF is represented by the presence of wound amylase in drains [22].

Once PCF appears, it is known that between 60% and 80% of cases will heal with "conservative treatments" [23]. Conventionally, a broad-spectrum antibiotic therapy is set up, along with compressive wound care, and enteral nutritional support through a nasogastric tube. Although they are not formally supported by the evidence, these treatments appear to be plausible and somehow even obvious [23,24]. Surgical repair remains the most effective and rapid way to close PCF, which, if left untreated, can favor deep neck infections and carotid blowout syndrome [5,25]. A recent multicenter study has even shown an independent association between PCF and the development of distant metastases, but the authors did not include in their model the delayed start of adjuvant treatments [26].

In the present review, we have shown that additional non-surgical strategies, such as HBOT, VAC, or botulinum toxin therapy, might yield an overall satisfactory PCF closure rate. Even though no side effects were reported with these strategies, we think that this result is heavily weakened by the lack of a control group, the fact that confounding factors, such as preoperative comorbidities or previous RT, were not evaluated, and the very low number of cases available. Furthermore, we strongly believe that these strategies should be reserved only in very particular cases and, whenever judged to be clinically necessary, prompt surgical closure should be performed [1,5].

HBOT is based on the favorable effects of repetitive periods of hyperoxia (and subsequent hypoxia) on the wound healing process and mainly thanks to the production of the vascular endothelial growth factor (VEGF) by macrophages [27]. The treatment is quite safe, even though some side effects were reported, including reversible myopia, barotrauma in the form of tympanic membrane perforation, tracheobronchial symptoms (from a simple cough to pneumothorax), and even seizures [28]. While the use of HBOT has become a cornerstone in other fields of head and neck surgery, such as in the case of mandibular osteonecrosis [29], we retrieved no satisfactory study for PCF treatment. In addition, HBOT for treating PCF raises some questions, such as the yet unassessed cost-benefit ratio, or the risk of promoting tumor progression, since oxygen was shown to promote cellular and vascular proliferation in wounds [30]. However, according to a review of the literature conducted some years ago, this latter risk remains more theoretical than clinically meaningful [31].

The efficacy of NPWT/VAC therapy for all kinds of head and neck wounds has been recently reviewed in an excellent paper [32]. One problem is the definition of the outcome. For example, one study using NPWT considered "success" the mere formation of granulation tissue in the PCF tract, without specifying any further [33]. Another issue arises from the difficulty to understand when NPWT can be applied non-invasively or when it needs to be placed in the operating room along with open surgical wound revision [34–37], or even by an endoscopic insertion [38]. Not all the patients of the considered articles were, therefore, included for this study. In two papers, for example, for some patients of the cohorts, an explicitly invasive surgical procedure was associated with VAC [10,11]. Furthermore, maintaining the necessary hermetic seal is notably difficult because of the proximity of the PCF to the tracheal stoma, whose secretions also complicate VAC adherence to the skin [11]. On the other hand, NPWT has got very few side effects other than pain/discomfort [39], or hemorrhage if vessels are not properly protected [40]. Regarding costs, it was shown they are comparable to those of conventional wound dressing, because of the need for fewer dressing changes and a shorter duration of hospitalization [41].

Botulinum toxin therapy represents one of the many pharmacological strategies to reduce salivary flow, which is a major culprit in PCF formation and persistence [6 bomeli]. This molecule has been extensively used in the treatment of sialorrhea for many neurological syndromes [42–45]. Botulinum toxin starts to reduce the salivary secretion from 72 h after the periparotid infiltration and it has a more noticeable effect after 5 to 7 days [46]; its action is reversible and it lasts about 2–4 months, and with minimal systemic side effects [47]. A study conducted some years ago demonstrated, by the use of 99 mTc pertechnetate scintigraphy, a reduction of up to 80% total salivary flow of secretion. However, it should be noted that some residual flow remains nonetheless important against oral cavity infections and xerostomia [48]. In addition, botulinum toxin use for PCF is currently off-label, and a comprehensive and written informed consent to the procedure should be obtained (as done by one [13] of the two aforementioned studies). Another potentially useful antisecretory drug would be constituted by scopolamine patches, which, however, are not free from anticholinergic side effects (e.g., blurred vision and urinary retention) [49,50]. However, in our literature search anticholinergic drugs were reported for the treatment of neurological chronic drooling [51,52], or for the prevention of sialocele or the treatment of salivary fistulas following parotid surgery [53,54], while no mention as a possible treatment for PCF was found. For the sake of completeness, we found that successful use of combination treatments, such as scopolamine + botulinum toxin for a post-parotidectomy fistula [55], or scopolamine + NPWT for treating an entero-cutaneous fistula after esophagectomy [56], was also presented in case reports.

The possible role of previous RT as a risk factor is well known since many years: the scientific evidence has been strengthened by several meta-analyses, even though some studies have shown contradictory results [1,15,57]. Furthermore, it has been shown that chemo-radiotherapy increases the risk of developing a PCF compared to radiotherapy alone [16]. It should be recalled that the group receiving salvage RT may receive more extensive procedures because of the higher recurrent T/N stage and the need for larger resection margins, and this latter aspect can increase, by itself, the risk of complications [58]. Since the publication of the aforementioned meta-analyses, it has become almost imperative to reinforce pharyngeal closure with a vascularized flap and many choices are available (pectoralis major flap, supraclavicular artery island flap, fasciocutaneous free flaps, mammary artery, perforator propeller flap, latissimus dorsi flaps, or facial artery-based cutaneous island flap) [59–62]. In a large multicenter study conducted by the American Academy of Otolaryngology-Head & Neck Surgery, vascularized tissue augmentation was shown to significantly reduce the overall fistula rate and fistula requiring reoperation, but, also, to possibly impair speech and swallowing outcomes [63].

Limitations of our study include the heterogeneity in terms of elapsed time from PCF diagnosis and the start of the therapy, in terms of indications, and in the definition of the outcome. For instance, Steffen et al. reported six patients with PCF and treated with botulinum toxin, speaking only of "improvement of the patients' conditions", and without mentioning the fistula closure [64]. Another issue arises from the lack of a control group: only the study by Neovius et al. had a reference group, but the authors did not make any statistical comparison between the two cohorts [8]. The diffuse underreporting (of comorbidities, of previous RT, etc.) of all of the available studies is the major reason for the low level of evidence of the present work. In addition, since it is based mostly on case series/reports, it is very probable that the success rate is high for the simple fact that only successful treatments have been reported (i.e., publication bias). Moreover, concomitant or subsequent multiple non-surgical treatments would not allow us to draw any conclusion on what, in the end, has helped in the healing process, such cases are, therefore, not useful for comparison against other surgical or single non-surgical treatments. Hopefully the present review will prompt future research in this field and we suggest that a basic set of clinical information must be reported with these treatments if we want to draw stronger clinical conclusions.

5. Conclusions

The outcomes of non-surgical strategies for expediting the closure of PCF seem apparently promising, but they are derived from only a few non-randomized and retrospective studies. The very low level of evidence available does not currently justify the use of these strategies in the current clinical management of PCF and further well-designed and exhaustive studies are needed in this field of head and neck surgery.

Author Contributions: Conceptualization, L.G.L. and O.G.; methodology, L.G.L. and G.L.; validation, G.M. and O.G.; formal analysis, G.L.; investigation, L.G.L. and G.L.; resources, L.G.L. and G.L.; data curation, L.G.L. and G.L.; writing—original draft preparation, L.G.L. and G.L.; writing—review and editing, G.M. and O.G.; visualization, L.G.L., G.L., G.M. and O.G. All authors have read and agreed to the published version of the manuscript.

Funding: This research received no external funding.

Data Availability Statement: The data presented in this study are available upon reasonable request from the corresponding author.

Conflicts of Interest: The authors declare no conflict of interest.

References

1. Paydarfar, J.A.; Birkmeyer, N.J. Complications in Head and Neck Surgery: A meta-analysis of postlaryngectomy pharyngocutaneous fistula. *Arch. Otolaryngol. Head Neck Surg.* **2006**, *132*, 67–72. [CrossRef]
2. Cavalot, A.L.; Gervasio, C.F.; Nazionale, G.; Albera, R.; Bussi, M.; Staffieri, A.; Ferrero, V.; Cortesina, G. Pharyngocutaneous Fistula as a Complication of Total Laryngectomy: Review of the Literature and Analysis of Case Records. *Otolaryngol. Neck Surg.* **2000**, *123*, 587–592. [CrossRef] [PubMed]
3. Kiong, K.L.; Tan, N.C.; Skanthakumar, T.; Teo, C.E.; Soo, K.C.; Tan, H.K.; Roche, E.; Yee, K.; Iyer, N.G. Salivary fistula: Blue dye testing as part of an algorithm for early diagnosis. *Laryngoscope* **2017**, *2*, 363–368. [CrossRef] [PubMed]
4. Friedman, M.; Venkatesan, T.K.; Yakovlev, A.; Lim, J.W.; Tanyeri, H.M.; Caldarelli, D.D. Early Detection and Treatment of Postoperative Pharyngocutaneous Fistula. *Otolaryngol. Neck Surg.* **1999**, *121*, 378–380. [CrossRef]
5. Khoo, M.J.W.; Ooi, A.S.H. Management of postreconstructive head and neck salivary fistulae: A review of current practices. *J. Plast. Reconstr. Aesthet. Surg.* **2021**, *74*, 2120–2132. [CrossRef]
6. Bomeli, S.R.; Desai, S.C.; Johnson, J.T.; Walvekar, R.R. Management of salivary flow in head and neck cancer patients—A systematic review. *Oral Oncol.* **2008**, *44*, 1000–1008. [CrossRef] [PubMed]
7. Liberati, A.; Altman, D.G.; Tetzlaff, J.; Mulrow, C.; Gøtzsche, P.C.; Ioannidis, J.P.A.; Clarke, M.; Devereaux, P.; Kleijnen, J.; Moher, D. The PRISMA statement for reporting systematic reviews and meta-analyses of studies that evaluate healthcare interventions: Explanation and elaboration. *BMJ* **2009**, *339*, b2700. [CrossRef]
8. Neovius, E.B.; Lind, M.G.; Lind, F.G. Hyperbaric oxygen therapy for wound complications after surgery in the irradiated head and neck: A review of the literature and a report of 15 consecutive patients. *Head Neck* **1997**, *19*, 315–322. [CrossRef]
9. Abu Eta, R.; Eviatar, E.; Gavriel, H. Hyperbaric oxygen therapy as an alternative to surgery for non-healing pharyngocutaneous fistula. *Eur. Arch. Oto-Rhino-Laryngol.* **2016**, *273*, 3857–3861. [CrossRef]
10. Andrews, B.T.; Smith, R.B.; Hoffman, H.T.; Funk, G.F. Orocutaneous and Pharyngocutaneous Fistula Closure Using a Vacuum-Assisted Closure System. *Ann. Otol. Rhinol. Laryngol.* **2008**, *117*, 298–302. [CrossRef] [PubMed]
11. Loaec, E.; Vaillant, P.-Y.; Bonne, L.; Marianowski, R. Negative-pressure wound therapy for the treatment of pharyngocutaneous fistula. *Eur. Ann. Otorhinolaryngol. Head Neck Dis.* **2014**, *131*, 351–355. [CrossRef]
12. Teixeira, S.; Costa, J.; Bartosch, I.; Correia, B.; Álvaro, S. Management of Pharyngocutaneous Fistula with Negative-Pressure Wound Therapy. *J. Craniofac. Surg.* **2017**, *28*, e364–e367. [CrossRef]

13. Marchese, M.R.; Almadori, G.; Giorgio, A.; Paludetti, G. Post-surgical role of botulinum toxin-A injection in patients with head and neck cancer: Personal experience. *Acta Otorhinolaryngol. Ital.* **2008**, *28*, 13–16.
14. Guntinas-Lichius, O.; Eckel, H.E. Temporary Reduction of Salivation in Laryngectomy Patients with Pharyngocutaneous Fistulas by Botulinum Toxin A Injection. *Laryngoscope* **2002**, *112*, 187–189. [CrossRef]
15. Busoni, M.; Deganello, A.; Gallo, O. Fistola faringocutanea dopo laringectomia totale: Analisi dei fattori di rischio, della prognosi e delle modalità di trattamento. *Acta Otorhinolaryngol. Ital.* **2015**, *35*, 400–405. [CrossRef] [PubMed]
16. Sayles, M.; Grant, D.G. Preventing pharyngo-cutaneous fistula in total laryngectomy: A systematic review and meta-analysis. *Laryngoscope* **2014**, *124*, 1150–1163. [CrossRef]
17. Nesemeier, R.; Dunlap, N.; McClave, S.A.; Tennant, P. Evidence-Based Support for Nutrition Therapy in Head and Neck Cancer. *Curr. Surg. Rep.* **2017**, *5*, 18. [CrossRef]
18. Guimarães, A.V.; Aires, F.T.; Dedivitis, R.A.; Kulcsar, M.A.V.; Ramos, D.M.; Cernea, C.R.; Brandão, L.G. Efficacy of pectoralis major muscle flap for pharyngocutaneous fistula prevention in salvage total laryngectomy: A systematic review. *Head Neck* **2015**, *38*, E2317–E2321. [CrossRef] [PubMed]
19. Singh, R.; Karantanis, W.; Fadhil, M.; Dow, C.; Fuzi, J.; Robinson, R.; Jacobson, I. Meta-analysis on the rate of pharyngocutaneous fistula in early oral feeding in laryngectomy patients. *Am. J. Otolaryngol.* **2021**, *42*, 102748. [CrossRef] [PubMed]
20. Le Flem, M.; Santini, L.; Boulze, C.; Alshukry, A.; Giovanni, A.; Dessi, P.; Fakhry, N. Early oral hydration protects against pharyngocutaneous fistula after total laryngectomy or total pharyngolaryngectomy. *Head Neck* **2020**, *42*, 1902–1906. [CrossRef]
21. Crosetti, E.; Arrigoni, G.; Sprio, A.E.; Succo, G. "Fistula Zero" Project After Total Laryngectomy: The Candiolo Cancer Institute Experience. *Front. Oncol.* **2021**, *11*, 690703. [CrossRef]
22. Morton, R.P.; Mehanna, H.; Hall, F.T.; McIvor, N.P. Prediction of pharyngocutaneous fistulas after laryngectomy. *Otolaryngol. Neck Surg.* **2007**, *136*, s46–s49. [CrossRef]
23. De Zinis, L.O.R.; Ferrari, L.; Tomenzoli, D.; Premoli, G.; Parrinello, G.; Nicolai, P. Postlaryngectomy pharyngocutaneous fistula: Incidence, predisposing factors, and therapy. *Head Neck* **1999**, *21*, 131–138. [CrossRef]
24. Mäkitie, A.A.; Irish, J.; Gullane, P.J. Pharyngocutaneous fistula. *Curr. Opin. Otolaryngol. Head Neck Surg.* **2003**, *11*, 78–84. [CrossRef]
25. Powitzky, R.; Vasan, N.; Krempl, G.; Medina, J. Carotid Blowout in Patients with Head and Neck Cancer. *Ann. Otol. Rhinol. Laryngol.* **2010**, *119*, 476–484. [CrossRef] [PubMed]
26. Davies, J.C.; Hugh, S.; Rich, J.T.; de Almeida, J.R.; Gullane, P.J.; Orsini, M.; Eskander, A.; Monteiro, E.; Mimica, X.; McGill, M.; et al. Association of Pharyngocutaneous Fistula with Cancer Outcomes in Patients After Laryngectomy. *JAMA Otolaryngol. Neck Surg.* **2021**, *47*, 1027–1034. [CrossRef] [PubMed]
27. Tandara, A.A.; Mustoe, T.A. Oxygen in Wound Healing—More than a Nutrient. *World J. Surg.* **2004**, *28*, 294–300. [CrossRef]
28. Tibbles, P.M.; Edelsberg, J.S. Hyperbaric-Oxygen Therapy. *N. Engl. J. Med.* **1996**, *334*, 1642–1648. [CrossRef]
29. Wang, C.; Schwaitzberg, S.; Berliner, E.; Zarin, D.A.; Lau, J. Hyperbaric Oxygen for Treating Wounds. *Arch. Surg.* **2003**, *138*, 272–279. [CrossRef]
30. Marx, R.E.; Ehler, W.J.; Tayapongsak, P.; Pierce, L.W. Relationship of oxygen dose to angiogenesis induction in irradiated tissue. *Am. J. Surg.* **1990**, *160*, 519–524. [CrossRef]
31. Moen, I.; Stuhr, L.E.B. Hyperbaric oxygen therapy and cancer—A review. *Target. Oncol.* **2012**, *7*, 233–242. [CrossRef]
32. Mir, A.; Guys, N.; Bs, K.A.; Svider, P.F.; Rayess, H.; Zuliani, G.; Raza, S.N.; Lin, H. Negative Pressure Wound Therapy in the Head and Neck: An Evidence-Based Approach. *Laryngoscope* **2019**, *129*, 671–683. [CrossRef] [PubMed]
33. Rosenthal, E.L.; Blackwell, K.E.; McGrew, B.; Carroll, W.R.; Peters, G.E. Use of negative pressure dressings in head and neck reconstruction. *Head Neck* **2005**, *27*, 970–975. [CrossRef] [PubMed]
34. Inatomi, Y.; Kadota, H.; Yoshida, S.; Kamizono, K.; Shimamoto, R.; Fukushima, S.; Miyashita, K.; Matsuo, M.; Yasumatsu, R.; Tanaka, S.; et al. Utility of negative-pressure wound therapy for orocutaneous and pharyngocutaneous fistula following head and neck surgery. *Head Neck* **2020**, *42*, 103–110. [CrossRef] [PubMed]
35. Asher, S.A.; White, H.N.; Illing, E.A.; Carroll, W.R.; Magnuson, J.S.; Rosenthal, E.L. Intraluminal Negative Pressure Wound Therapy for Optimizing Pharyngeal Reconstruction. *JAMA Otolaryngol. Neck Surg.* **2014**, *140*, 143–149. [CrossRef]
36. Johnston, J.; Mariano, F.; Vokes, D. Negative pressure dressing around the airway. *N. Z. Med. J.* **2013**, *126*, 24045317.
37. Yang, Y.-H.; Jeng, S.-F.; Hsieh, C.-H.; Feng, G.-M.; Chen, C.C. Vacuum-assisted closure for complicated wounds in head and neck region after reconstruction. *J. Plast. Reconstr. Aesthet. Surg.* **2013**, *66*, e209–e216. [CrossRef]
38. Steinbichler, T.B.; Wolfram, D.; Runge, A.; Hartl, R.; Dejaco, D.; Rauchenwald, T.; Pototschnig, C.; Riechelmann, H.; Schartinger, V.H. Modified vacuum-assisted closure (EndoVAC) therapy for treatment of pharyngocutaneous fistula: A case series and a review of the literature. *Head Neck* **2021**, *43*, 2377–2384. [CrossRef]
39. Waldie, K. Pain associated with negative pressure wound therapy. *Br. J. Nurs.* **2013**, *22*, S15–S21. [CrossRef] [PubMed]
40. Reiter, M.; Harréus, U. Vacuum assisted closure in the management of wound healing disorders in the head and neck: A retrospective analysis of 23 cases. *Am. J. Otolaryngol.* **2013**, *34*, 411–415. [CrossRef] [PubMed]
41. Braakenburg, A.; Obdeijn, M.C.; Feitz, R.; Van Rooij, I.A.L.M.; Van Griethuysen, A.J.; Klinkenbijl, J.H.G. The Clinical Efficacy and Cost Effectiveness of the Vacuum-Assisted Closure Technique in the Management of Acute and Chronic Wounds: A Randomized Controlled Trial. *Plast. Reconstr. Surg.* **2006**, *118*, 390–397. [CrossRef] [PubMed]
42. Shehee, L.; O'Rourke, A.; Garand, K.L. The Role of Radiation Therapy and Botulinum Toxin Injections in the Management of Sialorrhea in Patients with Amyotrophic Lateral Sclerosis: A Systematic Review. *J. Clin. Neuromuscul. Dis.* **2020**, *21*, 205–221. [CrossRef]

43. Ruiz-Roca, J.A.; Pons-Fuster, E.; Lopez-Jornet, P. Effectiveness of the Botulinum Toxin for Treating Sialorrhea in Patients with Parkinson's Disease: A Systematic Review. *J. Clin. Med.* **2019**, *8*, 317. [CrossRef] [PubMed]
44. Ng, L.; Khan, F.; Young, C.A.; Galea, M. Symptomatic treatments for amyotrophic lateral sclerosis/motor neuron disease. *Cochrane Database Syst. Rev.* **2017**, *2017*, CD011776. [CrossRef]
45. Walshe, M.; Smith, M.; Pennington, L. Interventions for drooling in children with cerebral palsy. *Cochrane Database Syst. Rev.* **2012**, *11*, CD008624. [CrossRef]
46. Corradino, B.; Di Lorenzo, S.; Mossuto, C.; Costa, R.P.; Moschella, F. Botulinum toxin in preparation of oral cavity for microsurgical reconstruction. *Acta Oto-Laryngol.* **2010**, *130*, 156–160. [CrossRef] [PubMed]
47. Lee, D.; Lee, Y.; Park, H.; Lee, J.W.; Cha, W. Intraoperative botulinum toxin injection for superficial partial parotidectomy: A prospective pilot study. *Clin. Otolaryngol.* **2021**, *46*, 998–1004. [CrossRef]
48. Corradino, B.; Di Lorenzo, S.; Moschella, F.; Bartolo, C.; Sara, D.L.; Francesco, M. Botulinum Toxin A for Oral Cavity Cancer Patients: In Microsurgical Patients BTX Injections in Major Salivary Glands Temporarily Reduce Salivary Production and the Risk of Local Complications Related to Saliva Stagnation. *Toxins* **2012**, *4*, 956–961. [CrossRef]
49. Lewis, D.W.; Fontana, C.; Mehallick, L.K.; Everett, Y. Transdermal Scopolamine for Reduction Of Drooling In Developmentally Delayed Children. *Dev. Med. Child Neurol.* **2008**, *36*, 484–486. [CrossRef]
50. Talmi, Y.P.; Zohar, Y.; Finkelstein, Y.; Laurian, N. Reduction of Salivary Flow with Scopoderm Tts. *Ann. Otol. Rhinol. Laryngol.* **1988**, *97*, 128–130. [CrossRef]
51. Reid, S.M.; Westbury, C.; Guzys, A.T.; Reddihough, D.S. Anticholinergic medications for reducing drooling in children with developmental disability. *Dev. Med. Child Neurol.* **2020**, *62*, 346–353. [CrossRef] [PubMed]
52. Varley, L.P.; Denieffe, S.; O'Gorman, C.; Murphy, A.; Gooney, M. A systematic review of noninvasive and invasive sialorrhoea management. *J. Clin. Nurs.* **2019**, *28*, 4190–4206. [CrossRef]
53. Mantsopoulos, K.; Goncalves, M.; Iro, H. Transdermal scopolamine for the prevention of a salivary fistula after parotidectomy. *Br. J. Oral Maxillofac. Surg.* **2018**, *56*, 212–215. [CrossRef] [PubMed]
54. Send, T.; Bertlich, M.; Eichhorn, K.W.; Bootz, F.; Jakob, M. Management and Follow-up Results of Salivary Fistulas Treated with Botulinum Toxin. *Laryngoscope* **2019**, *129*, 403–408. [CrossRef]
55. Dessy, L.; Mazzocchi, M.; Monarca, C.; Onesti, M.; Scuderi, N. Combined transdermal scopolamine and botulinum toxin A to treat a parotid fistula after a face-lift in a patient with siliconomas. *Int. J. Oral Maxillofac. Surg.* **2007**, *36*, 949–952. [CrossRef]
56. Suzuki, S.; Aihara, R.; Ooki, T.; Matsumura, N.; Wada, W.; Mogi, A.; Hosouchi, Y.; Nishida, Y.; Sakai, M.; Sohda, M.; et al. Successful treatment of enterocutaneous fistula after esophagectomy with scopolamine ointment and negative pressure wound therapy: A case report. *Surg. Case Rep.* **2020**, *6*, 177. [CrossRef]
57. Wang, M.; Xun, Y.; Wang, K.; Lu, L.; Yu, A.; Guan, B.; Yu, C. Risk factors of pharyngocutaneous fistula after total laryngectomy: A systematic review and meta-analysis. *Eur. Arch. Oto-Rhino-Laryngol.* **2020**, *277*, 585–599. [CrossRef]
58. Deganello, A.; Gallo, O.; De Cesare, J.M.; Ninu, M.B.; Gitti, G.; Campora, L.D.; Radici, M.; Campora, E.D. Supracricoid partial laryngectomy as salvage surgery for radiation therapy failure. *Head Neck* **2008**, *30*, 1064–1071. [CrossRef] [PubMed]
59. Alam, D.S.; Vivek, P.P.; Kmiecik, J. Comparison of voice outcomes after radial forearm free flap reconstruction versus primary closure after laryngectomy. *Otolaryngol. Neck Surg.* **2008**, *139*, 240–244. [CrossRef] [PubMed]
60. Patel, U.A.; Keni, S.P. Pectoralis Myofascial Flap during Salvage Laryngectomy Prevents Pharyngocutaneous Fistula. *Otolaryngol. Neck Surg.* **2009**, *141*, 190–195. [CrossRef]
61. Higgins, K.M.; Ashford, B.; Erovic, B.; Yoo, J.; Enepekides, D.J. Temporoparietal fascia free flap for pharyngeal coverage after salvage total laryngectomy. *Laryngoscope* **2011**, *122*, 523–527. [CrossRef] [PubMed]
62. Frisch, T. Versatility of the facial artery myomucosal island flap in neopharyngeal reconstruction. *Head Neck* **2016**, *39*, E29–E33. [CrossRef] [PubMed]
63. Microvascular Committee of the American Academy of Otolaryngology-Head & Neck Surgery. Salvage laryngectomy and laryngopharyngectomy: Multicenter review of outcomes associated with a reconstructive approach. *Head Neck* **2019**, *41*, 16–29. [CrossRef] [PubMed]
64. Steffen, A.; Hasselbacher, K.; Heinrichs, S.; Wollenberg, B. Botulinum toxin for salivary disorders in the treatment of head and neck cancer. *Anticancer Res.* **2014**, *34*, 6627–6632.

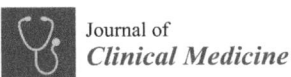

Article

Accumulation of Experience and Newly Developed Devices Can Improve the Safety and Voice Outcome of Total Thyroidectomy for Graves' Disease

Cheng-Hsun Chuang [1], Tzu-Yen Huang [1], Tzer-Zen Hwang [2,3], Che-Wei Wu [1], I-Cheng Lu [4], Pi-Ying Chang [5], Yi-Chu Lin [1], Ling-Feng Wang [1], Chih-Chun Wang [2,3], Ching-Feng Lien [2,3], Gianlorenzo Dionigi [6,7], Chih-Feng Tai [1,*] and Feng-Yu Chiang [2,3,*]

[1] Department of Otorhinolaryngology-Head and Neck Surgery, Kaohsiung Medical University Hospital, Faculty of Medicine, College of Medicine, Kaohsiung Medical University, No. 100 Tzyou First Road, Kaohsiung 807, Taiwan; 18chengxun@gmail.com (C.-H.C.); tyhuang.ent@gmail.com (T.-Y.H.); cwwu@kmu.edu.tw (C.-W.W.); reddust0113@yahoo.com.tw (Y.-C.L.); lifewang@kmu.edu.tw (L.-F.W.)

[2] Department of Otolaryngology-Head and Neck Surgery, E-Da Hospital, No. 1, Yida Road, Jiaosu Village, Yanchao District, Kaohsiung 824, Taiwan; tzhwang@hotmail.com.tw (T.-Z.H.); ccw5969@yahoo.com.tw (C.-C.W.); lien980206@yahoo.com.tw (C.-F.L.)

[3] School of Medicine, College of Medicine, I-Shou University, Kaohsiung 824, Taiwan

[4] Department of Anesthesiology, Kaohsiung Municipal Siaogang Hospital, Kaohsiung Medical University Hospital, Faculty of Medicine, College of Medicine, Kaohsiung Medical University, Kaohsiung 807, Taiwan; u9251112@gmail.com

[5] Department of Anesthesiology, Kaohsiung Municipal Tatung Hospital, Kaohsiung Medical University Hospital, Faculty of Medicine, College of Medicine, Kaohsiung Medical University, Kaohsiung 801, Taiwan; annabelle69@gmail.com

[6] Division of General Surgery, Endocrine Surgery Section, Istituto Auxologico Italiano IRCCS, 20095 Milan, Italy; gianlorenzo.dionigi@unimi.it

[7] Department of Pathophysiology and Transplantation, University of Milan, 20133 Milan, Italy

* Correspondence: cftai@kmu.edu.tw (C.-F.T.); fychiang@kmu.edu.tw (F.-Y.C.)

Abstract: Total thyroidectomy (TT) in patients with Graves' disease is challenging even for an experienced thyroid surgeon. This study aimed to investigate the accumulation of experience and applying newly developed devices on major complications and voice outcomes after surgery of a single surgeon over 30 years. This study retrospectively reviewed 90 patients with Graves' disease who received TT. Forty-six patients received surgery during 1990–1999 (Group A), and 44 patients received surgery during 2010–2019 (Group B). Major complications rates were compared between Group A/B, and objective voice parameters were compared between the usage of energy-based devices (EBDs) within Group B. Compared to Group B, Group A patients had higher rates of recurrent laryngeal nerve palsy (13.0%/1.1%, $p = 0.001$), postoperative hypocalcemia (47.8%/18.2%, $p = 0.002$), and postoperative hematoma (10.9%/2.3%, $p = 0.108$). Additionally, Group A had one permanent vocal cord palsy, four permanent hypocalcemia, and one thyroid storm, whereas none of Group B had these complications. Group B patients with EBDs had a significantly better pitch range ($p = 0.015$) and jitter ($p = 0.035$) than those without EBDs. To reduce the major complications rate, inexperienced thyroid surgeons should remain vigilant when performing TT for Graves' disease. Updates on surgical concepts and the effective use of operative adjuncts are necessary to improve patient safety and voice outcome.

Keywords: Graves' disease; total thyroidectomy; major complications; voice outcome; experience and newly developed devices; energy-based device (EBD)

1. Introduction

Graves' disease is the most common cause of persistent hyperthyroidism. The annual prevalence rate is approximately 20 to 30 cases per 100,000 individuals, and the lifetime prevalence rates in women and men are 3% and 0.5%, respectively [1]. Depending on the preferences and clinical features of the patient, treatment for Graves' disease may include anti-thyroid drugs, radioactive iodine therapy, and thyroidectomy [2].

The suggested indications for surgical treatment of Graves' disease include large goiters, lesions causing tracheal compression, moderate-to-severe ophthalmopathy, current pregnancy or breastfeeding, poor control of hyperthyroidism after radio-iodine ablation or after anti-thyroid drug therapy, and suspected malignancy of a coexisting nodule [3]. In the literature, two surgical managements for Graves' disease can be considered—subtotal or total thyroidectomy (TT). Subtotal thyroidectomy leaves 4 to 7 g of thyroid and provides patients with adequate thyroid function without requiring thyroxin replacement. Another advantage is that the procedure reduces the risk of hypoparathyroidism [4]. However, in a study of 415 consecutive Graves' disease patients treated by subtotal thyroidectomy with a mean thyroid remnant weight of 5.1 g, 28.7% (119 patients) had persistent or recurrent hyperthyroidism, over 50% had hypothyroidism, and 19.3% achieved an euthyroid state [5]. Furthermore, a second surgery for recurrence may be more difficult than a first surgery owing to distortion of tissue planes by scar tissue formation and may have a higher risk of injury to the recurrent laryngeal nerve (RLN) and parathyroid glands (PGs) [6]. Therefore, TT is a preferred surgical treatment option because of several advantages, including (1) low recurrence rate, (2) rapid and reliable control of hyperthyroidism and its related symptoms, (3) radical resection of coexisting malignant thyroid tumor, (4) optimal release of airway compression, (5) absence of side-effects such as those in radio-iodine and anti-thyroid drug therapy, and (6) possible elimination of further progression of ophthalmopathy [7–9].

Compared to patients with euthyroid multiple nodular goiters, TT for Graves' disease patients has significantly higher rates of vocal cord palsy, postoperative hypocalcemia (PH), and hematoma requiring reoperation [10]. Graves' disease patients tend to have a larger thyroid size and an adhesive thyroid capsule to the surrounding neck structure, Palestini et al. [11] reported that voice changes or neck discomfort were reported by 29% and 8% of patients after thyroidectomy for Graves' disease patients. Therefore, high levels of surgical experience and technical knowledge may have important roles in lowering the occurrence of the major complications and preventing voice impairment. To the best of our knowledge, this study is the first to investigate the surgical performance on major complications and voice outcome after TT for Graves' disease of a single surgeon over 30 years.

2. Materials and Methods

This retrospective study enrolled patients with Graves' disease who had received TT performed by a single thyroid surgeon (F.-Y.C.) within a 30 year period (1990–2019) in Kaohsiung Medical University Hospital. The surgeon performs more than 200 thyroid surgeries every year, and the surgical complications in recent years are presented in [12,13]. Ethical approval of this study was obtained from the Kaohsiung Medical University Hospital Institutional Review Board (KMUHIRB-E(II)-20200026). The surgeries were divided into two groups according to the time of surgery: Group A included 46 consecutive patients who had received TT during 1990–1999, and Group B included 44 consecutive patients who had received TT during 2010–2019. Thyroid surgeries with or without energy-based device (EBD) assistance in Group B were evaluated; in this study, the Ligasure^{TM} small jaw (Medtronic, Covidien, CO, USA) was applied as the EBD in Graves' disease surgery.

The surgical indications for patients with Graves' disease included refractory hyperthyroidism, suspected thyroid malignancy, local compression symptoms caused by Graves' disease, and Graves' ophthalmopathy. A different surgical strategy for preserving RLNs and PGs was used in each group. In Group A, all RLNs were identified and preserved by visualization alone, and preferably at least one PG was autotransplanted. In Group B, RLNs were routinely identified and preserved by visualization with the adjunct of intermittent intraoperative neuromonitoring (IONM), and PGs were preserved in situ whenever possible. Autotransplantation was the least preferred option for devascularized PGs.

In both groups of patients, vocal cord mobility was video-recorded with a flexible laryngo-fiberscope before and after surgery. If vocal cord palsy occurred, the patient was followed up until complete recovery of vocal cord function. An RLN palsy was considered permanent if vocal cord dysfunction persisted longer than 6 months after surgery. The RLN palsy rate was based on the number of nerves at risk.

Preoperative and postoperative (12, 24, 48, and 72 h after surgery) serum ionized calcium (iCa) levels were measured in each group. Normal iCa was defined as the mean (± 2SD) preoperative iCa. In Group A, PH was defined as iCa under 4.0 mg/dL in at least two measurements. In Group B, PH was defined as iCa under 4.2 mg/dL in at least two measurements. Permanent PH was defined as a persistent PH that required treatment with calcium supplements more than 12 months after surgery [13]. Postoperative hematoma was defined as progressive neck swelling that required emergent surgical intervention.

Objective voice analysis included the Multidimensional Voice Program (model 5105, version 3.1.7; KayPENTAX, NJ, USA) and Voice Range Profile (model 4326, version 3.3.0; KayPENTAX, NJ, USA). Objective voice parameters were obtained, including maximum pitch frequency (Fmax), minimum pitch frequency (Fmin), pitch range (PR), mean fundamental frequency (Mean F0), jitter, shimmer, and noise-to-harmonic ratio (NHR). The PR was defined as the number of semitones between Fmax and Fmin.

All patients received anti-thyroid drugs and were controlled to euthyroid state before surgery, and no patients in the two groups were given Lugol's solution preoperatively.

Variables were analyzed by the t-test and chi-square test performed using SPSS (version 18.0 for windows; SPSS Inc., Chicago, IL, USA). A two-tailed p value less than 0.05 was considered statistically significant.

3. Results

Table 1 shows the demographic and clinical characteristics of the patients. There was no significant difference in gender, age, or pathology results between Group A and Group B. Among the patients in Group B, 3 of 7 patients having a malignant pathology result received radioactive iodine treatment, and none of the 7 patients received re-intervention or had cancer recurrence. However, the two groups significantly differed in the number of patients with at least one PG autotransplantation; forty (87.0%) patients in Group A and twenty-two (50.0%) patients in Group B had at least one PG autotransplantation ($p = 0.001$).

Table 1. Demographic and clinical characteristics of Group A and Group B.

	Group A (46 Patients)	Group B (44 Patients)	p Value
Gender			0.697
Women	35	35	
Men	11	9	
Age (Year, Mean ± SD)	35.8 ± 13.8	40.8 ± 14.1	0.096
Pathology			0.489
Benign (%)	41 (89.1)	37 (84.1)	
Malignancy (%)	5 (10.9)	7 (15.9)	
PG autotransplantation * (%)	40 (87.0)	22 (50.0)	0.001

* The number of patients with at least one parathyroid gland (PG) autotransplantation.

Table 2 compares the major complication rates in the two groups. The RLN palsy rate was significantly higher in Group A compared to Group B (13.0% vs. 1.1%, $p = 0.001$). Group A had 11 temporary palsies and one permanent palsy while Group B had only one temporary RLN palsy. Group A also had a significantly higher PH rate compared to Group B (47.8% vs. 18.2%, $p = 0.002$). Additionally, Group A had 18 (39.1%) patients with temporary PH and 4 (8.7%) patients with permanent PH, whereas Group B only had 8 (18.2%) patients with temporary PH and no patients with permanent PH.

Five (10.9%) patients in Group A and one (2.3%) patient in Group B developed postoperative hematoma, which showed no significant difference ($p = 0.108$). Only one patient in Group A had a thyroid storm.

Table 2. Major complications of total thyroidectomy in Graves' Disease.

	Group A (46 Patients)	Group B (44 Patients)	p Value
RLN palsy [a,b] (%)	12/92 (13.0)	1/88 (1.1)	
Temporary (%)	11 (11.9)	1 (1.1)	0.001
Permanent (%)	1 (1.1)	0 (0.0)	
Postoperative hypocalcemia (%)	22/46 (47.8)	8/44 (18.2)	
Temporary (%)	18 (39.1)	8 (18.2)	0.002
Permanent (%)	4 (8.7)	0 (0.0)	
Postoperative hematoma (%)	5/46 (10.9)	1/44 (2.3)	0.108
Thyroid storm (%)	1/46 (2.2)	0/44 (0.0)	0.323

[a] Recurrent laryngeal nerve (RLN) palsy was considered permanent if vocal cord dysfunction persisted longer than 6 months after surgery. The incidence was based on the number of RLNs at risk. [b] No occurrence of bilateral RLN palsy.

Table 3 compares the changes in objective voice parameters between preoperative and 6 week postoperative periods in Group B with (n = 22) or without (n = 22) EBD assistance. The patients that received surgery with EBDs had a significantly lower proportion of PR decrease >30% (40.9% vs. 9.1%, $p = 0.015$) and Jitter increase >30% (63.6% vs. 31.8%, $p = 0.035$) compared to the without-EBD group.

Table 3. Six-week postoperative objective voice analysis in Group B with or without EBD.

	Without EBD (22 Patients)	With EBD (22 Patients)	p Value
Fmin decrease > 30%	2 (9.1)	3 (13.6)	0.635
Fmax decrease > 30%	10 (45.5)	5 (22.7)	0.112
PR decrease > 30%	9 (40.9)	2 (9.1)	0.015 *
Mean F0 decrease > 30%	2 (9.1)	2 (9.1)	1.000
Jitter increase > 30%	14 (63.6)	7 (31.8)	0.035 *
Shimmer increase > 30%	6 (27.3)	5 (22.7)	0.728
NHR increase > 30%	5 (22.7)	3 (13.6)	0.434

Abbreviation: EBD = Energy-based devices; Fmin = Minimum frequency; Fmax = Maximum frequency; PR = Pitch range; Mean F0 = Mean fundamental frequency; NHR = Noise-harmonic ratio. * $p < 0.05$ was considered statistically significant.

4. Discussion

In comparison with Group A, Group B showed less incidence of major complications, particularly RLN palsy and PH. In Group B, surgery with EBD assistance showed better voice outcomes. Surgical experience, updates on surgical concepts, and effective use of operative adjuncts show a strong association to the surgical performance after TT in patients with Graves' disease.

Duclos et al. [14] reported a permanent RLN palsy rate of 2.08% in 2357 patients under thyroid procedures, and the patients' thyroid disease consisted of 69.8% (n = 1645) non-toxic nodule, 10.7% (n = 253) hyperthyroidism, 9.7% (n = 228) Grave's disease, and 9.8% (n = 231) malignant neoplasm. In the group of Graves' patients, the permanent RLN palsy rate was 3.5%. They demonstrated that the successful RLN preservation may be challenging even for experienced, high-volume surgeons. Wagner and Seiler also reported that, after thyroidectomy, patients with Graves' disease had a higher rate of permanent RLN palsy compared to those with euthyroid nodular goiter (4% vs. 1.7%, respectively) [15]. All Group A patients in this study had received surgery performed by a single surgeon in his first decade of clinical practice. The RLN palsy rate reached as high as 13.0% when the surgeon had a relatively low experience level and did not use innovative surgical techniques such as IONM. Although the RLN was visually identified in all cases in Group A, 11 temporary palsies and one permanent palsy occurred. In other words, the visual integrity of the RLN is not consistent with the functional preservation, especially the temporary nerve injuries. In contrast, the RLN palsy rate decreased to 1.1% in Group B patients who received the surgeon's third decade of practice and with the aid of IONM. The comparison suggests that the accumulated experience of the surgeon and the assistance of IONM provided the accuracy in identifying RLN, understood the mechanism of nerve injury, and improved the surgical technique, which resulted in a reduced RLN palsy rate in Group B.

Patients with thyroiditis do not have abnormal perceptual vocal evaluation or acoustic findings compared with controls [16]; however, the mass effect of Graves' disease can be a negative factor for patients' voice. Voice changes or neck discomfort were not uncommon after thyroidectomy for Graves' disease patients [11]. For better surgical field exposure, Ko et al. [17] reported U-shape muscle flap (USMF) surgical methods and included two patients with large Graves' disease in that study. They concluded that voice and swallowing functions after USMF are comparable to those obtained by the midline approach. Liu et al. [12] reported a 1000 neuro-monitored thyroidectomies series compared the surgical outcomes between the EBD group (Ligasure) and conventional group, including 23 patients with Graves' disease. The EBD group had overall lower surgical complication rates in comparison with the conventional group. Effective hemostasis helps to avoid excessive muscle retraction and reduce the injury of the extralaryngeal muscles, thereby avoiding the influence of the extralaryngeal muscles on the fine control of voice production after thyroid surgery. In the current study, applying EBDs in modern thyroid surgery for Graves' disease brought a better objective voice outcome in PR and Jitter. The continuous developments of novel nerve monitoring and hemostasis devices can further change the surgical procedures; in addition, the anti-adhesive material/technique also show great potential for improving surgical outcomes.

PH is one of the most common complications after TT [18], particularly in Graves' disease [19–21]. Graves' disease patients usually have a large thyroid volume and a vigorous vessel supply. Dissecting the thyroid lobe in a narrow space is susceptible to bleeding and increases the risk of PG damage due to poor visualization, especially in procedures performed by low-volume surgeons [22]. In a study of 42 Graves' disease patients, Nair et al. [20] reported temporary and permanent hypocalcemia in 42.85% and 9.52% of patients, respectively. Similarly, in another study of 165 Graves' disease patients, Guo et al. [21] reported temporary and permanent hypocalcemia in 18.8% and 3.6% of patients, respectively. In the current study, Group A patients treated by the surgeon in his first decade of practice had high rates of temporary and permanent PH (39.1% and 8.7%, respectively). In Group B, the improved outcomes on the temporary and permanent PH rates (18.2% and 0.0%, respectively) may be attributable to improvements in surgical technique and strategies for preserving PG function. In Group A patients, we preferred the strategy of at least one PG autotransplantation, which in the 1990s, was believed to have a low risk of permanent hypoparathyroidism [23,24]. Our current principles of intraoperative PG management is in situ preservation, and the procedures include (1) division of individual blood vessels near the thyroid gland to avoid interference with the blood supply to PGs, (2) careful inspection of the thyroid capsule to determine whether PGs had adhered to the capsule, (3) routine check of PG blood supply with stabbing test (stabbing PG with a 23 G needle to check if fresh blood flowed out) or nick test (incision made on PG capsule with fine scissors to check if fresh blood flowed out) when a disturbance of blood supply was suspected, and (4) PG autotransplantation only in the case of devascularization [13].

Weiss et al. reported a 1.34% postoperative hematoma rate and a 0.32% mortality rate in 150,012 thyroid surgery patients [25]. The thyroid gland is a highly vascularized organ [26], particularly in Graves' disease. Hematoma is reported in a large proportion of

Graves' disease patients who undergo thyroid surgeries [27]. In the current study, Group A had a higher hematoma rate compared with Group B, but the difference was not statistically significant (10.5% vs. 2.3%, $p = 0.108$). Some studies have reported that the use of EBDs decreases the occurrence of hematoma after thyroidectomy [28,29]. However, others have shown that hematoma does not significantly differ between EBDs and the conventional clamp-and-tie technique [30–32]. Therefore, the advantage of EBDs needs further study in a high volume of Graves' disease patients.

Surgeon performance can be evaluated by the occurrence of postoperative complications, and the experience of surgeons can be roughly estimated by their age or their years of surgical practice. For young surgeons, the importance of education and training to gain experience is obvious [33]. To achieve the best results, surgeons need time to acquire the necessary technical background and to master routine procedures [34,35]. Experts typically reach their peak performance after approximately 10 years of experience in their specialty [36]. However, the surgical performance of older surgeons might decline over time due to mental fatigue from performing repetitive procedures, physiological factors, lack of updated knowledge, and poor adherence to principles of evidence-based medicine and new techniques, all of which can contribute to reduced safety and poor treatment outcomes [14,37].

According to some studies, thyroid surgeries performed by experienced surgeons tend to have low complication rates, short lengths of hospital stay [38,39], and low costs of treating complications [39]. However, defining an experienced thyroid surgeon is difficult and requires the consideration of factors other than age, years of practice, and number of thyroidectomy procedures performed [33]. For example, Duclos et al. demonstrated high rates of complications after thyroidectomy in procedures performed by inexperienced surgeons and older surgeons [14]. Generally, an experienced thyroid surgeon can be defined as a surgeon who has (1) has at least 10 years of experience in thyroid surgery, (2) an average annual volume of 100 thyroidectomies with a low complication rate [40], and (3) familiarity with new technologies, e.g., IONM and EBDs. This study showed that, as surgeon experience increases, the rate of major postoperative complication rates in TT for Graves' disease decreases.

Talent and experience are insufficient to ensure a safe surgery if a surgeon lacks the motivation and willingness to progress [41]. To maintain a high level of performance for the rest of their careers, surgeons must continuously evaluate the quality of the care they deliver and update their surgical concepts. As the result in this study, we suggest that the inexperienced surgeons should improve the technique to safely preserve the function of RLN and PGs in regular thyroid surgeries before performing operations on Graves' disease patients.

This study had some limitations. As this was not a prospective or randomized study, bias resulting from comparisons of patients treated in different periods and by different techniques and instruments was unavoidable. However, the data were collected from a single surgeon over his 30 years of experience in performing surgery in patients with Graves' disease. This study was indeed comparing the different experience levels with surgical performance from the same surgeon. The description about "peak performance" in this article is the general situation of the surgeon's career. However, in the development of thyroid surgery, the progress in IONM and EBDs in the past decade was too remarkable, which had a very positive impact on the surgical outcomes. Therefore, accumulation of surgical experience and the utilization of newly developed devices are the indispensable factors for thyroid surgeons in this era to improve patient safety. This was also the specific reason for choosing the two time periods (Group A and Group B) for comparison.

5. Conclusions

TT for Graves' disease is a challenging procedure with a high rate of major complications. To reduce the major complications rate, inexperienced thyroid surgeons should remain vigilant when performing total thyroidectomy for Graves' disease. It is also suggested that inexperienced surgeons should improve the technique to safely preserve the function of RLN and PGs in regular thyroid surgeries before performing operations on Graves' disease patients. Updates on surgical concepts and the effective use of operative adjuncts (i.e., EBD) are necessary to improve patient safety and functional outcomes.

Author Contributions: Supervision—T.-Z.H., C.-W.W., L.-F.W. and G.D.; materials—I.-C.L. and F.-Y.C.; data collection and processing—P.-Y.C., C.-C.W., C.-F.L. and C.-F.T.; analysis and interpretation—C.-H.C., T.-Y.H., C.-W.W., Y.-C.L. and G.D.; literature Search—C.-H.C., T.-Y.H., C.-F.T. and F.-Y.C.; writing manuscript—All authors. All authors have read and agreed to the published version of the manuscript.

Funding: This study was supported by grants from Kaohsiung Medical University Hospital, Kaohsiung Medical University (KMUH108-8M48, KMUH109-9M44, KMUH110-0R51), Kaohsiung Municipal Siaogang Hospital/Kaohsiung Medical University Research Center grants (KMHK-DK(C)110009, I-109-04, H-109-05, I-108-02), and Ministry of Science and Technology (MOST 110-2314-B-037-104-MY2, MOST 110-2314-B-037-120), Taiwan.

Institutional Review Board Statement: The study was conducted according to the guidelines of the Declaration of Helsinki and approved by the Kaohsiung Medical University Hospital Institutional Review Board (KMUHIRB-E(II)- 20200026).

Informed Consent Statement: Patient consent was waived. The study has minimal risks and the potential risk level to the study subjects is not beyond the level of nonparticipants. In addition, the rights of the study subjects are not affected.

Data Availability Statement: The original contributions presented in the study are included in the article. Further inquiries can be directed to the corresponding authors.

Acknowledgments: The authors gratefully acknowledge the technical assistance provided by Hui-Chun Chen (clinical nurse specialist, Department of Nursing, KMUH).

Conflicts of Interest: The authors declare no conflict of interest.

References

1. Smith, T.J.; Hegedüs, L. Graves' disease. *N. Engl. J. Med.* **2016**, *375*, 1552–1565. [CrossRef] [PubMed]
2. Burch, H.B.; Cooper, D.S. Management of Graves disease: A review. *JAMA* **2015**, *314*, 2544–2554. [CrossRef] [PubMed]
3. The American Thyroid Association and American Association of Clinical Endocrinologists Taskforce on Hyperthyroidism and Other Causes of Thyrotoxicosis; Bahn, R.S.; Burch, H.B.; Cooper, D.S.; Garber, J.R.; Greenlee, M.C.; Klein, I.; Laurberg, P.; McDougall, I.P.; Montori, V.M.; et al. Hyperthyroidism and other causes of thyrotoxicosis: Management guidelines of the American Thyroid Association and American Association of Clinical Endocrinologists. *Thyroid* **2011**, *21*, 593–646. [CrossRef] [PubMed]
4. Ross, D.S.; Burch, H.B.; Cooper, D.S.; Greenlee, M.C.; Laurberg, P.; Maia, A.L.; Rivkees, S.A.; Samuels, M.; Sosa, J.A.; Stan, M.N. 2016 American Thyroid Association guidelines for diagnosis and management of hyperthyroidism and other causes of thyrotoxicosis. *Thyroid* **2016**, *26*, 1343–1421. [CrossRef] [PubMed]
5. Lin, Y.-S.; Lin, J.-D.; Hsu, C.-C.; Yu, M.-C. The long-term outcomes of thyroid function after subtotal thyroidectomy for Graves' hyperthyroidism. *J. Surg. Res.* **2017**, *220*, 112–118. [CrossRef] [PubMed]
6. Shaha, A.R. Revision thyroid surgery–technical considerations. *Otolaryngol. Clin. N. Am.* **2008**, *41*, 1169–1183. [CrossRef] [PubMed]
7. Wilhelm, S.M.; McHenry, C.R. Total thyroidectomy is superior to subtotal thyroidectomy for management of Graves' disease in the United States. *World J. Surg.* **2010**, *34*, 1261–1264. [CrossRef]
8. Bartalena, L.; Tanda, M.; Piantanida, E.; Lai, A.; Pinchera, A. Relationship between management of hyperthyroidism and course of the ophthalmopathy. *J. Endocrinol. Investig.* **2004**, *27*, 288–294. [CrossRef]
9. Barczyński, M.; Konturek, A.; Hubalewska-Dydejczyk, A.; Gołkowski, F.; Nowak, W. Randomized clinical trial of bilateral subtotal thyroidectomy versus total thyroidectomy for Graves' disease with a 5-year follow-up. *Br. J. Surg.* **2012**, *99*, 515–522. [CrossRef]
10. Rubio, G.A.; Koru-Sengul, T.; Vaghaiwalla, T.M.; Parikh, P.P.; Farra, J.C.; Lew, J.I. Postoperative outcomes in Graves' disease patients: Results from the nationwide inpatient sample database. *Thyroid* **2017**, *27*, 825–831. [CrossRef]
11. Palestini, N.; Grivon, M.; Durando, R.; Freddi, M.; Odasso, C.; Robecchi, A. Thyroidectomy for Graves' hyperthyroidism. *Ann. Ital. Chir.* **2007**, *78*, 405–412. [PubMed]

12. Liu, C.-H.; Wang, C.-C.; Wu, C.-W.; Lin, Y.-C.; Lu, I.; Chang, P.-Y.; Lien, C.-F.; Wang, C.-C.; Hwang, T.-Z.; Huang, T.-Y. Comparison of surgical complications rates between LigaSure small jaw and clamp-and-tie hemostatic Technique in 1,000 neuro-monitored thyroidectomies. *Front. Endocrinol.* **2021**, *12*, 313. [CrossRef] [PubMed]
13. Chiang, F.Y.; Lee, K.D.; Tae, K.; Tufano, R.P.; Wu, C.W.; Lu, I.C.; Chang, P.Y.; Lin, Y.C.; Huang, T.Y. Comparison of hypocalcemia rates between LigaSure and clamp-and-tie hemostatic technique in total thyroidectomies. *Head Neck* **2019**, *41*, 3677–3683. [CrossRef] [PubMed]
14. Duclos, A.; Peix, J.L.; Colin, C.; Kraimps, J.L.; Menegaux, F.; Pattou, F.; Sebag, F.; Touzet, S.; Bourdy, S.; Voirin, N.; et al. Influence of experience on performance of individual surgeons in thyroid surgery: Prospective cross sectional multicentre study. *BMJ* **2012**, *344*, d8041. [CrossRef] [PubMed]
15. Wagner, H.; Seiler, C. Recurrent laryngeal nerve palsy after thyroid gland surgery. *Br. J. Surg.* **1994**, *81*, 226–228. [CrossRef] [PubMed]
16. Hamdan, A.-l.; Nassar, J.; El-Dahouk, I.; Al Zaghal, Z.; Jabbour, J.; Azar, S.T. Vocal characteristics in patients with thyroiditis. *Am. J. Otolaryngol.* **2012**, *33*, 600–603. [CrossRef]
17. Ko, H.-Y.; Lu, I.-C.; Chang, P.-Y.; Wang, L.-F.; Wu, C.-W.; Yu, W.-H.V.; Hwang, T.Z.; Wang, C.C.; Huang, T.-Y.; Chiang, F.-Y. U-shaped strap muscle flap for difficult thyroid surgery. *Gland Surg.* **2020**, *9*, 372. [CrossRef]
18. Bergenfelz, A.; Jansson, S.; Kristoffersson, A.; Martensson, H.; Reihner, E.; Wallin, G.; Lausen, I. Complications to thyroid surgery: Results as reported in a database from a multicenter audit comprising 3,660 patients. *Langenbecks Arch. Surg.* **2008**, *393*, 667–673. [CrossRef] [PubMed]
19. Thomusch, O.; Machens, A.; Sekulla, C.; Ukkat, J.; Lippert, H.; Gastinger, I.; Dralle, H. Multivariate analysis of risk factors for postoperative complications in benign goiter surgery: Prospective multicenter study in Germany. *World J. Surg.* **2000**, *24*, 1335–1341. [CrossRef]
20. Nair, C.G.; Babu, M.J.; Menon, R.; Jacob, P. Hypocalcaemia following total thyroidectomy: An analysis of 806 patients. *Indian J. Endocrinol. Metab.* **2013**, *17*, 298–303. [CrossRef]
21. Kwon, H.; Kim, J.K.; Lim, W.; Moon, B.I.; Paik, N.S. Increased risk of postoperative complications after total thyroidectomy with Graves' disease. *Head Neck* **2019**, *41*, 281–285. [CrossRef] [PubMed]
22. Thomas, G.; McWade, M.A.; Paras, C.; Mannoh, E.A.; Sanders, M.E.; White, L.M.; Broome, J.T.; Phay, J.E.; Baregamian, N.; Solorzano, C.C.; et al. Developing a Clinical Prototype to Guide Surgeons for Intraoperative Label-Free Identification of Parathyroid Glands in Real Time. *Thyroid* **2018**, *28*, 1517–1531. [CrossRef] [PubMed]
23. Shaha, A.R.; Jaffe, B.M. Parathyroid preservation during thyroid surgery. *Am. J. Otolaryngol.* **1998**, *19*, 113–117. [CrossRef]
24. Olson Jr, J.A.; DeBenedetti, M.K.; Baumann, D.S.; Wells Jr, S.A. Parathyroid autotransplantation during thyroidectomy. Results of long-term follow-up. *Ann. Surg.* **1996**, *223*, 472. [CrossRef] [PubMed]
25. Weiss, A.; Lee, K.C.; Brumund, K.T.; Chang, D.C.; Bouvet, M. Risk factors for hematoma after thyroidectomy: Results from the nationwide inpatient sample. *Surgery* **2014**, *156*, 399–404. [CrossRef]
26. Adam, M.A.; Thomas, S.; Youngwirth, L.; Hyslop, T.; Reed, S.D.; Scheri, R.P.; Roman, S.A.; Sosa, J.A. Is There a Minimum Number of Thyroidectomies a Surgeon Should Perform to Optimize Patient Outcomes? *Ann Surg.* **2017**, *265*, 402–407. [CrossRef]
27. Rosato, L.; Avenia, N.; Bernante, P.; De Palma, M.; Gulino, G.; Nasi, P.G.; Pelizzo, M.R.; Pezzullo, L. Complications of thyroid surgery: Analysis of a multicentric study on 14,934 patients operated on in Italy over 5 years. *World J. Surg.* **2004**, *28*, 271–276. [CrossRef]
28. Moran, K.; Grigorian, A.; Elfenbein, D.; Schubl, S.; Jutric, Z.; Lekawa, M.; Nahmias, J. Energy vessel sealant devices are associated with decreased risk of neck hematoma after thyroid surgery. *Updates Surg.* **2020**, *72*, 1135–1141. [CrossRef]
29. Petrakis, I.E.; Kogerakis, N.E.; Lasithiotakis, K.G.; Vrachassotakis, N.; Chalkiadakis, G.E. LigaSure versus clamp-and-tie thyroidectomy for benign nodular disease. *Head Neck J. Sci. Spec. Head Neck* **2004**, *26*, 903–909. [CrossRef]
30. Yao, H.S.; Wang, Q.; Wang, W.J.; Ruan, C.P. Prospective clinical trials of thyroidectomy with LigaSure vs conventional vessel ligation: A systematic review and meta-analysis. *Arch. Surg.* **2009**, *144*, 1167–1174. [CrossRef]
31. Ramouz, A.; Rasihashemi, S.Z.; Safaeiyan, A.; Hosseini, M. Comparing postoperative complication of LigaSure Small Jaw instrument with clamp and tie method in thyroidectomy patients: A randomized controlled trial [IRCT2014010516077N1]. *World J. Surg. Oncol.* **2018**, *16*, 154. [CrossRef] [PubMed]
32. Kuboki, A.; Nakayama, T.; Konno, W.; Goto, K.; Nakajima, I.; Kanaya, H.; Hirabayashi, H.; Haruna, S.-i. New technique using an energy-based device versus conventional technique in open thyroidectomy. *Auris Nasus Larynx* **2013**, *40*, 558–562. [CrossRef] [PubMed]
33. Reznick, R.K.; MacRae, H. Teaching surgical skills—Changes in the wind. *N. Engl. J. Med.* **2006**, *355*, 2664–2669. [CrossRef] [PubMed]
34. Ramsay, C.R.; Grant, A.M.; Wallace, S.A.; Garthwaite, P.; Monk, A.; Russell, I. Statistical assessment of the learning curves of health technologies. *Health Technol. Assess.* **2001**, *5*, 1–79. [CrossRef] [PubMed]
35. Carty, M.J.; Chan, R.; Huckman, R.; Snow, D.; Orgill, D.P. A detailed analysis of the reduction mammaplasty learning curve: A statistical process model for approaching surgical performance improvement. *Plast. Reconstr. Surg.* **2009**, *124*, 706–714. [CrossRef] [PubMed]
36. Anders Ericsson, K. Deliberate practice and acquisition of expert performance: A general overview. *Acad. Emerg. Med.* **2008**, *15*, 988–994. [CrossRef]

37. Choudhry, N.K.; Fletcher, R.H.; Soumerai, S.B. Systematic review: The relationship between clinical experience and quality of health care. *Ann. Intern. Med.* **2005**, *142*, 260–273. [CrossRef]
38. Sosa, J.A.; Mehta, P.J.; Wang, T.S.; Boudourakis, L.; Roman, S.A. A population-based study of outcomes from thyroidectomy in aging Americans: At what cost? *J. Am. Coll. Surg.* **2008**, *206*, 1097–1105. [CrossRef]
39. Sosa, J.A.; Bowman, H.M.; Tielsch, J.M.; Powe, N.R.; Gordon, T.A.; Udelsman, R. The importance of surgeon experience for clinical and economic outcomes from thyroidectomy. *Ann. Surg.* **1998**, *228*, 320. [CrossRef]
40. Stavrakis, A.I.; Ituarte, P.H.; Ko, C.Y.; Yeh, M.W. Surgeon volume as a predictor of outcomes in inpatient and outpatient endocrine surgery. *Surgery* **2007**, *142*, 887–899. [CrossRef]
41. Wallace, J.E.; Lemaire, J.B.; Ghali, W.A. Physician wellness: A missing quality indicator. *Lancet* **2009**, *374*, 1714–1721. [CrossRef]

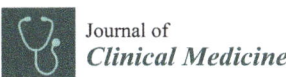

Article

Olfactory Neuroblastomas: What Actually Happens in the Long-Term?

Konstantinos Mantsopoulos [1,*], Michael Koch [1], Heinrich Iro [1] and Jannis Constantinidis [2]

[1] Department of Otorhinolaryngology, Head and Neck Surgery, University of Erlangen–Nürnberg, 91054 Erlangen, Germany; michael.koch@uk-erlangen.de (M.K.); heinrich.iro@uk-erlangen.de (H.I.)
[2] 1st Department of Otolaryngology, Head & Neck Surgery, Aristotle University of Thessaloniki, 54636 Thessaloniki, Greece; janconst@otenet.gr
* Correspondence: konstantinos.mantsopoulos@uk-erlangen.de; Tel.: +49-(0)9131-8533156; Fax: +49-(0)9131-8533833

Citation: Mantsopoulos, K.; Koch, M.; Iro, H.; Constantinidis, J. Olfactory Neuroblastomas: What Actually Happens in the Long-Term? J. Clin. Med. 2022, 11, 2288. https://doi.org/10.3390/jcm11092288

Academic Editors: Luca Giovanni Locatello, Oreste Gallo and Eng Ooi

Received: 12 March 2022
Accepted: 18 April 2022
Published: 20 April 2022

Publisher's Note: MDPI stays neutral with regard to jurisdictional claims in published maps and institutional affiliations.

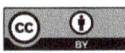

Copyright: © 2022 by the authors. Licensee MDPI, Basel, Switzerland. This article is an open access article distributed under the terms and conditions of the Creative Commons Attribution (CC BY) license (https://creativecommons.org/licenses/by/4.0/).

Abstract: Objective: The aim of this study was to investigate the long-term oncologic outcome and review the state of the art in the management of olfactory neuroblastomas. Material and Methods: The records of all patients treated for olfactory neuroblastomas in two academic departments between 1975 and 2012 were evaluated retrospectively. Data on epidemiological parameters were collected (age, gender), along with staging (Kadish, Morita), histologic grading (Hyams), time and form of treatment, locoregional control, and disease-specific and overall survival. Patients with other malignant diseases, distant metastases of olfactory neuroblastomas at the time of initial diagnosis, a follow-up time of less than 5 years, or insufficient clinical-pathological data were excluded from further analysis. Results: In total, 53 cases made up our final study sample (26 men, 27 women; male–female ratio 0.96:1). Their mean age was 48.6 years (range: 10–84 years). The mean follow-up time was 137.5 months (4–336 months, SD: 85.0). A total of 5 out of 53 study cases (9.4%) showed metastatic involvement of the neck at the time of initial presentation. Local recurrence was detected in 8/53 (15.1%) and regional recurrence in 7/53 of our study cases (13.2%). Three patients (42.8%) from the group of cases with surgery as the sole form of management (7/53, 13.2%) died due to the disease. The cumulative disease-specific survival and overall survivalfor the whole group of patients were 88.6% and 63.6%, respectively. The cumulative disease-specific survival stratified by Kadish A/B vs. Kadish C/D as well as Hyams I/II vs. Hyams III/IV showed superior results for limited tumors, albeit without significance, and low-grade tumors (highly significant difference). Conclusion: Craniofacial or sometimes solely endoscopically controlled resection can warrant resection of the olfactory neuroblastoma with wide margins. However, locoregional failures and distant metastases can occur after a long period of time. The non-negligible incidence of regional recurrences, partly in unusual localizations, leads us to consider the need to identify the "recurrence-friendly" cases and to perform individualized elective irradiation of the neck in cases with high-risk features.

Keywords: olfactory neuroblastoma; esthesioneuroblastoma; Kadish; Hyams; recurrence; survival; endoscopic surgery

1. Introduction

The neuroectodermal malignancy of olfactory neuroblastoma (ON), which was discovered less than 100 years ago and initially named "*esthesioneuroepitheliome olfactif*" [1], has an incidence of about 0.4 cases per million and accounts for 3–6% of all sinonasal malignancies [2]. The vague symptomatic and demanding anatomic localization ("rhino-neurosurgical border"), the extremely variable and hardly predictable biologic behavior [3–5] (cases with slow evolution and late recurrences as well as aggressive and metastatic forms with fulminant behavior already at onset [6,7]) in combination with the extremely low prevalence constitute the challenging profile of this lesion. In our view, almost no other malignant entity in the head and neck region is complicated by such a large number of open, controversial clinical and surgical issues: the various staging systems [4,8–14] (as well as the absence of an official AJCC (The American Joint Committee on Cancer)/UICCC (Union internationale contre le cancer) staging system [11]); the debatable prognostic role [13,15–17]; the subjectivity as well as the sampling dependence [18] of histopathology-based Hyams grading; the possibility of reducing therapeutic invasiveness (single-modality surgical treatment) in carefully selected "low-risk" cases [19]; the role of local irradiation as well as elective nodal irradiation of a cN0 neck in "low-risk" lesions [7,20,21], e.g., in teenagers and young adults [6]; and the ideal imaging modality for the follow-up [22] as well as the long-term course of the disease [12,23] dominate the relevant literature. In the last three decades, the establishment of endoscopically controlled approaches (as the first or sole surgical step in tumors confined to the nasal cavity) as well as new irradiation modalities (e.g., intensity-modulated radiation therapy) opened new horizons in the "quality-of-life"-oriented but still oncologically sufficient management of these tumors [24,25].

The aim of this study was to present the experience of two academic centers in the long-term outcome of patients with ON over a period of 42 years (1975–2017) with a minimum follow-up of 5 years as well as review the state of the art in the relevant literature regarding the aforementioned controversial clinical and therapeutic issues of this demanding entity. The motivation behind this study lay in the need to optimize our patient counseling by enriching it with long-term feedback and perhaps by thoroughly reconsidering our management philosophy.

2. Materials and Methods

This study was performed at two academic tertiary referral centers (Department of Otorhinolaryngology, Head and Neck Surgery, University of Erlangen–Nuremberg, Erlangen, Germany and Department of Otorhinolaryngology, Head and Neck Surgery, University of Thessaloniki, Thessaloniki, Greece). The records of all patients treated curatively for ON before 2012 were studied retrospectively. Patients with other malignant diseases, distant metastases of ON at the time of initial diagnosis, a follow-up time of less than 5 years, or insufficient clinical-pathological data were excluded from further analysis. Data was collected on epidemiological parameters (age, gender), staging (Kadish [8], modified Kadish–Morita [26]), histologic profile (Hyams [13]), time and form of management, locoregional control, and disease-specific and overall survival. The specimens of all cases managed before introduction of Hyams' grading in 1988 [13] were evaluated retrospectively for histopathologic grading from an experienced head and neck pathologist in our department. Staging was performed using information from patients' surgical archives or imaging data (CT and/or MRI). The five-year overall survival estimate (OS) was defined as the percentage of patients who were still alive within 5 years divided by the total number of patients. The five-year disease-specific survival rate estimate (DSS) was defined using the time from the date of diagnosis to death from the cancer or from complications of treatment. Regional recurrence was defined as histologically confirmed ON in the neck after completion of initial treatment. DSS and OS were calculated using the Kaplan–Meier method. Univariate comparisons between subgroups were performed using the Log-Rank test. The association of 5-year-DSS with Kadish–Morita staging, Hyams grading, and initial N status was examined by means of multivariate linear regression analysis. A p-value < 0.05 indicated statistical significance. SPSS for Windows v. 25.0 (SPSS, Inc., Chicago, IL, USA) was used for statistical analysis. Approval was obtained from the institutional review boards of both hospitals.

3. Results

In total, 53 cases made up our final study sample (26 men, 27 women; male–female ratio 0.96:1). Their mean age was 48.6 years (range: 10–84 years). The mean follow-up time was 137.5 months (4–336 months, SD: 85.0). Detailed information on patients' demographics, tumor characteristics, treatment form, and oncologic outcome is given in Tables 1 and 2. A total of 5 out of 53 study cases (9.4%) showed metastatic involvement of the neck at the time of initial presentation. Local recurrence was detected in 8/53 (15.1%) and regional recurrence in 7/53 of our study cases (13.2%). Three patients (42.8%) from the group of cases with surgery as the sole form of management (7/53, 13.2%) died of the disease. The cumulative 5-year-DSS and OS for the whole group of patients were 88.6% and 63.6%, respectively Figures 1 and 2. The cumulative DSS stratified by Kadish A/B vs. Kadish C/D as well as Hyams I/II vs. Hyams III/IV showed superior results for limited tumors, albeit without significance, and low-grade tumors (highly significant difference, Table 3, Figures 3 and 4). Multivariate linear regression analysis showed that among the examined factors (Kadish–Morita staging, Hyams grading, initial N status), only Hyams grading was an independent prognostic for survival ($p = 0.05$). The 5-year-DSS was significantly higher in the group of patients treated in the 2001–2017 period compared to the patients treated in the 1975–2000 period (100% vs. 72.2%, $p = 0.002$).

Table 1. Patient, tumor, and treatment characteristics of all patients of our study sample (ESS: endoscopic sinus surgery, TFA: transfacial approach (lateral rhinotomy), BFC: bifrontal craniotomy, aRT: adjuvant irradiation, RCT: Radiochemotherapy, AND: alive and free of disease, AWD: alive with disease, DOD: dead because of disease, DAD: dead for non-disease-relevant reason).

ID	Gender	Age (y)	Stage (Kadish)	Stage (Kadish–Morita)	Histologic Grading (Hyams)	N Status	Treatment	Recurrence (After ... Months)	Outcome (Follow-Up in Months)
1	Female	10	B	B	IIII	N0	Neoadjuvant RCT + BFC	Local	AND (144)
2	Male	56	B	B	III	N0	Neoadjuvant RT + BFC	Local	DAD (259)
3	Female	22	C	D	IV	N3	Neoadjuvant RCT + BFC	No	DOD (4)
4	Female	38	C	C	III	N0	Neoadjuvant RT + TFA	Locoregional	DOD (21)
5	Male	59	A	A	II	N0	ESS	No	AND (199)
6	Male	54	B	B	I	N0	ESS	No	AND (156)
7	Female	63	B	B	II	N0	ESS	No	AND (120)
8	Female	77	B	B	IV	N0	TFA	Local	DOD (14)
9	Female	46	C	C	III	N0	BFC	No	AND (122)
10	Female	50	B	B	III	N0	BFC	Locoregional	DOD (8)
11	Male	50	C	C	III	N0	BFC	No	DOD (4)
12	Male	28	B	B	II	N0	ESS + aRT	No	AND (214)
13	Female	67	B	B	II	N0	ESS + aRT	No	DAD (131)
14	Male	16	B	B	III	N0	ESS + aRT	No	AND (141)
15	Male	52	B	D	III	N1	ESS + aRT	No	AND (124)
16	Male	36	C	C	III	N0	ESS + aRT	No	AND (208)
17	Male	48	C	C	III	N0	ESS + aRT	Regional	AND (189)
18	Female	55	C	C	III	N0	ESS + aRT	No	AND (154)
19	Female	41	C	C	III	N0	ESS + aRT	No	AND (115)
20	Male	71	B	B	III	N0	ESS + aRT	No	DAD (132)
21	Male	27	B	B	II	N0	ESS + aRT	Regional	AND (180)
22	Female	56	B	B	III	N0	ESS + aRT	No	AND (120)
23	Female	64	C	D	II	N1	ESS + BFC+ aRT	No	AND (205)
24	Female	62	C	C	I	N0	ESS + BFC+ aRT	No	AND (75)
25	Male	80	B	B	I	N0	ESS + BFC + aRT	No	DAD (143)
26	Male	57	A	A	II	N0	ESS + BFC + aRT	No	AND (264)
27	Female	53	B	B	II	N0	ESS + BFC + aRT	No	AND (300)
28	Male	32	C	C	III	N0	ESS + BFC + aRT	Local	DOD (26)
29	Male	15	B	B	II	N0	TFA + aRT	No	AND (288)
30	Male	51	B	B	I	N0	BFC + aRT	Local	AND (156)
31	Male	48	C	C	I	N0	BFC + aRT	No	AND (264)
32	Female	57	C	C	I	N0	BFC + aRT	No	AND (252)
33	Male	62	C	C	I	N0	BFC + aRT	No	DAD (117)
34	Female	38	B	B	II	N0	BFC + aRT	Regional	AND (192)
35	Female	31	B	B	II	N0	BFC + aRT	No	AND (180)

Table 1. Cont.

ID	Gender	Age (y)	Stage (Kadish)	Stage (Kadish–Morita)	Histologic Grading (Hyams)	N Status	Treatment	Recurrence (After... Months)	Outcome (Follow-Up in Months)
36	Female	84	B	B	II	N0	BFC + aRT	No	DAD (16)
37	Male	36	C	C	III	N0	BFC + aRT	No	AND (336)
38	Female	34	C	D	III	N3	BFC + aRT	Regional	AND (180)
39	Female	45	C	C	III	N0	BFC + aRT	No	AND (123)
40	Female	43	C	C	III	N0	BFC + aRT	No	AND (126)
41	Male	68	C	C	III	N0	BFC + aRT	Distant recurrence	AND (144)
42	Female	69	C	C	IV	N0	BFC + aRT	No	AND (259)
43	Female	17	B	B	III	N0	ESS + aRT	No	AND (96)
44	Male	51	C	C	III	N0	ESS + aRT	No	AND (84)
45	Male	24	C	C	IV	N0	ESS + BFC + aRT	No	AND (70)
46	Female	44	B	B	III	N0	ESS +aRT	No	AND (64)
47	Male	62	A	A	II	N0	ESS + aRT	No	AND (58)
48	Male	55	C	C	III	N2	Neoadjuvant RCT + ESS	No	AND (47)
49	Female	65	C	C	II	N0	ESS + BFC + aRT	No	AND (61)
50	Male	53	B	B	II	N0	ESS + aRT	No	AND (84)
51	Female	67	B	B	III	N0	ESS + aRT	No	AND (93)
52	Female	43	C	C	III	N0	ESS + BFC + aRT	Local, distant	AWD (104)
53	Male	47	B	B	III	N0	ESS + aRT	Regional	AND (124)

Table 2. Detailed information of all study patients and treatment characteristics.

Gender (n, %)	
Male	26 (49.1)
Female	27 (50.9)
Kadish [8] stage (n, %)	
A	3 (5.7)
B	25 (47.2)
C	25 (47.2)
Kadish–Morita [26] grading (n, %)	
A	3 (5.7)
B	24 (45.3)
C	22 (41.5)
D	4 (7.5)
Hyams [13] (n, %)	
I	7 (13.2)
II	1 (28.3)
III	26 (49.1)
IV	5 (9.4)
Nodal stage (n, %)	
N0	48 (90.6)
N+	5 (9.4)
Therapeutic approach (n, %)	
Surgery only	7 (13.2)
Surgery + adjuvant irradiation	41 (77.3)
Neoadjuvant R(C)T + surgery	5 (9.4)
Surgical approach (n, %)	
Endoscopic only	22 (41.5)
Endoscopic + open (craniofacial)	22 (41.5)
Open (craniofacial)	9 (17)

Table 3. Disease-specific survival estimates for all study patients stratified by Kadish–Morita stage and Hyams grading.

KERRYPNX	5-Year Disease-Specific Survival Estimates	p-Value
Kadish–Morita [26] stage		
A–B	92.6%	0.377
C–D	84.6%	
Hyams [13] grading		
I–II	100%	
III–IV	80.6%	0.32

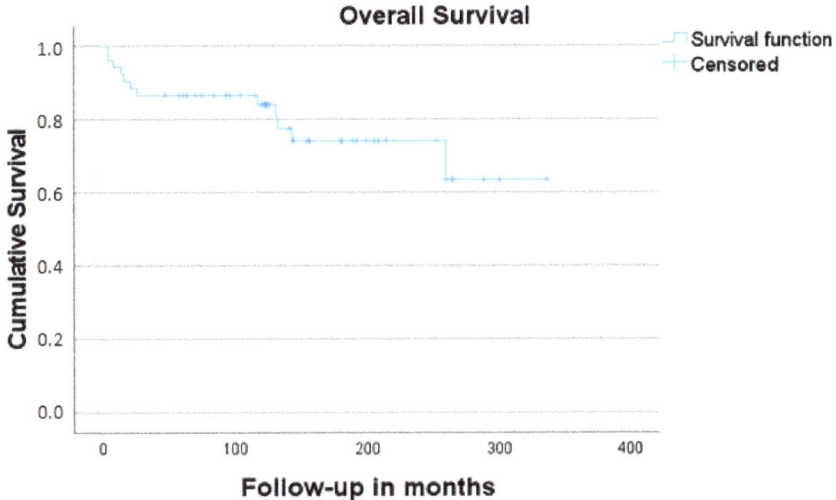

Figure 1. Overall survival estimates for all patients included in the study.

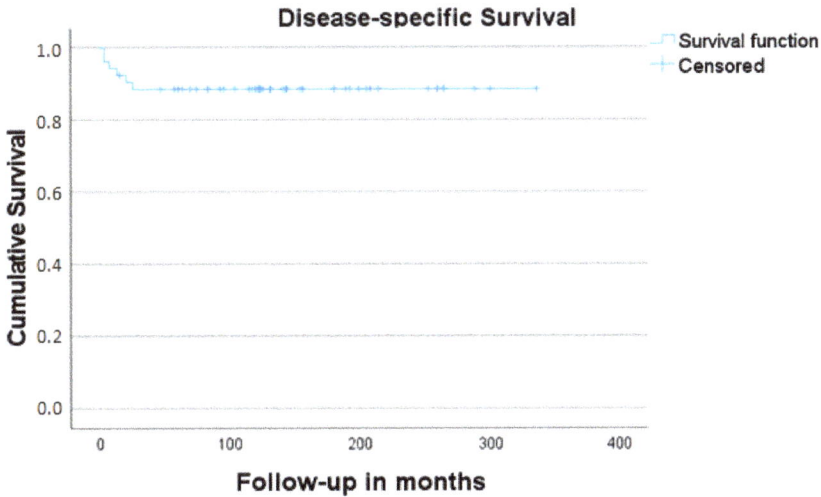

Figure 2. Disease-free survival estimates for all patients included in the study.

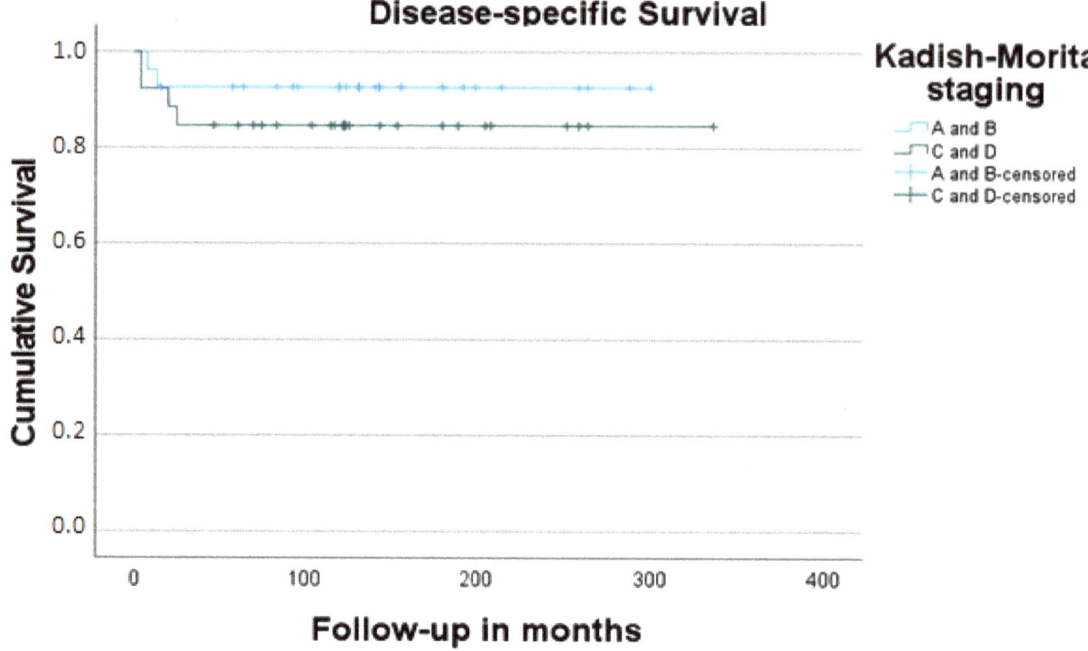

Figure 3. Estimated disease-free (D) survival stratified by Kadish–Morita stage.

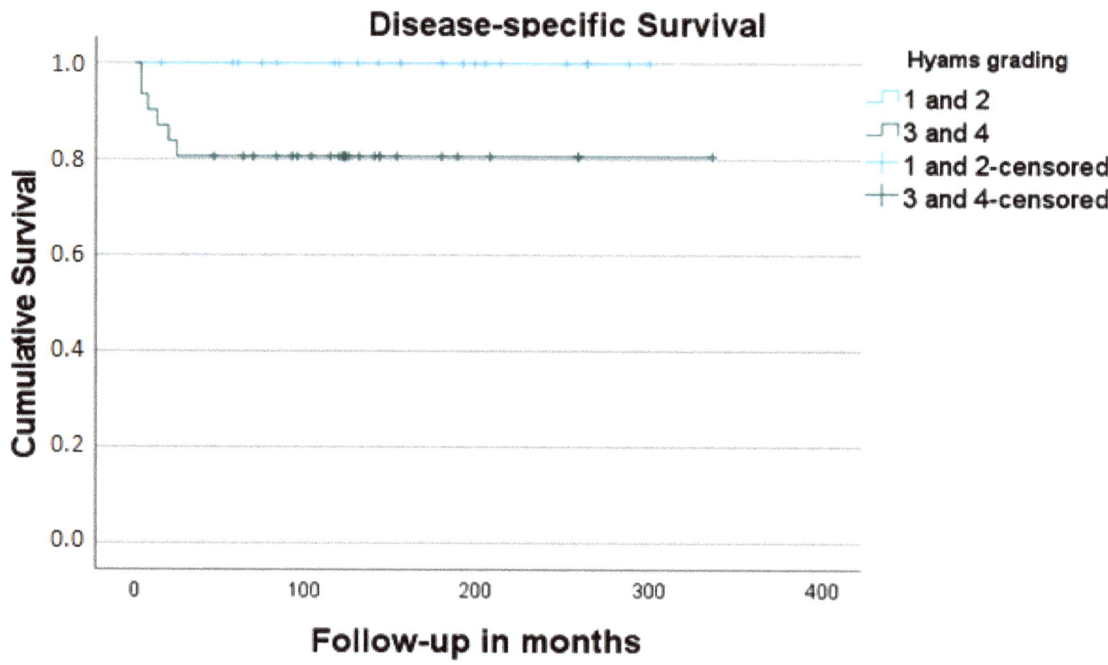

Figure 4. Estimated disease-free survival stratified by histologic grading (Hyams).

4. Discussion

A thorough search of the relevant literature reveals that prospective data remain elusive because of the extremely low incidence of this entity [27]. The increased incidence in the literature of recent years mirrors the improved diagnostic capacity and underlines the necessity for well-designed treatment algorithms [28]. The first issue to deal with is the form of management of the primary tumor. A review of the literature, as well as an investigation of our data, revealed a shift of paradigm from the "gold standard" of craniofacial resection in recent decades of the last century to the continuously increasing performance of endoscopic resection (as a sole or adjunct approach), with some centers even employing endoscopic techniques for the resection of selected tumors with intracranial extension (Figures 5 and 6) [29,30]. In any case, a multimodal approach (surgery with adjuvant irradiation) is thought to be the "gold standard" for high-risk cases (e.g., R1 situation, advanced Kadish stages, aggressive Hyams subtypes) in treatment protocols intended to cure. While the role of chemotherapy is not well defined [30], it could, however, play a role in neoadjuvant settings for locally advanced tumorous lesions [19,31] and cases with primary distant metastases or distant recurrences [32]. Several literature reports point out the possibility of surgery as the sole form of treatment in very carefully selected cases [19]. Examining the subgroup of our study patients with surgery as the sole form of management (6/42, 14.3%), we saw that three patients (50%) died of the disease (among them, one with Kadish stage C and one with Hyams IV). Meerwein et al. saw a potential reduction in therapeutic invasiveness (surgery as a single-modality treatment) in cases with the following profile: limited local tumor extension (Kadish stage A–B), absence of brain involvement, Hyams grade up to III, and microscopically clear surgical margins (based on a definitive histopathological workup) [19]. An investigation of our data revealed a shift of paradigm in the treatment of these tumors following the development and expansion of the spectrum of endoscopic surgery for this indication three decades ago. It seems that surgery alone could only be an equal alternative to multimodal treatment in carefully selected patients with a lack of risk factors and after a thorough discussion of each case with an interdisciplinary tumor board.

A reasonable treatment algorithm should be based on thorough knowledge of the biologic (metastatic) behavior of the disease. In this context, Koch et al. detected local recurrences in 23% of their study cases [3]. Similarly, Constantinidis et al. found local recurrences in 19.2% of their patient sample [33]. In our study, local recurrence was detected in 8/53 of the study cases (15.1%). The vast majority of these cases (7/8) had a Kadish stage higher than B and a Hyams grade higher than III. Three cases were managed (in the first years of the study) by means of neoadjuvant radio(chemo)therapy and two with adjuvant irradiation after primary surgery. Reasonably, local recurrence reflects a highly aggressive form of the disease, with the majority of the cases (4/8) dying within a short period of time (8–26 months) after the initial diagnosis of the tumor.

According to the relevant literature, 5–8% of patients with ON show metastatic involvement of the neck at the time of initial presentation [3,34,35]. In our study sample, regional involvement at the time of the first diagnosis was almost 10%. This percentage scale is certainly below the "20% law" for elective treatment of the regional lymphogenous network that was described by Weiss et al. [36], pointing to the fact that a possible "wait-and-scan" policy without management of the lymphatic stations might be sufficient in the majority of cases. However, this percentage does not justify complacency and makes a thorough scan of the neck within the initial diagnostic workout inevitable. Admittedly, the involvement of the neck gains much more importance in the form of regional recurrence at a later stage in the course of disease, with an incidence as high as 25% [34]. The incidence of this parameter in our long-term analysis (7/53, 13.2%) was almost the same as that seen in a systematic review by Naples et al. [12]. A careful investigation of this subgroup of patients revealed the consistent presence of "high-risk" tumor characteristics, namely higher Kadish stages (three cases with Kadish stage B and three with C) and advanced Hyams grades (higher than II) in all cases. Six out of these seven cases had received irradiation of the primary lesion (neoadjuvant in one case with Kadish stage C and Hyams grade III, adjuvant in the remaining five cases). In two cases, the regional failure was combined with local relapse, and the disease showed massive progression with subsequent distant metastases and the patient's death after 8 and 21 months after initial diagnosis. In the remaining five cases with solitary regional recurrences, the mean time to regional recurrence was 83 months (68–96 months). Our data showed that management of the invaded lymph nodes by means of neck dissection with adjuvant radio (chemo) therapy could achieve an acceptable long-term oncologic result (Table 1).

The ongoing controversy in the management of a clinically negative neck in ON [7] is reflected, among others, in a popular radiation oncology textbook that states, on the one hand, that "the available data do not justify routine elective nodal treatment", but recommends in another Section, 123 pages later, that "with advanced-stage disease, cervical lymph nodes should be initially managed by irradiation, radical neck dissection, or a combination of both" [37]. Elective neck irradiation was not administered routinely to a cN0 neck in either of the departments involved in the present study. However, as patients with regional recurrences tend to have higher mortality [12] (worse survival outcomes) and given that "prevention is the best treatment", our aforementioned observations sustain the reasonability of elective neck management (e.g., irradiation) in specific cases in which risk-stratified adjuvant irradiation of the primary tumor site is indicated [38]. In other words, if a local finding has such aggressive features that it has to be irradiated, then a cN0 neck will probably also have to be irradiated, as both the primary tumor and the regional lymphatic network belong to the same case of a "high-risk" profile! Eighteen years ago, Constantinidis et al. pointed to the frequent development of regional recurrences, sometimes long after initial therapy, independent of any type of aggressive therapy [33]. Another interesting observation was that in 2/7 cases with regional recurrence, the positive lymph node was localized in the retro- and parapharyngeal space (Figure 7). The already described rather rare tendency of the olfactory neuroepithelium tumor cells to metastasize in the lymphatic network of the retro- and parapharyngeal space [39,40] necessitates radiologic vigilance both in the initial staging and in the follow-up. In a relevant literature report [39], as well as in one of our cases, the pathologic changes in the lymph nodes, in retrospect, were already present on the first images of the axial datasets and were initially overlooked on routine MRI evaluation of the neck. Potential involvement of the retro- or parapharyngeal lymph nodes (Figure 7) has both a clinical relevance as well as a radiologic implication: First of all, it seems reasonable that primary management of the cN0 neck, if indicated, has to take the form of irradiation, as an elective neck dissection alone cannot easily address the (in case of recurrence frequently usually involved) retro- and parapharyngeal space without a significant increase in surgical morbidity [41]. Secondly, it gives computer tomography, MRI, or FDG-PET/CT the lead over ultrasound in the imaging of the neck. Considering the fact that an N+ situation changes the stage to Kadish–Morita D [26], worsens the prognosis [12,35], and definitively justifies adjuvant irradiation in the initial phase [42], it cannot be emphasized enough that a thorough initial scan of the patient is of major importance.

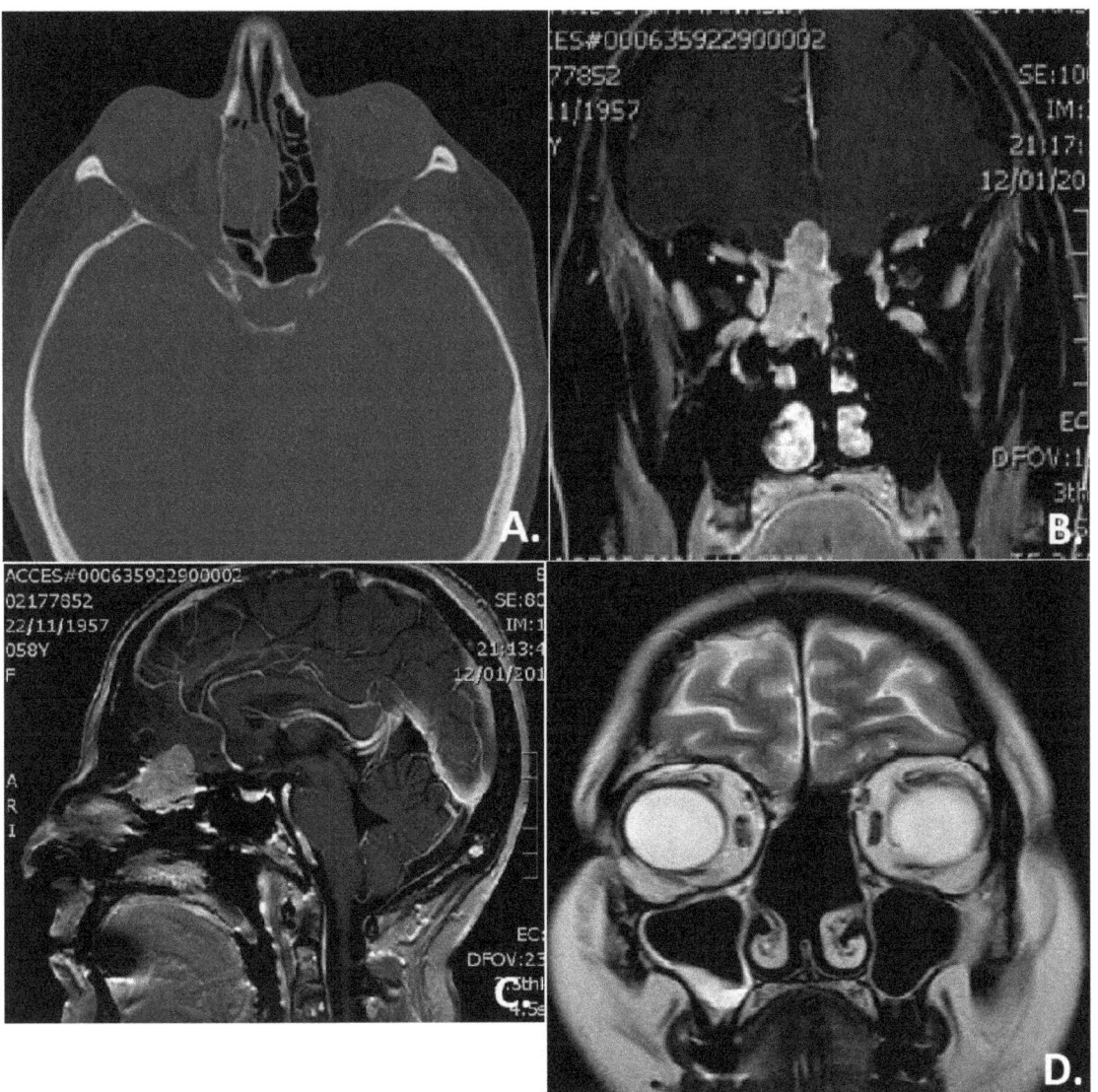

Figure 5. Imaging of a patient with an olfactory neuroblastoma. (**A**) Computed tomography (axial section) shows involvement of the ethmoid cells on the right side. (**B**) Magnetic resonance imaging (coronal section) and (**C**) sagittal section shows a marked "nodular" intracranial extension of the tumor. (**D**) Follow-up: magnetic resonance imaging (coronal section) without sign of local recurrence on follow-up.

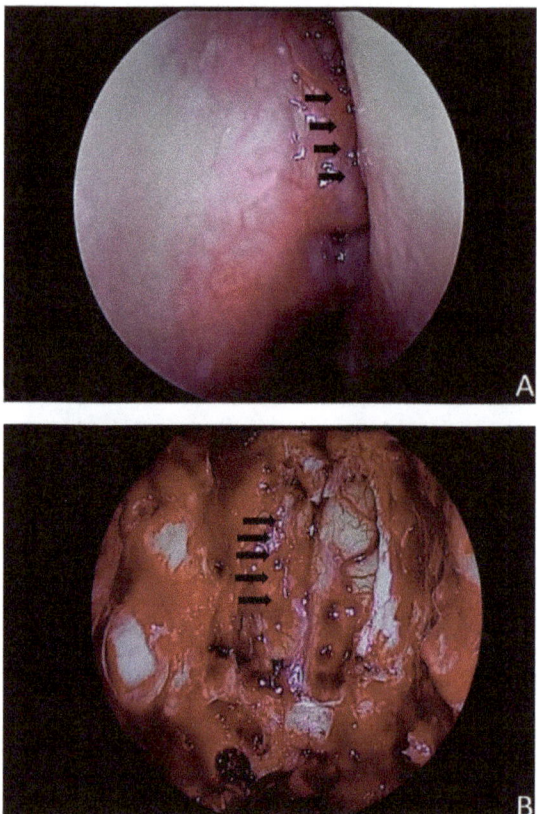

Figure 6. Intraoperative photos of the same case with olfactory neuroblastoma. (**A**) Endoscopic picture of the tumorous lesion (black arrows) in the right nasal cavity. (**B**) Surgical situs after sole endoscopic resection of the olfactory neuroblastoma, bilateral resection of the olfactory bulbs, and the remaining intracranial portion of the tumor (black arrows).

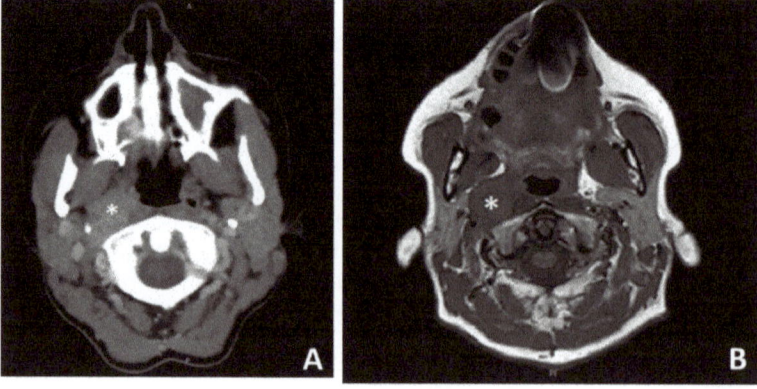

Figure 7. Axial contrast-enhanced computed tomography (**A**) and T1-weighted MRI (**B**) of a patient with regional recurrence in the right parapharyngeal space (white asterisk) 68 months after initial craniofacial resection and adjuvant irradiation in olfactory neuroblastoma Kadish–Morita stage B/Hyams grade III.

5. Conclusions

Firstly, the survival analysis of our study showed superior cumulative DSS for limited lesions (no significance) and low-grade tumors (highly significant). A review of the relevant literature reveals a more consistent position concerning the prognostic importance of the Kadish staging system [19] but more variability concerning the prognostic impact of the histologic grading [16]. Secondly, a statistically better survival was detected in the group of patients being treated in the latter study period (with cases of advanced stage as well as a higher grade being homogeneously distributed in both study groups), pointing to the positive impact of the increasing experience in the oncologic outcome of our cases. Thirdly, the non-negligible incidence of regional recurrences, partly in unusual localizations (e.g., retro- and parapharyngeal space), leads us to consider the need for identifying the "recurrence-friendly" cases and for primary elective irradiation of the neck in cases with high-risk features. Interestingly, the present long-term study confirms the reliability of the results of an analysis of one of the involved departments 18 years ago [33]. Last but not least, individualization of this indication with consideration of other factors (e.g., age) is needed.

Author Contributions: Conceptualization, K.M., M.K., H.I. and J.C.; Formal analysis, K.M. and J.C.; Funding acquisition, K.M. and H.I.; Investigation, K.M. and J.C.; Methodology, K.M., H.I. and J.C.; Project administration, K.M., M.K., H.I. and J.C.; Resources, K.M., M.K., H.I. and J.C.; Software, K.M.; Supervision, K.M. and J.C.; Validation, K.M. and J.C.; Visualization, K.M., M.K. and H.I.; Writing—original draft, K.M. and J.C.; Writing—review & editing, K.M., M.K., H.I. and J.C. All authors have read and agreed to the published version of the manuscript.

Funding: The APC was funded by the Friedrich-Alexander Universität Erlangen-Nürnberg.

Institutional Review Board Statement: Approval was obtained from the institutional review boards of the academic departments conducting the study.

Data Availability Statement: The data presented in this study are available on request from the corresponding author.

Conflicts of Interest: The authors declare no conflict of interest.

References

1. Berger, L.L.R.; Richard, D. L'esthesioneuroepithe liome olfactif. *Bull. Assoc. Fr. Etud. Cancer* **1924**, *13*, 410–421.
2. Ferlito, A.; Rinaldo, A.; Rhys-Evans, P.H. Contemporary clinical commentary: Esthesioneuroblastoma: An update on management of the neck. *Laryngoscope* **2003**, *113*, 1935–1938. [CrossRef]
3. Koch, M.; Constantinidis, J.; Dimmler, A.; Strauss, C.; Iro, H. Long-term experiences in the therapy of esthesioneuroblastoma. *Laryngorhinootologie* **2006**, *85*, 723–730. [CrossRef]
4. Dulguerov, P.; Calcaterra, T. Esthesioneuroblastoma: The UCLA experience 1970–1990. *Laryngoscope* **1992**, *102*, 843–849. [CrossRef]
5. Rimmer, J.; Lund, V.J.; Beale, T.; Wei, W.I.; Howard, D. Olfactory neuroblastoma: A 35-year experience and suggested follow-up protocol. *Laryngoscope* **2014**, *124*, 1542–1549. [CrossRef]
6. Dumont, B.; Lemelle, L.; Cordero, C.; Couloigner, V.; Bernard, S.; Cardoen, L.; Brisse, H.J.; Jehanno, N.; Fréneaux, P.; Helfre, S.; et al. Esthesioneuroblastoma in children, adolescents and young adults. *Bull. Cancer* **2020**, *107*, 934–945. [CrossRef]
7. Demiroz, C.; Gutfeld, O.; Aboziada, M.; Brown, D.; Marentette, L.J.; Eisbruch, A. Esthesioneuroblastoma: Is there a need for elective neck treatment? *Int. J. Radiat. Oncol. Biol. Phys.* **2011**, *81*, e255–e261. [CrossRef]
8. Kadish, S.; Goodman, M.; Wang, C.C. Olfactory neuroblastoma. A clinical analysis of 17 cases. *Cancer* **1976**, *37*, 1571–1576. [CrossRef]
9. Biller, H.F.; Lawson, W.; Sachdev, V.P.; Som, P. Esthesioneuroblastoma: Surgical treatment without radiation. *Laryngoscope* **1990**, *100*, 1199–1201. [CrossRef]
10. Foote, R.L.; Morita, A.; Ebersold, M.J.; Olsen, K.D.; Lewis, J.E.; Quast, L.M.; Ferguson, J.A.; O'Fallon, W.M. Esthesioneuroblastoma: The role of adjuvant radiation therapy. *Int. J. Radiat. Oncol. Biol. Phys.* **1993**, *27*, 835–842. [CrossRef]
11. Sun, M.; Wang, K.; Qu, Y.; Zhang, J.; Zhang, S.; Chen, X.; Wang, J.; Wu, R.; Zhang, Y.; Yi, J.; et al. Proposal of a TNM classification-based staging system for esthesioneuroblastoma: More precise prediction of prognosis. *Head Neck* **2021**, *43*, 1097–1104. [CrossRef]
12. Naples, J.G.; Spiro, J.; Tessema, B.; Kuwada, C.; Kuo, C.L.; Brown, S.M. Neck recurrence and mortality in esthesioneuroblastoma: Implications for management of the N0 neck. *Laryngoscope* **2016**, *126*, 1373–1379. [CrossRef]
13. Hyams, V.J. Olfactory neuroblastoma. In *Tumors of the Upper Respiratory Tract and Ear*; Hyams, V.J.B.J., Michaels, L., Eds.; Armed Forces Institute of Pathology: Washington, DC, USA, 1988; pp. 240–248.

14. Koka, V.N.; Julieron, M.; Bourhis, J.; Janot, F.; Le Ridant, A.M.; Marandas, P.; Luboinski, B.; Schwaab, G. Aesthesioneuroblastoma. *J. Laryngol. Otol.* **1998**, *112*, 628–633. [CrossRef]
15. Lund, V.J.; Howard, D.; Wei, W.; Spittle, M. Olfactory neuroblastoma: Past, present, and future? *Laryngoscope* **2003**, *113*, 502–507. [CrossRef]
16. Zafereo, M.E.; Fakhri, S.; Prayson, R.; Batra, P.S.; Lee, J.; Lanza, D.C.; Citardi, M.J. Esthesioneuroblastoma: 25-year experience at a single institution. *Otolaryngol. Head Neck Surg.* **2008**, *138*, 452–458. [CrossRef]
17. Diaz, E.M., Jr.; Johnigan, R.H., III; Pero, C.; El-Naggar, A.K.; Roberts, D.B.; Barker, J.L.; DeMonte, F. Olfactory neuroblastoma: The 22-year experience at one comprehensive cancer center. *Head Neck* **2005**, *27*, 138–149. [CrossRef]
18. Platek, M.E.; Merzianu, M.; Mashtare, T.L.; Popat, S.R.; Rigual, N.R.; Warren, G.W.; Singh, A.K. Improved survival following surgery and radiation therapy for olfactory neuroblastoma: Analysis of the SEER database. *Radiat. Oncol.* **2011**, *6*, 41. [CrossRef]
19. Meerwein, C.M.; Nikolaou, G.; Binz, G.H.A.; Soyka, M.B.; Holzmann, D. Surgery as Single-Modality Treatment for Early-Stage Olfactory Neuroblastoma: An Institutional Experience, Systematic Review and Meta-analysis. *Am. J. Rhinol. Allergy* **2021**, *35*, 525–534. [CrossRef]
20. Jiang, W.; Mohamed, A.S.R.; Fuller, C.D.; Kim, B.Y.S.; Tang, C.; Gunn, G.B.; Hanna, E.Y.; Frank, S.J.; Su, S.Y.; Diaz, E.; et al. The role of elective nodal irradiation for esthesioneuroblastoma patients with clinically negative neck. *Pract. Radiat. Oncol.* **2016**, *6*, 241–247. [CrossRef]
21. Yin, Z.Z.; Luo, J.W.; Gao, L.; Yi, J.L.; Huang, X.D.; Qu, Y.; Wang, K.; Zhang, S.P.; Xiao, J.P.; Xu, G.Z.; et al. Spread patterns of lymph nodes and the value of elective neck irradiation for esthesioneuroblastoma. *Radiother. Oncol.* **2015**, *117*, 328–332. [CrossRef]
22. Zlochower, A.B.; Steinklein, J.M. Doing Great with DOTATATE: Update on GA-68 DOTATATE Positron Emission Tomography/Computed Tomography and Magnetic Resonance Imaging for Evaluation of Sinonasal Tumors. *Top. Magn. Reason. Imaging* **2021**, *30*, 151–158. [CrossRef]
23. Ow, T.J.; Hanna, E.; Roberts, D.B.; Levine, N.B.; El-Naggar, A.K.; Rosenthal, D.; Demonte, F.; Kupferman, M.E. Optimization of long-term outcomes for patients with esthesioneuroblastoma. *Head Neck* **2014**, *36*, 524–530. [CrossRef]
24. Casiano, R.R.; Numa, W.A.; Falquez, A.M. Endoscopic resection of esthesioneuroblastoma. *Am. J. Rhinol.* **2001**, *15*, 271–279. [CrossRef]
25. Gallia, G.L.; Reh, D.D.; Salmasi, V.; Blitz, A.M.; Koch, W.; Ishii, M. Endonasal endoscopic resection of esthesioneuroblastoma: The Johns Hopkins Hospital experience and review of the literature. *Neurosurg. Rev.* **2011**, *34*, 465–475. [CrossRef]
26. Morita, A.; Ebersold, M.J.; Olsen, K.D.; Foote, R.L.; Lewis, J.E.; Quast, L.M. Esthesioneuroblastoma: Prognosis and management. *Neurosurgery* **1993**, *32*, 706–714, discussion 14–15. [CrossRef]
27. Liermann, J.; Syed, M.; Held, T.; Bernhardt, D.; Plinkert, P.; Jungk, C.; Unterberg, A.; Rieken, S.; Debus, J.; Herfarth, K.; et al. Advanced Radiation Techniques in the Treatment of Esthesioneuroblastoma: A 7-Year Single-Institution's Clinical Experience. *Cancers* **2018**, *10*, 457. [CrossRef]
28. Yin, Z.; Wang, Y.; Wu, Y.; Zhang, X.; Wang, F.; Wang, P.; Tao, Z.; Yuan, Z. Age distribution and age-related outcomes of olfactory neuroblastoma: A population-based analysis. *Cancer Manag. Res.* **2018**, *10*, 1359–1364. [CrossRef]
29. Ramakrishna, R.; Kim, L.J.; Bly, R.A.; Moe, K.; Ferreira, M., Jr. Transorbital neuroendoscopic surgery for the treatment of skull base lesions. *J. Clin. Neurosci.* **2016**, *24*, 99–104. [CrossRef]
30. Nichols, A.C.; Chan, A.W.; Curry, W.T.; Barker, F.G.; Deschler, D.G.; Lin, D.T. Esthesioneuroblastoma: The massachusetts eye and ear infirmary and massachusetts general hospital experience with craniofacial resection, proton beam radiation, and chemotherapy. *Skull Base* **2008**, *18*, 327–337. [CrossRef]
31. Eden, B.V.; Debo, R.F.; Larner, J.M.; Kelly, M.D.; Levine, P.A.; Stewart, F.M.; Cantrell, R.W.; Constable, W.C. Esthesioneuroblastoma. Long-term outcome and patterns of failure—The University of Virginia experience. *Cancer* **1994**, *73*, 2556–2562. [CrossRef]
32. Porter, A.B.; Bernold, D.M.; Giannini, C.; Foote, R.L.; Link, M.J.; Olsen, K.D.; Moynihan, T.J.; Buckner, J.C. Retrospective review of adjuvant chemotherapy for esthesioneuroblastoma. *J. Neurooncol.* **2008**, *90*, 201–204. [CrossRef]
33. Constantinidis, J.; Steinhart, H.; Koch, M.; Buchfelder, M.; Schaenzer, A.; Weidenbecher, M.; Iro, H. Olfactory neuroblastoma: The University of Erlangen-Nuremberg experience 1975–2000. *Otolaryngol. Head Neck Surg.* **2004**, *130*, 567–574. [CrossRef]
34. Zanation, A.M.; Ferlito, A.; Rinaldo, A.; Gore, M.R.; Lund, V.J.; McKinney, K.A.; Suárez, C.; Takes, R.P.; Devaiah, A. When, how and why to treat the neck in patients with esthesioneuroblastoma: A review. *Eur. Arch. Otorhinolaryngol.* **2010**, *267*, 1667–1671. [CrossRef]
35. Banuchi, V.E.; Dooley, L.; Lee, N.Y.; Pfister, D.G.; McBride, S.; Riaz, N.; Bilsky, M.H.; Ganly, I.; Shah, J.P.; Kraus, D.H.; et al. Patterns of regional and distant metastasis in esthesioneuroblastoma. *Laryngoscope* **2016**, *126*, 1556–1561. [CrossRef]
36. Weiss, M.H.; Harrison, L.B.; Isaacs, R.S. Use of decision analysis in planning a management strategy for the stage N0 neck. *Arch. Otolaryngol. Head Neck Surg.* **1994**, *120*, 699–702. [CrossRef]
37. *Principles and Practice of Radiation Oncology*, 5th ed.; Lippincott Williams & Wilkins: Philadelphia, PA, USA, 2008.
38. Managing Esthesioneuroblastoma—An Expert's Guide. ERS Webinar Autumn Series. 2021. Available online: https://www.youtube.com/watch?v=6Mgl-p5-Dxo (accessed on 1 February 2022).
39. Zollinger, L.V.; Wiggins, R.H., III; Cornelius, R.S.; Phillips, C.D. Retropharyngeal lymph node metastasis from esthesioneuroblastoma: A review of the therapeutic and prognostic implications. *AJNR Am. J. Neuroradiol.* **2008**, *29*, 1561–1563. [CrossRef]
40. Kim, H.J.; Kim, J.; Yoon, J.H. Retropharyngeal lymph node metastasis from olfactory neuroblastoma: A report of two cases. *Eur. Arch. Otorhinolaryngol.* **2006**, *263*, 778–782. [CrossRef]

41. Teshima, M.; Otsuki, N.; Shinomiya, H.; Morita, N.; Furukawa, T.; Morimoto, K.; Nakamura, T.; Hashikawa, K.; Kiyota, N.; Sasaki, R.; et al. Impact of retropharyngeal lymph node dissection in the surgical treatment of hypopharyngeal cancer. *Head Neck* **2019**, *41*, 1738–1744. [CrossRef]
42. Sun, M.; Wang, K.; Qu, Y.; Zhang, J.; Zhang, S.; Chen, X.; Wang, J.; Wu, R.; Zhang, Y.; Yi, J.; et al. Long-term analysis of multimodality treatment outcomes and prognosis of esthesioneuroblastomas: A single center results of 138 patients. *Radiat. Oncol.* **2020**, *15*, 219. [CrossRef]

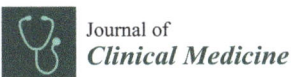

Brief Report

Post-Laryngectomy Voice Prosthesis Changes by Speech-Language Pathologists: Preliminary Results

Stéphane Hans [1], Grégoire Vialatte de Pemille [1], Robin Baudouin [1], Aude Julien-Laferriere [1], Florent Couineau [1], Lise Crevier-Buchman [1], Marta P. Circiu [1] and Jérôme R. Lechien [1,2,3,*]

[1] Department of Otorhinolaryngology and Head and Neck Surgery, Foch Hospital, School of Medicine, UFR Simone Veil, Université Versailles Saint-Quentin-en-Yvelines (Paris Saclay University), F-92150 Paris, France; prhans.foch@gmail.com (S.H.); g.vialatte-de-pemille@hopital-foch.com (G.V.d.P.); robin.baudouin@aol.fr (R.B.); ajlaferriere@gmail.com (A.J.-L.); florentcouineau@gmail.com (F.C.); lise.buchman1@gmail.com (L.C.-B.); mp.circiu@gmail.com (M.P.C.)

[2] Department of Human Anatomy and Experimental Oncology, Faculty of Medicine, UMONS Research Institute for Health Sciences and Technology, University of Mons (UMons), B-7000 Mons, Belgium

[3] Department of Otorhinolaryngology and Head and Neck Surgery, Elsan Polyclinic of Poitiers, F-86000 Poitiers, France

* Correspondence: jerome.lechien@umons.ac.be

Abstract: Background: In the present study, we assess the feasibility and success outcomes of voice prosthesis (VP) changes when performed by a speech-language pathologist (SLP). Methods: Patients treated with total laryngectomy (TL) from January 2020 to December 2020 were prospectively recruited from our medical center. Patients benefited from tracheoesophageal puncture. The VP changes were performed by the senior SLP and the following data were collected for each VP change: date of placement; change or removal; VP type and size; reason for change or removal; and use of a washer for periprosthetic leakage. A patient-reported outcome questionnaire including six items was proposed to patients at each VP change. Items were assessed with a 10-point Likert-scale. Results: Fifty-two VP changes were performed by the senior SLP during the study period. The mean duration of the SLP consultation, including patient history, examination and VP change procedure, was 20 min (range: 15–30). The median prosthesis lifetime was 88 days. The main reasons for VP changes were transprosthetic ($n = 34$; 79%) and periprosthetic ($n = 7$; 21%) leakages. SLP successfully performed all VP changes. He did not change one VP, but used a periprosthetic silastic to stop the periprosthetic leakages. In two cases, SLP needed the surgeon's examination to discuss the following indication: implant mucosa inclusion and autologous fat injection. The patient satisfaction was high according to the speed and the quality of care by the SLP. Conclusions: The delegation of VP change from the otolaryngologist–head and neck surgeon to the speech-language pathologist (SLP) may be achieved without significant complications. The delegation of VP change procedure to SLP may be interesting in some rural regions with otolaryngologist shortages.

Keywords: total laryngectomy; cancer; voice; voice prosthesis; otolaryngology; head neck surgery; speech language therapists

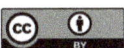

1. Introduction

Total laryngectomy (TL) is a common oncological surgery in head and neck surgery. The post-TL voice rehabilitation is challenging for both patients and practitioners due to the complex nature of patient presentation and the involvement of many motivational and oncological factors [1,2]. To date, tracheoesophageal speech is considered the gold standard for post-TL voice rehabilitation [1,2]. The mean voice prosthesis (VP) lifetime ranges from 3 to 6 months, which supports the need of adequate follow-up and VP changes 3. In most countries, the VP changes are performed by physicians because it is considered as a medical act.

In the present study, we assessed the feasibility and success outcomes of VP changes when performed by a speech-language pathologist (SLP).

2. Materials and Methods

2.1. Ethical Consideration

The local institutional review board approved the study protocol (APHP-HEGP-2018). A waiver of informed consent of participants was granted because participant data were protected and anonymized.

2.2. Subjects and Setting

Patients treated with TL from January 2020 to December 2020 were prospectively recruited from our medical center. Patients benefited from a tracheoesophageal puncture and 1-month post-TL VP. The surgeon used the Provox® 2 type prosthesis (Atos Medical AB, Hörby, Sweden). Patients were followed by an experienced otolaryngologist and SLP for the voice rehabilitation and the oncological follow-up. The first VP change was performed by the senior SLP (GD) who was supervised by the senior head and neck surgeon (SH). The rest of the VP changes were performed by the same SLP without surgeon supervision. However, the surgeon was called in the case of problems.

2.3. Practitioner and Patient Outcomes

The following outcomes were considered: gender; age; primary tumor site; cTNM classification; primary treatment; TL indication (primary, salvage, second primary, and dysfunctional larynx); surgical characteristics (e.g., neck dissection and flap reconstruction); driving distance to the hospital; and survival outcome. The following data were collected for each VP change: date of placement; change or removal; VP type and size; reason for change or removal; and use of a washer for periprosthetic leakage.

A patient-reported outcome questionnaire including 6 items was proposed to patients at each VP change. Items were assessed with a 10-point Likert-scale.

3. Results

Ten patients completed the evaluations. The epidemiological and clinical outcomes of patients are available in Table 1. There were eight males and two females, respectively. The median age was 63.2 yo (range of 48–79 yo). TL was performed for the following indications: low-grade cricoid chondrosarcoma ($n = 2$), recurrent laryngeal cancer after radiation ($n = 3$), or chemoradiation ($n = 5$).

Table 1. Characteristics of patients followed by the speech therapist.

Patient Number	Age (year)	Gender	Comorbidities	Initial Treatment	Indications	cTNM	VP (nb)	Complications
1	75	F	Tobacco	RT	Rec. LSCC	T3N0	4	-
2	79	M	Tobacco	RT	Rec. LSCC	T2N0	3	-
3	64	M	Tobacco, HTA	CRT	Rec. LSCC	T3N1	5	-
4	58	M	HTA	-	CS	-	7	-
5	61	F	Tobacco	CRT	Rec. LSCC	T3N0	4	-
6	68	M	Tobacco HTA	CRT	Rec. LSCC	T2N1	4	-
7	57	M	Tobacco	RT	Rec. LSCC	T1N0	4	-
8	48	M	Tobacco	CRT	Rec. LSCC	T3N0	5	-
9	52	M	Tobacco	CRT	Rec. LSCC	T3N0	3	-
10	70	M	-	-	CS	-	4	-

Abbreviations: CS = chondrosarcoma; RT: radiation therapy; CRT = chemoradiation; F/M = female/male; HTA = hypertension; m = minutes; Rec. LSCC = recurrent laryngeal squamous cell carcinoma; VP = Voice prosthesis; nb: number of prosthesis during the study period.

Fifty-two VP changes were performed by the senior SLP during the study period. The mean duration of the SLP consultation, including patient history, examination, and VP change procedure, was 20 min (range: 15–30). The median prosthesis lifetime was 88 days. The main reasons for VP changes were transprosthetic ($n = 34$; 79%) and periprosthetic ($n = 7$; 21%) leakages. SLP successfully performed all VP changes. He did not change one VP, but used a periprosthetic silastic to stop the periprosthetic leakages. In two cases, the SLP needed the surgeon's examination to discuss the following indications: implant mucosa inclusion and autologous fat injection.

The patient satisfaction was high according to the speed and the quality of care by the SLP (Table 2).

Table 2. Responses to questionnaires.

Questions/Answers	1	2–3	4–5	6–7	8–9	10
Early appointement	39 (93)	2 (5)	1 (2)	-	-	-
Speed and availability of practitioner	39 (93)	2 (5)	1 (2)	-	-	-
Quality of care	40 (96)	1 (2)	1 (2)			
Voice prosthesis change speed	39 (93)	-	2 (5)	-	1 (2)	-
Discomfort during change	32 (75)	4 (10)	4 (10)		2 (5)	
Speech therapist for voice prosthesis change in the future	40 (95)	1 (5)	1 (5)	-	-	-

The numbers in brackets are %. Forty-two patients completed a 10-point evaluation of quality and speed of care, ranging from 1 (very high satisfaction) to 10 (very low satisfaction).

4. Discussion

Voice rehabilitation after TL is an important postoperative issue for the patient quality of life [3–5]. In practice, the VP change is a simple procedure that is usually performed by residents or board-certified physicians. In this study, we reported adequate SLP and patient-reported outcome perception about the SLP-related VP change. The delegation of some clinical tasks from the otolaryngologist–head and neck surgeon to the SLP is a current topical issue that may be associated with many advantages.

First, it is commonly accepted that the development of post-TL tracheoesophageal speech involves important speech rehabilitation work and adequate follow-up for the management of VP leakage, which may be time-consuming for the physician [4]. Currently, the number and the availability of otolaryngologists in rural areas may be limited in some European regions regarding some government hospital reforms that led to significant reductions in medical centers and physicians [6,7]. In our country, the shortage of otolaryngologists in rural regions may lead to patient proposition of post-TL esophageal speech rather than tracheoesophageal speech to limit the need of post-TL care [8]. In that way, the availability of SLPs in the management of VP changes may, therefore, be an advantage for the patient accessibility to health care and follow-up. Second, in some world regions, SLPs already perform routine videolaryngostroboscopy, which was associated with the enhancement of the SLP role in the decision-making process in voice restoration [9]. According to the voice rehabilitation process, SLPs know their patients well, and a trusting relationship may develop throughout the rehabilitation sessions. In the present study, more than 90% of patients reported a high rate of satisfaction outcomes about the SLP-VP change procedure, which may be explained by the trusting relationship between the SLP and patient and the feasibility of the procedure.

The delegation of VP changes to SLP makes particular sense in our country because SLPs have been able to prescribe respiratory or phonatory rehabilitation equipment for TL patients for the past 4 years (law of 30 March 2017). Interestingly, a recent Italian study reported that physicians were not opposed to the delegation of this task to other health professionals, which strengthens the need of debate about this task delegation issue.

The primary limitations of the present study are the low number of procedures performed by the SLP (42 procedures) and the low number of patients, which limited the realization of statistical analysis. The lack of use of validated patient-reported outcome questionnaires assessing the VP change procedure is an additional limitation. To the best of our knowledge, there is no similar study available in the literature, which is the main strength of this preliminary study.

5. Conclusions

The VP change is a feasible procedure for SLP associated with few complications, rare need of physician intervention and adequate patient-reported outcome perception. Future controlled studies are needed to compare VP change outcomes between physicians and SLPs and to evaluate its cost-effectiveness.

Author Contributions: Conceptualization, G.V.d.P. and A.J.-L.; methodology, S.H. and J.R.L.; validation, R.B., J.R.L., F.C., L.C.-B., M.P.C. and S.H.; formal analysis, S.H.; investigation, A.J.-L., L.C.-B. and M.P.C. resources, G.V.d.P. and A.J.-L.; writing—original draft preparation, S.H. and J.R.L. writing—review and editing, J.R.L. All authors have read and agreed to the published version of the manuscript.

Funding: This research received no external funding.

Institutional Review Board Statement: The local institutional review board approved the study protocol (APHP-HEGP-2018). A waiver of informed consent of participants was granted because participant data were protected and anonymized.

Informed Consent Statement: Informed consent was obtained from all subjects involved in the study.

Data Availability Statement: Data are available upon request.

Conflicts of Interest: The authors declare no conflict of interest.

References

1. Mayo-Yáñez, M.; Cabo-Varela, I.; Suanzes-Hernández, J.; Calvo-Henríquez, C.; Chiesa-Estomba, C.; González-Botas, J.H. Use of double flange voice prosthesis for periprosthetic leakage in laryngectomised patients: A prospective case-crossover study. *Clin. Otolaryngol.* **2020**, *45*, 389–393. [CrossRef] [PubMed]
2. Luu, K.; Chang, B.A.; Valenzuela, D.; Anderson, D. Primary versus secondary tracheoesophageal puncture for voice rehabilitation in laryngectomy patients: A systematic review. *Clin. Otolaryngol.* **2018**, *43*, 1250–1259. [CrossRef] [PubMed]
3. Tang, C.G.; Sinclair, C.F. Voice Restoration After Total Laryngectomy. *Otolaryngol. Clin. N. Am.* **2015**, *48*, 687–702. [CrossRef] [PubMed]
4. Maniaci, A.; Lechien, J.R.; Caruso, S.; Nocera, F.; Ferlito, S.; Iannella, G.; Grillo, C.M.; Magliulo, G.; Pace, A.; Vicini, C.; et al. Quality of Life After Total LaryngectomyVoice-Related Quality of Life After Total Laryngectomy: Systematic Review and Meta-Analysis. *J. Voice* **2021**, in press. [CrossRef] [PubMed]
5. Peabody, J.W.; DeMaria, L.; Smith, O.; Hoth, A.; Dragoti, E.; Luck, J. Large-Scale Evaluation of Quality of Care in 6 Countries of Eastern Europe and Central Asia Using Clinical Performance and Value Vignettes. *Glob. Health Sci. Pract.* **2017**, *5*, 412–429. [CrossRef] [PubMed]
6. Straume, K.; Shaw, D.M. Effective physician retention strategies in Norway's northernmost county. *Bull. World Health Organ.* **2010**, *88*, 390–394. [CrossRef] [PubMed]
7. Mérol, J.C.; Swierkosz, F.; Urwald, O.; Nasser, T.; Legros, M. Acoustic comparison of esophageal versus tracheoesophageal speech. *Rev. Laryngol. Otol. Rhinol.* **1999**, *120*, 249–252.
8. Pilsworth, S. Routine use of nasendoscopy to enhance the speech and language therapist'sdecision- making process in surgical voice restoration. *Otolaryngol. Head Neck Surg.* **2011**, *145*, 86–90. [CrossRef] [PubMed]
9. Parrilla, C.; Longobardi, Y.; Paludetti, G.; Marenda, M.E.; D'Alatri, L.; Bussu, F.; Scarano, E.; Galli, J. A one-year time frame for voice prosthesis management. What should the physician expect? Is it an overrated job? *Acta Otorhinolaryngol. Ital.* **2020**, *40*, 270–276. [CrossRef] [PubMed]

Post-Operative Infections in Head and Neck Cancer Surgery: Risk Factors for Different Infection Sites

Giancarlo Pecorari, Giuseppe Riva *, Andrea Albera, Ester Cravero, Elisabetta Fassone, Andrea Canale and Roberto Albera

Division of Otorhinolaryngology, Department of Surgical Sciences, University of Turin, 10126 Turin, Italy
* Correspondence: giuseppe.riva84@gmail.com; Tel.: +39-011-633-7030

Abstract: Background: Post-operative infections in head and neck cancer (HNC) surgery represent a major problem and are associated with an important increase in mortality, morbidity, and burden on the healthcare system. The aim of this retrospective observational study was to evaluate post-operative infections in HNC surgery and to analyze risk factors, with a specific focus on different sites of infection. Methods: Clinical data about 488 HNC patients who underwent surgery were recorded. Univariate and multivariate analyses were performed to identify risk factors for post-operative infections. Results: Post-operative infections were observed in 22.7% of cases. Respiratory and surgical site infections were the most common. Multiple site infections were observed in 3.9% of cases. Considering all infection sites, advanced stage, tracheotomy, and higher duration of surgery were risk factors at multivariate analysis. Median hospital stay was significantly longer in patients who had post-operative infection (38 vs. 9 days). Conclusions: Post-operative infections may negatively affect surgical outcomes. A correct identification of risk factors may help the physicians to prevent post-operative infections in HNC surgery.

Keywords: head and neck surgery; head and neck cancer; post-operative infection; surgical site infection; pneumonia; bacteremia; urinary tract infection

1. Introduction

Healthcare-associated infections (HAIs) are reported to be associated with an important increase in mortality, morbidity, and burden on the healthcare system, especially in the post-operative setting. In the clinical practice, the most frequent types of HAIs are: surgical site infection (SSI), bloodstream infection, respiratory infection, and urinary tract infection [1].

Post-operative HAIs in head and neck cancer (HNC) surgery represent a critical problem and may affect oncological results. Indeed, they can determine a delay in adjuvant radiotherapy (RT) and/or chemotherapy (CT) [2]. Despite the use of prophylactic antibiotics and the best pre- and post-operative care, HAIs incidence is still high due to the expanding microbial resistance [3].

SSIs following head and neck oncological surgery are the main post-operative HAIs and range from 10 to 50% [2–21]. Respiratory infection after HNC surgery ranges between 7 and 40%, urinary tract infection between 2.1 and 6.1%, and bacteremia from 0.7 to 13.8% [2,22–27]. HAIs are associated with prolonged hospitalization, readmission rates, poor cosmetic results and mortality [2,3,18,22,24,27]. Consequently, direct costs rise [25].

Risk factors for SSIs have been analyzed in a number of studies and included higher American Society of Anesthesiologists (ASA) score, comorbidities, smoking, alcohol consumption, previous RT or CT, advanced tumor stage, longer duration of surgery, blood loss and/or anemia, hypoalbuminemia and/or malnutrition (weight loss), presence of tracheotomy, flap reconstruction, and clean-contaminated surgery [4,6,10–12,14–21,28]. Although different authors analyzed these risk factors, significant disagreements with heterogeneous results exist in the literature.

Only a few studies investigated risk factors for respiratory infections and identified age, chronic obstructive pulmonary disease (COPD), tumor stage, smoking, weight loss as significant factors for infections occurrence [2,22–24,27]. Only two studies evaluated risk factors for infections from different sites considered together (all HAIs) [2,22]. In particular, previous radiotherapy, anemia, salvage surgery, tracheotomy, longer surgery duration, microvascular reoperation < 72 h, and flap loss were identified as risks factors for HAIs [2,22]. Finally, to the best of our knowledge, risk factors for multiple site infections have never been investigated.

The aim of this retrospective observational study was to evaluate post-operative infections in HNC surgery and to analyze risk factors identifying the patients at higher risk, with a specific focus on different sites of infection.

2. Materials and Methods

The study sample included 488 patients who underwent HNC surgery at our Division between January 2015 and May 2022. Inclusion criteria were: age > 18 years, and surgery for cancer of oral cavity, pharynx, larynx, paranasal sinuses, salivary glands. Minor procedures, such as biopsies, were excluded from the study. The study was conducted in accordance with the Declaration of Helsinki and approved by the Institutional Review Board (protocol code 0021433, date of approval 26 February 2021). All the patients were contacted and provided written informed consent.

We collected the following clinical data: age, sex, tumor site, smoking, alcohol consumption, body mass index (BMI), comorbidities (allergies, diabetes mellitus, COPD, chronic kidney disease—CKD, cirrhosis), chronic systemic corticosteroid and/or immunosuppressive therapy, tumor node metastasis (TNM) stage, previous RT and/or CT for head and neck cancer, American Society of Anesthesiologists (ASA) score, type of surgical procedure (clean or clean-contaminated surgery), flap reconstruction, tracheotomy, duration of surgery, presence of peripherally inserted central catheter (PICC) or other central venous catheter (CVC), presence of nasogastric feeding tube, post-operative Intensive Care Unit (ICU) stay, pre- and postoperative hemoglobin (Hb), hospitalization length, and site of the infection (surgical site, respiratory system, urinary system, bloodstream, other sites). Antibiotic prophylaxis was performed in clean-contaminated surgery. Intravenous amoxicillin with clavulanic acid 2.2 g was usually used during surgical procedure and every 8 h for at least 3 days after surgery. Intravenous clarithromycin 500 mg was administered to patients who were allergic to amoxicillin.

HAIs are defined according to the United States Centers for Disease Control and Prevention (CDC) guidelines, until the 30th post-operative day [1].

All statistical analyses were carried out using the Statistical Package for Social Sciences, version 20.0 (IBM Corporation, Armonk, NY, USA). The Kolmogorov–Smirnov test demonstrated a non-Gaussian distribution of variables, so non-parametric tests were used. A descriptive analysis of all data was performed, and they were reported as medians and interquartile range (IQR), or percentages. The Mann–Whitney U test was used to assess differences between groups in the mean of continuous variables, while the Chi-squared test was used for categorical variables. Logistic regression (forced entry method) was used for multivariate analysis. If less than 10 cases per each variable were present, multivariate analysis was not performed because of insufficient statistical power. A $p < 0.05$ was considered statistically significant.

3. Results

Median age was 66 years (IQR 15 years). Fifty-one percent of patients was older than 65 years. Median BMI was 24.44 (IQR 5.31). Tables 1 and 2 report patient and tumor characteristics. In particular, 226 (46.3%) patients had an ASA score of 1 or 2, while 262 (53.7%) cases had an ASA score of 3 or 4. Tumors were diagnosed in early stage (I–II) in 53.2% of cases, whereas 46.8% of patients had an advanced tumor (stage III–IV).

Table 1. Patients' characteristics.

Patient and Tumor Characteristics	N° (%)
Sex	
Male	381 (78.1)
Female	107 (21.9)
BMI	
Low (<18.5)	24 (4.9)
Normal (18.5–25)	246 (50.4)
High (>25)	218 (44.7)
Smoking	
Never	104 (21.3)
Former	211 (43.2)
Active	173 (35.5)
Alcohol consumption *	243 (49.8)
Allergies **	99 (20.3)
COPD	64 (13.1)
Cirrhosis	13 (2.7)
CKD	18 (3.7)
Diabetes mellitus	64 (13.1)
Previous transplantation ***	6 (1.2)
Chronic systemic corticosteroid therapy ****	16 (3.3)
Immunosuppression	3 (0.6)
Previous radiation therapy	118 (24.2)
Previous chemotherapy	71 (14.5)
ASA score	
1	44 (9.0)
2	187 (38.3)
3	235 (48.2)
4	22 (4.5)

* Refers to current alcohol consumption (>2 drinks per day for men and >1 drink per day for women). ** Refers to any type of allergy (environmental, drugs, foods) proven by prick tests and/or serological exams. *** Three patients had solid organ transplantation and underwent immunosuppression, while three patients had stem cell transplantation. **** For allergic diseases (13 cases; prednisone 5–10 mg per day for more than 30 days/year) or previous solid organ transplantation (3 cases; prednisone 25 mg per day). BMI, body mass index; COPD, chronic obstructive pulmonary disease; CKD, chronic kidney disease; ASA, American Society of Anesthesiologists.

Table 2. Tumor characteristics.

Patient and Tumor Characteristics	N° (%)
Tumor site	
Nasal cavities and paranasal sinuses	36 (7.4)
Nasopharynx	1 (0.2)
Oral cavity	145 (29.6)
Oropharynx	57 (11.7)

Table 2. *Cont.*

Patient and Tumor Characteristics	N° (%)
Larynx	177 (36.3)
Hypopharynx	23 (4.7)
Salivary glands	37 (7.6)
Unknown primary	12 (2.5)
T	
0	28 (5.7)
1	199 (40.8)
2	102 (20.9)
3	93 (19.1)
4	66 (13.5)
N	
0	344 (70.5)
1	44 (9.0)
2	76 (15.6)
3	24 (4.9)
Stage	
I	190 (38.9)
II	70 (14.3)
III	94 (19.3)
IV	134 (27.5)

T, tumor; N, node.

Surgical treatments are highlighted in Table 3. Eighty-one (16.6%) patients went to ICU after surgery. ICU stay ranged between 1 and 3 days. Surgery was classified as clean in 83 (17.0%) cases and clean-contaminated in 405 (83%) cases. PICC/CVC was used in 190 (38.9%) patients, while nasogastric feeding tube was positioned in 269 (55.1%) cases.

Table 3. Surgical procedures.

Surgery	N° (%)
Ethmoido-maxillectomy	6 (12.3)
Partial maxillectomy	25 (51.2)
Subtotal/total maxillectomy	10 (2.0)
Partial glossectomy	43 (8.8)
Hemiglossectomy	27 (5.5)
Subtotal/total glossectomy	8 (1.6)
Glossectomy with mandibulectomy	10 (2.0)
Oral floor cancer removal	16 (3.3)
Cheek mucosa cancer removal	10 (2.0)
Lip cancer removal	11 (2.3)
Retromolar trigone cancer removal	9 (1.8)
Partial pharyngectomy	43 (8.8)
Cordectomy	65 (13.3)
Partial laryngectomy	41 (8.4)
Total laryngectomy/pharyngolaryngectomy	82 (16.8)
Parotidectomy	31 (6.4)
Submandibular gland cancer removal	2 (0.4)
Neck dissection	263 (53.9)
Reconstruction with pedicled flap	70 (14.3)
Reconstruction with free flap	30 (6.1)
Tracheotomy	242 (49.6)

Median duration of surgery was 195 min (IQR 210 min), and median hospital stay was 13 days (IQR 21 days). Median pre-operative Hb was 14.2 g/dL (IQR 2.0 g/dL), while it was 12.0 g/dL (IQR 2.8 g/dL) at first post-operative day.

Post-operative infections were observed in 111 (22.7%) patients, after a median time of 10 days (IQR 10.25 days). Respiratory infections were the most common (Figure 1). Moreover, multiple site infections were observed in 19 (3.9%) cases, with bacteremia and respiratory infection being the most frequent association. Other sites of infection included gastrointestinal tract (three cases) and male genital system (one case).

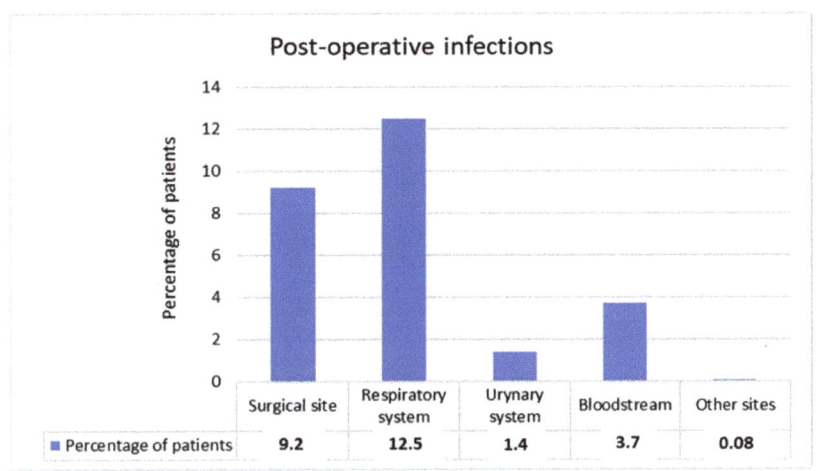

Figure 1. Sites of post-operative infections (percentages on 488 patients).

Significant risk factors for post-operative infection (all the sites) at univariate analyses were higher ASA score, advanced stage, longer duration of surgery, tracheotomy, clean-contaminated surgical procedure, flap reconstruction, ICU stay, lower post-operative Hb (first day after surgery), nasogastric feeding tube, and presence of PICC/CVC ($p < 0.05$). Median Hb at the days of infection diagnosis was 10.2 g/dL (IQR 2.4 g/dL), lower than levels at first post-operative day (1.8 g/dL lower on average). Table 4 reports the percentages of infections for each site and categorical risk factor, while Table 5 shows statistical significance for risk factors according to infection sites. Older patients had a higher risk of SSIs.

Table 4. Percentage of post-operative infection for each risk factor in different sites.

Risk Factors	All Infections	Surgical Site Infections	Respiratory Infections	Bloodstream	Multiple Site Infection
Age > 65 years (yes/no)	23.7/21.8	7.2/11.3	14.4/10.5	4.0/3.3	3.6/4.2
Sex (male/female)	23.8/18.7	9.7/7.5	12.9/11.2	3.9/2.8	4.2/2.8
Smoking (active/former or never)	25.4/21.3	11.5/7.9	12.1/12.7	4.6/3.2	4.0/3.8
Alcohol consumption	25.9/19.6	10.7/7.7	14.4/10.6	3.3/4.1	4.9/2.8
BMI (high/low or normal)	22.0/23.3	6.9/11.1	12.3/12.6	3.2/4.1	3.2/4.4
Allergies (yes/no)	28.3/21.3	11.1/8.7	15.1/11.8	5.0/3.3	3.0/4.1
COPD (yes/no)	21.9/22.9	10.9/8.9	12.5/12.5	1.6/4.0	4.7/3.8
Cirrhosis (yes/no)	30.8/22.5	7.7/9.3	15.4/12.4	7.7/3.6	0.0/4.0
CKD (yes/no)	11.1/23.2	5.5/9.4	0.0/12.9	5.5/3.6	0.0/4.0
Diabetes mellitus (yes/no)	26.6/22.2	9.4/9.2	18.7/11.5	3.1/3.8	6.2/3.5
Previous transplantation (yes/no)	33.3/22.6	0.0/9.3	0.0/12.6	16.7/3.5	0.0/3.9

Table 4. Cont.

Risk Factors	All Infections	Surgical Site Infections	Respiratory Infections	Bloodstream	Multiple Site Infection
Chronic corticosteroid therapy (yes/no)	37.5/22.2	6.2/9.3	18.7/12.3	6.2/3.6	0.0/4.0
Immunosuppression (yes/no)	33.3/22.7	0.0/9.3	0.0/12.6	0.0/3.7	0.0/3.9
Previous radiation therapy (yes/no)	17.8/24.3	7.6/9.7	10.2/13.2	5.1/3.2	5.9/3.2
Previous chemotherapy (yes/no)	26.8/22.1	8.4/9.3	16.9/11.7	8.4/2.9	8.4/3.1
ASA score (III–IV/I–II)	26.3/18.6	9.5/8.8	14.5/10.2	5.3/1.8	5.3/2.2
Stage (advanced/early)	36.1/10.8	13.5/5.4	20.4/5.4	5.6/1.9	6.1/1.9
PICC/CVC (yes/no)	36.8/13.7	13.7/6.4	21.0/7.0	8.4/1.0	7.9/2.0
Nasogastric feeding tube (yes/no)	35.3/7.3	15.2/1.8	18.6/5.0	5.6/1.4	6.3/0.9
Surgical procedure (clean-cont./clean)	26.7/3.6	11.1/0.0	14.6/2.4	4.4/0.0	4.7/0.0
Tracheotomy (yes/no)	39.2/6.5	14.5/4.1	22.7/2.4	7.0/0.4	7.4/0.4
Flap reconstruction (yes/no)	42.7/17.9	18.7/6.9	26.0/9.2	5.2/3.3	8.3/2.8
ICU stay (yes/no)	45.7/18.2	14.8/8.1	25.9/9.8	9.9/2.4	9.9/2.7

BMI, body mass index; COPD, chronic obstructive pulmonary disease; CKD, chronic kidney disease; ASA, American Society of Anesthesiologists; PICC, peripherally inserted central catheter; CVC, central venous catheter; ICU, intensive care unit.

Table 5. Risk factors for different sites of post-operative infections (p values at univariate analyses).

Risk Factors	All Infections	Surgical Site Infections	Respiratory Infections	Bloodstream	Multiple Site Infection
Age	0.839	*0.015 **	0.147	0.364	0.468
Sex	0.258	0.480	0.649	0.583	0.510
Smoking (active)	0.294	0.186	0.858	0.416	0.897
Alcohol consumption	0.095	0.261	0.205	0.644	0.235
BMI	0.565	0.140	0.685	0.807	0.865
Allergies	0.141	0.467	0.372	0.421	0.619
COPD	0.858	0.611	1.000	0.333	0.725
Cirrhosis	0.484	0.847	0.750	0.438	0.462
CKD	0.230	0.584	0.102	0.668	0.384
Diabetes mellitus	0.435	0.964	0.105	0.797	0.296
Previous transplantation	0.534	0.432	0.352	0.090	0.620
Chronic corticosteroid therapy	0.152	0.676	0.442	0.580	0.413
Immunosuppression	0.661	0.580	0.511	0.734	0.727
Previous radiation therapy	0.141	0.492	0.379	0.355	0.189
Previous chemotherapy	0.383	0.808	0.225	*0.021 **	*0.032 **
ASA score	*0.014 **	0.782	0.215	*0.001 **	*0.050 **
Tumor site	*0.008 **	0.458	0.536	0.985	0.893
Stage	*<0.001 **	*<0.001 **	*<0.001 **	0.105	*0.003 **
PICC/CVC	*<0.001 **	*0.007 **	*<0.001 **	*<0.001 **	*<0.001 **
Nasogastric feeding tube	*<0.001 **	*<0.001 **	*<0.001 **	*0.014 **	*0.002 **
Type of surgical procedure	*<0.001 **	*0.001 **	*0.002 **	*0.050 **	*0.044 **
Tracheotomy	*<0.001 **	*<0.001 **	*<0.001 **	*<0.001 **	*<0.001 **
Flap reconstruction	*<0.001 **	*<0.001 **	*<0.001 **	0.381	*0.012 **
Duration of surgery	*<0.001 **	*<0.001 **	*<0.001 **	*<0.001 **	*<0.001 **
ICU stay	*<0.001 **	0.057	*<0.001 **	*0.001 **	*0.002 **
Pre-operative Hb	0.440	0.855	0.255	0.801	0.993
Post-operative Hb (1st day)	*<0.001 **	*0.006 **	*<0.001 **	0.186	0.182

* $p < 0.05$ (Mann–Whitney U test for continuous variables and Chi-squared test for categorical variables). BMI, body mass index; COPD, chronic obstructive pulmonary disease; CKD, chronic kidney disease; ASA, American Society of Anesthesiologists; PICC, peripherally inserted central catheter; CVC, central venous catheter; ICU, intensive care unit; Hb, hemoglobin.

Multivariate analysis (logistic regression) was performed only considering all the infections, because there were too few cases for each infection site to perform statistical analysis. Since the presence of nasogastric feeding tube was significantly associated with the type of surgery (quite all the patients who underwent major clean-contaminated surgery had a feeding tube), it was removed from multivariate analysis. Significant risk factors for post-operative infection were advanced stage, tracheotomy, and longer duration of surgery ($p < 0.05$, Table 6).

Table 6. Multivariate analysis regarding risk factors for post-operative infection (all sites).

Risk Factor	*p*-Value
ASA score	0.227
Tumor site	0.652
Stage	*0.048* *
PICC/CVC	0.219
Type of surgical procedure	0.203
Tracheotomy	*0.039* *
Flap reconstruction	0.965
Duration of surgery	*0.001* *
ICU stay	0.402
Post-operative Hb (1st day)	0.224

* $p < 0.05$ (logistic regression). ASA, American Society of Anesthesiologists; PICC, peripherally inserted central catheter; CVC, central venous catheter; ICU, intensive care unit; Hb, hemoglobin.

Infections were observed in 10.9% and 36.0% of cases in patients with early (stage I–II) and advanced (stage III–IV) cancer, respectively ($p = 0.048$). Patients with tracheotomy had infection in 39.3% of cases, compared to 6.5% in those without tracheotomy ($p = 0.039$). Median duration of surgery was 320 and 150 min in patient with and without post-operative infection, respectively ($p = 0.001$). Median hospital stay was significantly longer in patients who had post-operative infection (38 vs. 9 days, $p < 0.001$, Figure 2).

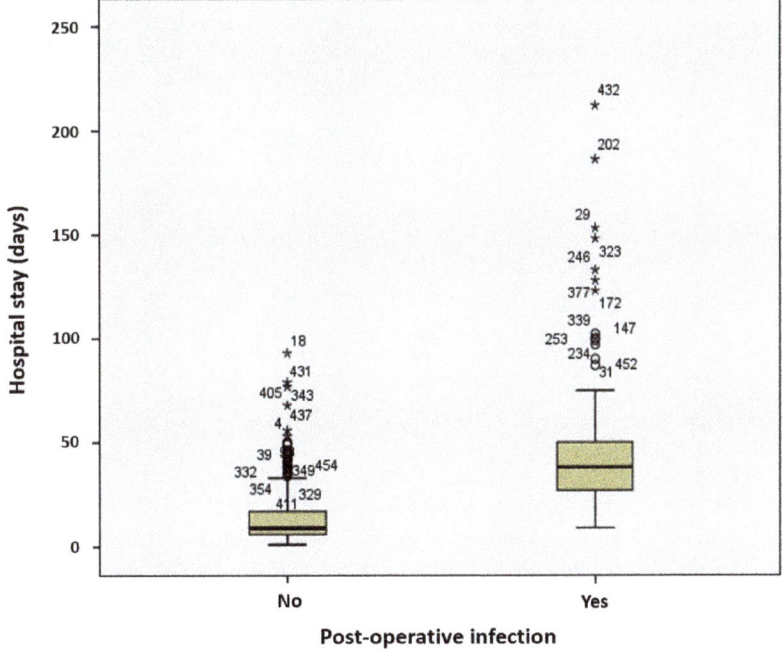

Figure 2. Median hospital stay according to infection status. Outliers are present in the figure as asterisks and circles.

4. Discussion

Post-operative infections represent an important issue in HNC surgery, leading to a longer hospital stay, a delay of adjuvant treatments, worse survival rates, and higher costs [2,25]. The increase of microbial resistance is worsening HAIs, reducing the efficacy of antibiotic prophylaxis. For example, methicillin-resistant Staphylococcus aureus (MRSA) has been emerging as a major cause of SSIs in HNC patients [3].

SSIs following HNC surgery are the main post-operative HAIs and range from 10 to 50% [2–21]. Respiratory infection, bacteremia, and urinary tract infection were observed in 7–40%, 2.1–6.1%, and 0.7–13.8% of cases, respectively [2,22–27]. Our study showed HAIs rates in agreement with the literature and located near lower range values. In particular, we observed SSIs in 9.2% of cases, respiratory infections in 12.5%, urinary tract infections in 1.4%, and bacteremia in 3.7%. Globally, we observed post-operative HAIs in 22.7% of patients. The heterogeneous results present in literature are due to different selection of patients in the studies. Indeed, some papers included only patients who underwent flap reconstruction, with a specific focus on free flaps. Since several studies identified flap reconstruction as a HAI risk factor, papers that included only patients who underwent reconstructive surgery reported a higher rate of post-operative infections [2,6,14].

Risk factors have been investigated for SSIs in several studies and for respiratory infections in some papers. However, there is no accordance among studies to identify the same risk factors. Concerning SSIs, the most reported risk factors were ASA score, comorbidities (e.g., diabetes mellitus), smoking, alcohol consumption, previous RT or CT, tumor stage, duration of surgery, blood loss and/or anemia, hypoalbuminemia and/or malnutrition (weight loss), tracheotomy, flap reconstruction, and clean-contaminated surgery [4,6,10–12,14–21,28]. Therefore, some variables related to the patient and others related to surgical procedure negatively impact on post-operative HAIs. In particular, malnutrition incidence in HNC patients ranges from 30% to 50% and together with surgical stress, lead to immunosuppression that results in a higher risk of infectious complications and a decrease in survival rates [19].

Our univariate analysis regrading all the infections showed that higher ASA score, tumor site (oral cavity and larynx/hypopharynx), advanced stage, presence of PICC/CVC or nasogastric feeding tube, clean-contaminated surgery, tracheotomy, flap reconstruction, higher duration of surgery, ICU stay, and lower post-operative Hb were potential risk factors. Multivariate analysis confirmed advanced stage, tracheotomy, and higher duration of surgery as risk factors for post-operative infections. The last two parameters were also identified as risk factors by Ramos-zayas et al. in a sample of 65 patients who underwent free flap reconstruction [2]. On the other hand, Tjoa et al. found that age > 65 years and clean-contaminated surgery were risk factors in a large sample of 715 patients who had flap reconstruction [22]. We did not find statistical significance for some clinical parameters, such as comorbidities, immunosuppression and previous RT and/or CT. Our data suggest that HNC surgery may be safe also for patients who underwent organ transplantation and were immunosuppressed. However, no definitive conclusion can be drawn because of small numbers.

Concerning infections of specific sites (surgical site, respiratory system, urinary tract, bloodstream), univariate analyses highlighted slightly different potential risk factors compare to all the infections. Our results about SSIs were in agreement with the literature. The main difference compared to all the infections was the lack of significance for ASA score, tumor site and ICU stay.

Respiratory infections had the same potential risk factors compared to SSIs, adding ICU stay. This is in agreement with the literature. Indeed, a recent meta-analysis showed a significant increase in the post-operative respiratory infections and sepsis in patients admitted to ICU compared with non-ICU setting [29].

Bacteremia and multiple site infections had similar risk factors. In particular, previous CT became significant, while post-operative anemia was not. Our study demonstrated that multiple site infections were more frequent in patients with higher ASA score, advanced tumor stage, previous CT, presence of PICC/CVC or nasogastric feeding tube, clean-contaminated surgery, tracheotomy, flap reconstruction, higher duration of surgery, and ICU stay.

According to literature, we found a longer hospitalization in patents with HAIs. In particular, median hospital stay was 38 days in patients who had post-operative infection, while it was 9 days in non-infected patients. As reported by Penel et al., post-operative infections with longer hospital stay lead to higher direct costs [25].

The strength of this study is the analysis of post-operative HAIs from different sites and the evaluation of multiple site infections. Indeed, at our knowledge, this is the first study that investigated risk factors for each site, including multiple infections. The main limit is the number of cases not sufficient for multivariate analysis for every infection site.

Further studies on large samples are mandatory to obtain reliable results from multivariate analyses. The exact identification of risk factors may help the physicians to prevent post-operative HAIs in HNC surgery.

5. Conclusions

Surgery represents one of the main treatments for HNC. However, post-operative infections may negatively affect surgical outcomes. Respiratory and surgical site infections are the most frequent infectious complications. Advanced stage, tracheotomy, and higher duration of surgery are risk factors considering all infection sites. Slight differences have been observed for specific anatomical sites. Future studies are necessary to identify risk factors exactly and thus help surgeons to reduce post-operative infections. In particular, higher attention should be paid to patients with greater risk, who may benefit from longer or different antibiotic prophylaxis.

Author Contributions: Conceptualization, G.P. and R.A.; methodology, G.R.; software, G.R.; validation, G.P. and G.R.; formal analysis, G.R.; investigation, G.R., E.C. and E.F.; data curation, G.R.; writing—original draft preparation, G.R. and E.C.; writing—review and editing, G.P., A.A., A.C. and R.A.; visualization, G.R.; supervision, R.A.; project administration, R.A. All authors have read and agreed to the published version of the manuscript.

Funding: This research received no external funding.

Institutional Review Board Statement: The study was conducted in accordance with the Declaration of Helsinki and approved by the Institutional Review Board of "AOU Città della Salute e della Scienza di Torino" (protocol code 0021433, date of approval 26 February 2021).

Informed Consent Statement: Informed consent was obtained from all subjects involved in the study.

Data Availability Statement: The data presented in this study are available on request from the corresponding author.

Conflicts of Interest: The authors declare no conflict of interest.

References

1. Horan, T.C.; Andrus, M.; Dudeck, M.A. CDC/NHSN surveillance definition of health care-associated infection and criteria for specific types of infections in the acute care setting. *Am. J. Infect. Control* **2008**, *36*, 309–332. [CrossRef]
2. Ramos-zayas, A.; López-medrano, F.; Urquiza-fornovi, I.; Zubillaga, I.; Gutiérrez, R.; Sánchez-aniceto, G.; Acero, J.; Almeida, F.; Galdona, A.; José Morán, M.; et al. The Impact of Healthcare-Associated Infections in Patients Undergoing Oncological Microvascular Head and Neck Reconstruction: A Prospective Multicentre Study. *Cancers* **2021**, *13*, 2109. [CrossRef]
3. Lin, S.; Melki, S.; Lisgaris, M.V.; Ahadizadeh, E.N.; Zender, C.A. Post-operative MRSA infections in head and neck surgery. *Am. J. Otolaryngol.* **2017**, *38*, 417–421. [CrossRef]
4. Park, S.Y.; Kim, M.S.; Eom, J.S.; Lee, J.S.; Rho, Y.S. Risk factors and etiology of surgical site infection after radical neck dissection in patients with head and neck cancer. *Korean J. Intern. Med.* **2016**, *31*, 162–169. [CrossRef]
5. Lee, J.I.; Kwon, M.; Roh, J.L.; Choi, J.; Choi, S.H.; Nam, S.; Kim, S. Postoperative hypoalbuminemia as a risk factor for surgical site infection after oral cancer surgery. *Oral Dis.* **2015**, *21*, 178–184. [CrossRef]
6. Wang, C.H.; Wong, Y.K.; Wang, C.P.; Wang, C.C.; Jiang, R.S.; Lai, C.S.; Liu, S.A. Risk factors of recipient site infection in head and neck cancer patients undergoing pectoralis major myocutaneous flap reconstruction. *Eur. Arch. Otorhinolaryngol.* **2015**, *272*, 3475–3482. [CrossRef]

7. Skitarelic, N.; Morovic, M.; Manestar, D. Antibiotic prophylaxis in clean-contaminated head and neck oncological surgery. *J. Craniomaxillofac. Surg.* **2007**, *35*, 15–20. [CrossRef]
8. Sato, J.; Goto, J.; Harahashi, A.; Murata, T.; Hata, H.; Yamazaki, Y.; Satoh, A.; Notani, K.I.; Kitagawa, Y. Oral health care reduces the risk of postoperative surgical site infection in inpatients with oral squamous cell carcinoma. *Support. Care Cancer* **2011**, *19*, 409–416. [CrossRef]
9. González-Márquez, R.; Rodrigo, J.P.; Nieto, C.S. Prognostic significance of postoperative wound infections after total laryngectomy. *Head Neck* **2012**, *34*, 1023–1027. [CrossRef]
10. Lee, D.H.; Kim, S.Y.; Nam, S.Y.; Choi, S.H.; Choi, J.W.; Roh, J.L. Risk factors of surgical site infection in patients undergoing major oncological surgery for head and neck cancer. *Oral Oncol.* **2011**, *47*, 528–531. [CrossRef]
11. Candau-Alvarez, A.; Linares-Sicilia, M.J.; Dean-Ferrer, A.; Pérez-Navero, J.L. Role of culture of postoperative drainage fluid in the prediction of infection of the surgical site after major oncological operations of the head and neck. *Br. J. Oral Maxillofac. Surg.* **2015**, *53*, 200–203. [CrossRef]
12. Kamizono, K.; Sakuraba, M.; Nagamatsu, S.; Miyamoto, S.; Hayashi, R. Statistical analysis of surgical site infection after head and neck reconstructive surgery. *Ann. Surg. Oncol.* **2014**, *21*, 1700–1705. [CrossRef] [PubMed]
13. Yang, C.H.; Chew, K.Y.; Solomkin, J.S.; Lin, P.Y.; Chiang, Y.C.; Kuo, Y.R. Surgical site infections among high-risk patients in clean-contaminated head and neck reconstructive surgery: Concordance with preoperative oral flora. *Ann. Plast. Surg.* **2013**, *71* (Suppl. S1), S55–S60. [CrossRef] [PubMed]
14. Karakida, K.; Aoki, T.; Ota, Y.; Yamazaki, H.; Otsuru, M.; Takahashi, M.; Sakamoto, H.; Miyasaka, M. Analysis of risk factors for surgical-site infections in 276 oral cancer surgeries with microvascular free-flap reconstructions at a single university hospital. *J. Infect. Chemother.* **2010**, *16*, 334–339. [CrossRef] [PubMed]
15. Cole, R.R.; Robbins, K.T.; Cohen, J.I.; Wolf, P.F. A predictive model for wound sepsis in oncologic surgery of the head and neck. *Otolaryngol. Head. Neck Surg.* **1987**, *96*, 165–171. [CrossRef]
16. Gan, C.; Wang, Y.; Tang, Y.; Wang, K.; Sun, B.; Wang, M.; Zhu, F. Risk factors for surgical site infection in head and neck cancer. *Support. Care Cancer* **2022**, *30*, 2735–2743. [CrossRef]
17. Penel, N.; Lefebvre, D.; Fournier, C.; Sarini, J.; Kara, A.; Lefebvre, J.L. Risk factors for wound infection in head and neck cancer surgery: A prospective study. *Head Neck* **2001**, *23*, 447–455. [CrossRef]
18. Goyal, N.; Emerick, K.S.; Deschler, D.G.; Lin, D.T.; Yarlagadda, B.B.; Rich, D.L.; Durand, M.L. Risk factors for surgical site infection after supraclavicular flap reconstruction in patients undergoing major head and neck surgery. *Head Neck* **2016**, *38*, 1615–1620. [CrossRef]
19. Son, H.J.; Roh, J.L.; Choi, S.H.; Nam, S.Y.; Kim, S.Y. Nutritional and hematologic markers as predictors of risk of surgical site infection in patients with head and neck cancer undergoing major oncologic surgery. *Head Neck* **2018**, *40*, 596–604. [CrossRef]
20. Hirakawa, H.; Hasegawa, Y.; Hanai, N.; Ozawa, T.; Hyodo, I.; Suzuki, M. Surgical site infection in clean-contaminated head and neck cancer surgery: Risk factors and prognosis. *Eur. Arch. Otorhinolaryngol.* **2013**, *270*, 1115–1123. [CrossRef]
21. Ogihara, H.; Takeuchi, K.; Majima, Y. Risk factors of postoperative infection in head and neck surgery. *Auris. Nasus. Larynx* **2009**, *36*, 457–460. [CrossRef]
22. Tjoa, T.; Rathi, V.K.; Goyal, N.; Yarlagadda, B.B.; Barshak, M.B.; Rich, D.L.; Emerick, K.S.; Lin, D.T.; Deschler, D.G.; Durand, M.L. Pneumonia, urinary tract infection, bacteremia, and Clostridioides difficile infection following major head and neck free and pedicled flap surgeries. *Oral Oncol.* **2021**, *122*, 105541. [CrossRef]
23. Damian, D.; Esquenazi, J.; Duvvuri, U.; Johnson, J.T.; Sakai, T. Incidence, outcome, and risk factors for postoperative pulmonary complications in head and neck cancer surgery patients with free flap reconstructions. *J. Clin. Anesth.* **2016**, *28*, 12–18. [CrossRef]
24. Liu, Y.; Di, Y.; Fu, S. Risk factors for ventilator-associated pneumonia among patients undergoing major oncological surgery for head and neck cancer. *Front. Med.* **2017**, *11*, 239–246. [CrossRef]
25. Penel, N.; Lefebvre, J.L.; Cazin, J.L.; Clisant, S.; Neu, J.C.; Dervaux, B.; Yazdanpanah, Y. Additional direct medical costs associated with nosocomial infections after head and neck cancer surgery: A hospital-perspective analysis. *Int. J. Oral Maxillofac. Surg.* **2008**, *37*, 135–139. [CrossRef]
26. Ong, S.K.; Morton, R.P.; Kolbe, J.; Whitlock, R.M.L.; McIvor, N.P. Pulmonary complications following major head and neck surgery with tracheostomy: A prospective, randomized, controlled trial of prophylactic antibiotics. *Arch. Otolaryngol.-Head Neck Surg.* **2004**, *130*, 1084–1087. [CrossRef] [PubMed]
27. Semenov, Y.R.; Starmer, H.M.; Gourin, C.G. The effect of pneumonia on short-term outcomes and cost of care after head and neck cancer surgery. *Laryngoscope* **2012**, *122*, 1994–2004. [CrossRef] [PubMed]
28. Liu, S.A.; Wong, Y.K.; Poon, C.K.; Wang, C.C.; Wang, C.P.; Tung, K.C. Risk factors for wound infection after surgery in primary oral cavity cancer patients. *Laryngoscope* **2007**, *117*, 166–171. [CrossRef]
29. Mashrah, M.A.; Aldhohrah, T.; Abdelrehem, A.; Sabri, B.; Ahmed, H.; Al-Rawi, N.H.; Yu, T.; Zhao, S.; Wang, L.; Ge, L. Postoperative care in ICU versus non-ICU after head and neck free-flap surgery: A systematic review and meta-analysis. *BMJ Open* **2022**, *12*, e053667. [CrossRef]

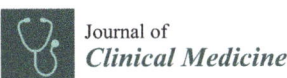

Review

Open Partial Laryngectomies: History of Laryngeal Cancer Surgery

Stéphane Hans [1], Robin Baudouin [1], Marta P. Circiu [1], Florent Couineau [1], Quentin Lisan [1], Lise Crevier-Buchman [1] and Jérôme R. Lechien [1,2,3,*]

[1] Department of Otorhinolaryngology and Head and Neck Surgery, Foch Hospital, School of Medicine, UFR Simone Veil, Université Versailles Saint-Quentin-en-Yvelines (Paris Saclay University), 92150 Suresnes, France
[2] Division of Laryngology and Broncho-Esophagology, EpiCURA Hospital, UMONS Research Institute for Health Sciences and Technology, University of Mons (UMons), 7000 Mons, Belgium
[3] Polyclinic of Poitiers—Elsan, 86000 Poitiers, France
* Correspondence: jerome.lechien@umons.ac.be

Abstract: Historically, surgery was the first-choice therapy for early, intermediate and advanced laryngeal squamous cell carcinoma (LSCC). Partial laryngeal surgery has evolved in recent decades and was influenced by many historic events and the development of new technologies. Partial laryngectomies may be performed by open, endoscopic or transoral robotic approaches. In this historic paper, we describe the evolution of open partial laryngectomy techniques, indications and surgical outcomes. Since the first partial laryngectomy in 1788, many U.S., U.K. and European surgeons, including Henry Sands, Jacob da Silva Solis-Cohen and Theodor Billroth, performed this surgical procedure under local anesthesia for tuberculosis, cancer or syphilis. Partial laryngectomy gained reputation in the medical community in 1888 due to the laryngeal cancer and death of the prince of Prussia, Frederick III. Frederick III's death represented the turning point in the history of partial laryngectomies, calling attention to the importance of semiotics, biopsy and early diagnosis in laryngeal cancers. Hemi-laryngectomy was indicated/proposed for lateral laryngeal tumors, while thyrotomy was indicated for cancers of the middle part of the vocal fold. The second landmark in the history of partial laryngectomies was the discovery of cocaine, novocaine and adrenaline and the related development of local anesthetic techniques, which, together with the epidemiological and hygienic advances of the 19th century, allowed for better perioperative outcomes. General anesthesia was introduced in the second part of the 20th century and further improved the surgical outcomes. The diagnosis of laryngeal cancer was improved with the development of X-rays and direct laryngoscopies. The 20th century was characterized by the development and improvement of vertical partial laryngectomy procedures and the development of horizontal partial laryngectomies for both supraglottic and glottic regions. The history and the evolution of these techniques are discussed in the present historical paper.

Keywords: larynx; laryngeal; cancer; partial laryngectomy; otolaryngology; head neck; surgery; history

1. Introduction

Head and neck squamous cell carcinoma is the sixth most common adult cancer worldwide, accounting for 5.3% of all cancers [1]. Among head and neck cancers, laryngeal squamous cell carcinoma (LSCC) is the second most prevalent carcinoma, corresponding to 211,000 new cases and 126,000 deaths per year worldwide [2,3]. The treatment of LSCC depends on tumor location, stage and patient comorbidities. Historically, surgery was the first-choice therapy for early, intermediate and advanced laryngeal squamous cell carcinoma (LSCC). Partial laryngeal surgery evolved over recent decades and was influenced by several historically important cases as well as by technological events. At present, partial laryngectomies may be performed through open, endoscopic or transoral robotic approaches. In this paper, we describe the evolution of the techniques, indications and surgical outcomes of partial laryngectomies.

The existing literature describes dozens of types of open partial laryngectomies. In our work, we choose to focus on a selection of publications that played an important role in illustrating two therapeutic extremes: the transoral approach and total laryngectomy. We also provide historical examples of partial laryngectomies to support examples. We learned about these delicate surgeries in the "School of Laënnec" in contact with professors Henri Laccourreye, Daniel Brasnu and Ollivier Laccourreye. Finally, we use the European Laryngological Society (ELS) classification for open partial horizontal laryngectomies (OPHL) [4].

2. The Pioneers

The first partial laryngectomy was carried out by the French surgeon Philippe-Jean Pelletan (1747–1829) in 1788 [5]. Philippe-Jean Pelletan proceeded to perform a midline thyrotomy to remove a laryngeal piece. The first partial laryngectomy performed for a laryngeal cancer was reported in 1863 by Henry B. Sands (1830–1888), who was a faculty surgeon at New York University [6]. The surgery consisted of a laryngeal fissure and extirpation of a laryngeal tumor in a patient who died two years after the surgery without evidence of recurrence [6]. In 1867, Jacob da Silva Solis-Cohen (1838–1927), a laryngologist from Philadelphia, published the first long-term follow-up (20 years) of a patient who underwent a median thyrotomy for a presumed laryngeal cancer. In that paper, the disease was still controlled 20 years after the surgery [7].

The first open hemi-laryngectomy was carried out in 1878 by Theodor Billroth (1829–1894), a few years after the first total laryngectomy (1873) [8]. At this time, total or partial laryngectomies were performed for three main types of chronic ulcerative laryngitis: tuberculosis, cancer and syphilis. The surgeries were not preceded by a biopsy because surgeons considered that biopsy increased the growth of cancer [9].

3. The Prince of Prussia

In January 1887, the prince of Prussia, Frederick III (1831–1888), was diagnosed with a laryngeal cancer, which was a milestone in the diagnosis and the evolution of the surgical treatment of laryngeal cancer [10,11]. The heir of the German Empire requested the expertise of Karl Gerhardt, who reported a thickening of the left vocal fold and prescribed thermal therapy at Bad Ems. On 15 May 1887, the doctor observed a left vocal fold movement impairment. The heir was examined by Ernst Von Bergmann (1836–1907), who clinically confirmed the possibility of laryngeal malignancy and proposed a laryngofissure. The family of the heir, especially his wife, the princess Victoria, requested a second opinion from Morell Mackenzie (1837–1892), an English laryngologist who suspected syphilis and performed a laryngeal biopsy. The pathological analysis was carried out by Rudolf Virchow (1821–1902), one of the leading physicians to Frederick III, who diagnosed "pachydermia". Based on this examination, the prince's relatives opposed the laryngectomy. Meanwhile, Emperor Guillaume I died, and Frederick III became Emperor. The reign of Frederick III lasted 99 days, and he died from the evolution of his laryngeal cancer on 15 June 1888. Before his death, physicians performed a tracheotomy and several additional biopsies that were all negative. According to the clinical evolution of the laryngeal disease, Rudolf Virchow and Heinrich W. Waldeyer (1836–1921) carried out an autopsy that supported the laryngeal cancer diagnosis. Because Frederick III was a politically important and valued person, the origin of his death led to debates and reflections regarding the importance of semiotics, biopsy and the early diagnosis of laryngeal cancer in the consideration of partial laryngectomies. The spread of these debates in Europe reinforced the importance of partial laryngectomies and several procedures were carried out in the U.K. (1894) and France (1895) by Sir Felix Semon (1849–1921) and Emile Jean Moure (1855–1941), respectively [8]. At this time, the discussions were focused on organ preservation via two main techniques: thyrotomy and Billroth's hemi-laryngectomy. However, the indications remained unclear.

The median thyrotomy was proposed for cancers of the middle part of the vocal cord without both anterior commissure invasion and laryngeal dysmotility. The lateral laryngeal tumors required hemi-laryngectomy. One of the first studies was published in 1897 by John Sendziak [12,13]. In this study, the author reported that the postoperative mortality rate and 3-year overall survival of midline thyrotomies (n = 88) were 9.8% and 8.7%, respectively, while total laryngectomies (n = 188) were associated with a postoperative mortality rate and overall survival of 44.7% and 5.85%, respectively [13]. At that time, many surgeons proposed palliative tracheotomy rather than partial or total laryngectomies.

4. The First Part of the 20th Century

4.1. The Influence of Hygiene and Anesthesia Development

At the end of the 19th century, patient anesthetization was performed with ether or chloroform. In the postoperative period, the prevalence of pneumonia, wound infections and other complications was high. The discovery of cocaine, novocaine and adrenaline led to the development of better local anesthetic techniques, and many laryngeal surgeries were, therefore, carried out under local anesthesia. At the same time, European progress in infectiology, hospital hygiene and epidemiology, achieved through the works of Ignace Semmelweis (1818–1865), Louis Pasteur (1822–1895) and Joseph Lister (1827–1912), led to better conditions in the operating room and better postoperative outcomes.

4.2. The Influence of X-rays

The discovery of X-rays in 1895 by Wilhelm Röntgen (1845–1923) is another event that significantly influenced partial laryngeal surgery. This discovery provided laryngologists and surgeons with a new imaging and exploration technique for the larynx. They performed profile images or frontal tomograms, allowing the visualization and characterization of both the epiglottis and the ventricle tumors. X-ray development improved the indications of partial laryngectomies because for more than 50 years, the surgical indications were based on palpation, indirect laryngoscopy and in-office biopsy under local anesthesia with cocaine.

4.3. Classifications and Laryngoscopy

The study of the location and extensions of laryngeal cancers developed during the second part of the 19th and throughout the 20th centuries. Emile Isambert (1827–1876) and Maurice Krishaber (1836–1883) reported two types of laryngeal cancers: the '*extrinsic laryngeal cancer*', with cervical nodes and poor prognosis, and the '*intrinsic laryngeal cancer*', without neck extension and better prognosis [14]. A few decades after this first classification, the laryngeal cancers were classified into subglottic, glottic or supraglottic according to the studies of Henri Rouvière (1876–1952) and others [15,16]. Laryngeal dissections led to a better understanding of the weak and resistant regions of the larynx and, therefore, the potential extension pathways of cancer [17]. At this time, the laryngeal examination was performed with the Garcia laryngeal mirror [18]. In 1895, Alfred Kirstein (1863–1922) performed the first direct laryngoscopy a few years before Gustav Killian (1860–1921), who also developed a laryngoscopy procedure (Figure 1) [19–21].

4.4. Vertical Partial Surgery

Many vertical partial surgery techniques appeared in the first part of the 20th century and were popularized by Chevalier Jackson (1865–1958), St. Clair Thomson (1859–1943) and others [16,22]. These approaches were developed to treat laryngeal cancer without requiring a total laryngectomy, which was seen as a mutilating approach. Three types of partial laryngectomy developed over time.

The first type consisted of thyrotomy with uni- or bilateral cordectomy, with potential extension to the arytenoid cartilage.

The second type was the vertical partial laryngectomy (fronto-lateral type) (Figure 2), which removed a part of the thyroid cartilage in the midline without cricoid cartilage resection. Described in 1956 by Leroux-Robert (1907–1998) [23], the fronto-lateral laryngectomy was indicated for cT1a tumors. This intervention included a monobloc resection of the affected vocal fold, the anterior commissure, the anterior part of the contralateral vocal fold and a part of the thyroid cartilage. To improve vocal function, glottic reconstruction was performed with repair of the false vocal fold [24]. To date, indications of fronto-lateral laryngectomy have decreased thanks to the development of transoral laser microsurgery. However, we currently use this vertical partial laryngectomy for tumors of the middle third of the vocal fold without involvement of the anterior commissure not exposed by TLM.

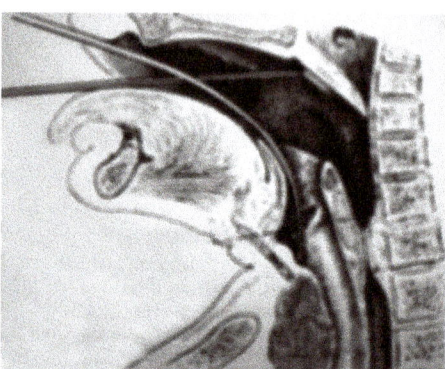

Figure 1. Killian laryngoscopy technique. This picture shows the technique of direct laryngoscopy developed by Killian.

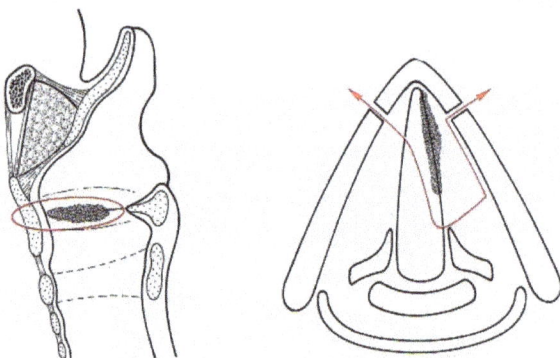

Figure 2. Fronto-lateral laryngectomy. Monobloc resection, removing a vertical fragment of the thyroid cartilage, of the entire vocal cord, of the anterior commissure and of the anterior part of the contralateral vocal cord.

The third type was hemi-laryngectomy, which was initially described by Billroth in 1878. This historical approach consisted of a median thyrotomy and the resection of the hemi-thyroid and hemi-cricoid laryngeal region affected by the tumor. Anything less than this resection was reported as a laryngofissure [9,16].

The postoperative outcomes of a vertical partial laryngectomy depended on the tumor location. Authors reported adequate outcomes for tumors limited to the middle third of the mobile vocal cord. They also noted that the closer the tumor was to the front or back of the vocal cord, the lower the chances of a successful surgery. [16]. The procedure was performed in Europe throughout the first part of the 20th century with the specification that the fixation of the arytenoid cartilage was a contraindication to partial laryngectomies [25,26]. The failure rate of vertical partial laryngectomies ranged from 2% to 18% for cT1 and from 4% to 24% for T2 laryngeal cancer. The failure rate was more than 40% if the vocal fold was fixed [16]. Since the spread of partial laryngectomy approaches in Europe in the first part of the 20th century, many modified approaches were reported with adequate outcomes [27]. However, the limitations of these techniques lay in the concept of relative independence of the two hemi-larynxes, which led to the advent of the horizontal laryngectomies.

5. The Second Part of the 20th Century

The second part of the 20th century included the development of horizontal partial laryngectomies, such as supraglottic laryngectomy (OPHL type I), glottic partial horizontal surgery (OPHL type IIa), and partial horizontal surgery of both glottic and supraglottic regions (OPHL type IIb) (Figure 3) [4]. We do not discuss supratracheal laryngectomies (OPHL type III) because they most often require a tracheotomy. In our opinion, the aim of a partial laryngectomy is to obtain the same local control as that obtained through a total laryngectomy, with oral swallowing (without a feeding tube), phonation and breathing without a tracheostomy.

5.1. The Horizontal Partial Supraglottic Laryngectomy (OPHL Type I)

The concept of the horizontal partial laryngectomy was based on Hajek's anatomical studies of the lymph node, which were developed through the studies of Henri Rouvière and Francois Baclesse (1896–1967) [28,29]. Initially, the first practical approaches for the resection of tumors of the supraglottic larynx and lateral pharyngeal wall were published by Wilfred Trotter (1872–1939) in a 1913 edition of *The Lancet* [30]. The techniques were then developed by a number of French surgeons [16], while the Uruguayan surgeon Justo M. Alonso (1886–1974) developed a voice-sparing supraglottic laryngectomy in 1947 [31]. Alonso's techniques were modified and spread worldwide by important laryngeal surgeons of the modern era, including Max L. Som (1904–1990), Joseph H. Ogura (1915–1983) and Jean Leroux-Robert [22,23] in France and Ettore Bocca in Italy [32]. The procedures evolved with the extension of the supraglottic laryngectomy to the base of the tongue, the arytenoid cartilage and the piriform sinus [4,33]. Preserving the mobility of one arytenoid unit was an important issue for supraglottic partial surgeries, while the postoperative course required a transient tracheostomy, feeding tube and hospital follow-up for nearly three weeks. Currently, these surgeries are still carried out but the development of transoral microsurgery or robotic approaches (early stages) or chemoradiotherapy (advanced stages) have reduced the indication of open partial laryngectomy.

5.2. The Horizontal Partial Glottic Laryngectomy (OPHL Type IIa)

The horizontal partial glottic surgery included several procedures classified according to the resection of the thyroid cartilage.

1. The first approach was developed by Tucker et al. (U.S.) [34] and consisted of a vertical resection of the thyroid cartilage preserving the posterior part of the thyroid wings. This approach was indicated for cT1–T2 laryngeal cancers with normal mobility of the vocal folds and was particularly interesting for tumors with an involvement of the anterior commissure.
2. The second approach is the supracricoid laryngectomy with crico-hyoido-epiglottopexy (CHEP) (Figure 4) [35–37]. In this procedure, the surgeon removes the thyroid cartilage; conserves the cricoid cartilage, hyoid bone and at least one arytenoid unit; and performs an epiglottopexy through a suture between the cricoid and hyoid (sure 4). At least one cricoarytenoid unit (cricoid, arytenoid, cricoarytenoid joint/muscles and the associated recurrent nerve) must be preserved for the functioning of the laryngeal sphincter. The technique was proposed by Majer and Rieder in 1957 and spread by Jean-Jacques Piquet et al. (1974), Henri Laccourreye and Daniel Brasnu under the name supracricoid laryngectomy with reconstruction by CHEP [37]. The indications were cT1–T2 tumors and some selected cT3 tumors with fixation of the vocal cord and

normal mobility of the arytenoid cartilage. This approach was particularly interesting for tumors with involvement of the anterior commissure.

Type 1: horizontal supraglottic laryngectomy

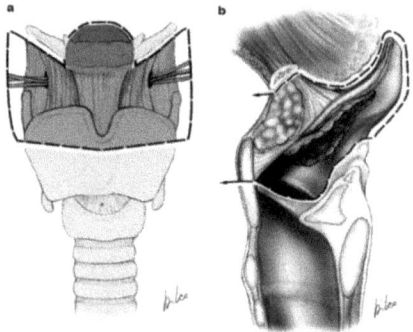

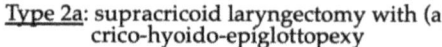

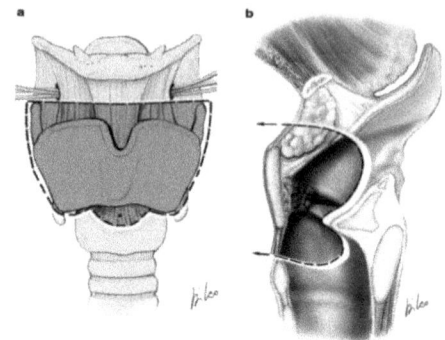

Type 2b: supracricoid laryngectomy with crico-hyoidopexy

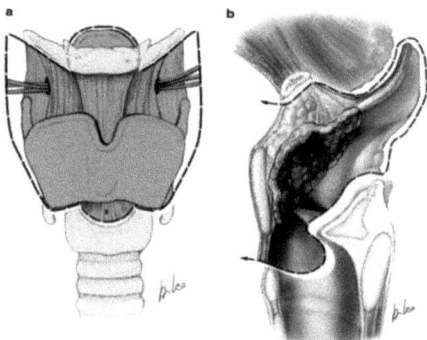

Type 3b: supratracheal laryngectomy with tracheo-hyoidopexy

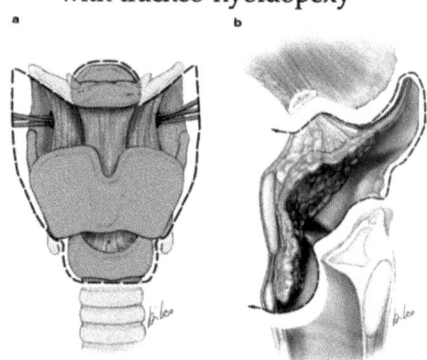

Figure 3. European Laryngological Society Classification of Open Partial Laryngectomies. Authors received the authorization of Pr. Marc Remacle to re-use the picture [4].

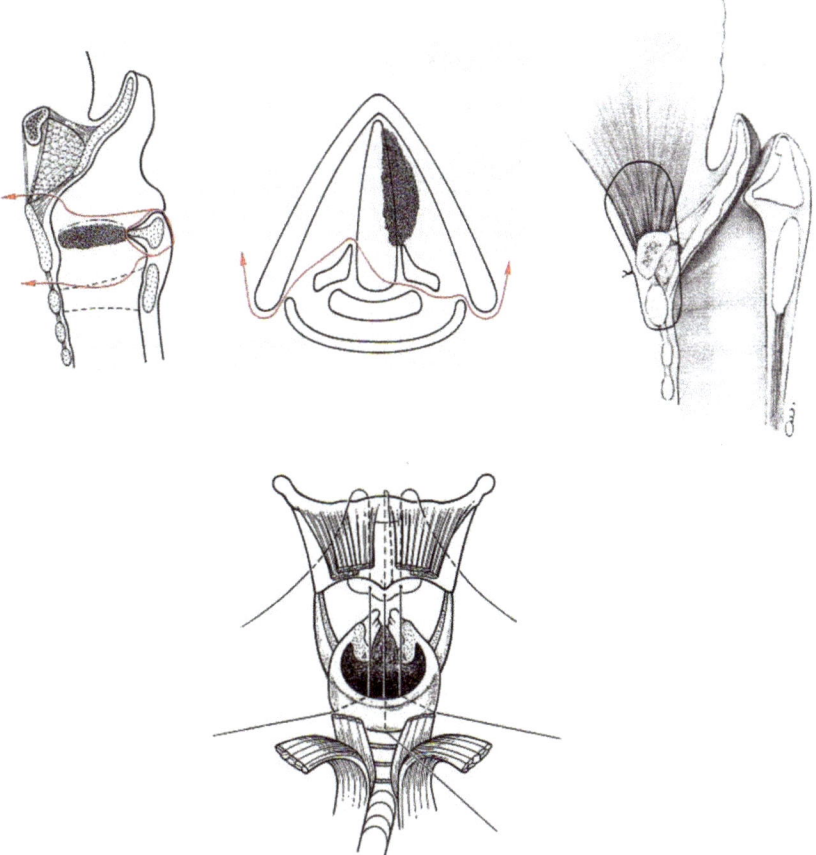

Figure 4. Supracricoid laryngectomy with crico-hyoido-epiglottopexy. Resection of the entire thyroid cartilage and both vocal folds with preservation of at least one arytenoid cartilage. Reconstruction: the closing of the larynx is carried out by an impaction between the cricoid cartilage, the epiglottis, the hyoid bone and the base of the tongue called a "crico-hyoido-epiglottopexy".

The postoperative evolution of these two types of surgery required a transient tracheostomy, feeding tube and hospital stay of 3–4 weeks. Such procedures were associated with adequate local and regional control rates for selected vocal fold tumors [34,36,37].

5.3. The Horizontal Partial Procedures for Glottic and Supraglottic Regions

In this group of partial laryngectomies, two main procedures may be described, depending on the type of resection of the thyroid cartilage.

1. The first approach consisted of a partial resection of the thyroid cartilage and was known as the three-quarter laryngectomy. This approach was developed by Bocca et al. in Italy (1971) [38] and Dedo in the U.S. (1975) [39].
2. Described in 1971 by Labayle and Bismuth [40], the second procedure consisted of a complete resection of the thyroid cartilage followed by a reconstruction through a crico-hyoido-pexy. The approach was called 'supracricoid laryngectomy with reconstruction by crico-hyoido-pexy' by Laccourreye and Brasnu [41].

Currently, both surgical approaches of the supraglottic and glottic regions are rarely carried out due to the increase in organ preservation protocols indicating chemotherapy and radiotherapy.

At the end of the 20th century, the 5-year local control rate and the 5-year laryngeal preservation rate of vocal cord cancers were 92–95% and 95–100%, respectively. For supraglottic cancers, the 5-year local control rate and the 5-year laryngeal preservation rate were 92–94% and 92–95%, respectively [42].

Many studies have demonstrated that vocal quality after a partial laryngectomy is related to the extent of the resection and the reconstruction methods. The spoken voice is called the "neoglottic substitution voice" after a partial vertical laryngectomy [24,43] and the "neolaryngeal substitution voice" after a supracricoid laryngectomy (OPHL type IIa/IIb) [44–46]. For open partial laryngectomies, the voice characteristics will depend on (i) the shape and nature of the remaining structures and the amount of effort and adaptation required to reach a vibrating neoglottic/neolaryngeal voicing sphincter; (ii) collateral constraints of external surgeries, such as a transient tracheostomy or nasogastric tube, that modify and lengthen the dynamics of vocal recovery; and (iii) for endoscopic surgeries, whether the physiological shape of the phonatory glottis is not modified. Thus, vocal rehabilitation aims to improve the closure of the neoglottis and the quality of the mucosal vibration with voice tone improvement (see *Laryngeal Cancer Surgery—Part II*). After a partial laryngectomy, voice rehabilitation is long and requires the patient's effort. In the case of vertical partial laryngectomies, many techniques (e.g., flap) have been developed to improve the voice [24,43]. According to our experience and the data in the literature, vocal progress is achievable even several months after a partial laryngectomy [45,46].

5.4. Evolution of Partial Laryngectomies over the Last Thirty Years

In the past thirty years, there has been a major transformation in the way we treat LSCC, including a decline in the use of open surgery as first-line treatment for a certain proportion of these tumors [47–49]. This evolution was made possible by several factors.

First, the incidence of LSCCs has decreased in most developed countries, partially as a result of public health agencies' efforts to decrease tobacco consumption. Second, advances in chemotherapy and radiation therapy (RT) have led to highly effective non-surgical regimens for patients with advanced laryngeal cancers, with the added advantage of laryngeal preservation in many cases. The Veterans Administration Study published in 1991 established the fact that the response to a neoadjuvant CT scan predicts the response of a tumor to RT. Patients with advanced tumors that responded either partially or completely to CT were treated with RT, and total laryngectomy was reserved for non-responders. This made it possible to preserve the larynx in a significant number of patients with locally advanced laryngeal cancer, while achieving local control and overall survival results equivalent to those achieved with initial total laryngectomy. By 2003, the results of the RTOG 93-11 trial, utilizing CCRT as initial treatment, were published, demonstrating a higher rate of laryngeal preservation with this protocol. Surgery was reserved for treatment failures. This concept changed the paradigm for management of advanced laryngeal cancer, greatly reducing the number of laryngectomies performed. While partial supracricoid laryngectomy has been employed for selected patients, total laryngectomy is the usual procedure for salvage *or* failure after nonsurgical treatment.

Third, technological advances with widespread availability, such as operating microscopes; endoscopes; lasers; image-guided surgery; and more recently, robotics, are transforming our surgical approaches, with transoral minimally invasive techniques greatly improving the postoperative course and functional outcomes for selected tumors (see *Laryngeal Cancer Surgery—Part II*).

5.5. Current Indications for Partial Laryngectomies

From our experience and recently published articles, the current indications for partial laryngectomies are laryngeal tumors with inadequate transoral exposure, certain tumors of the anterior commissure with vertical development (see *Laryngeal Cancer Surgery—Part II*) and selected salvage LSCCs, after radiation therapy failure. However, the experience of many contemporary surgeons with partial laryngectomy is quite limited. For the treatment of localized RT-resistant laryngeal cancer, the surgeon must be perfectly familiar with the type of extension of the tumor as well as with the indications for partial laryngectomies. Nevertheless, partial laryngectomy should be used with caution in patients requiring salvage surgical therapy for a recurrent or persistent laryngeal tumor. Recurrences after RT tend to be submucosal and difficult to evaluate. The only type of partial laryngectomies reported in the literature are the supracricoid partial laryngectomies [50,51]. In a systematic review, De Virgilio reported eleven papers (251 patients from 1990 to December 2017) with 2-year local control and 5-year overall survival rates of 92 and 70%, respectively. The larynx preservation rate was 85.2%. The decannulation rate was 92.1%, and the swallowing recovery rate was 96.5% (PEG dependance and the aspiration pneumonia rate were 3.5% and 6.4%, respectively) [51].

6. Conclusions

Throughout the 20th century, many surgical techniques were developed to avoid total laryngectomies. These procedures were developed through progress in anesthesiology, hygiene and infectiology, as well as due to the expertise of many laryngologists. These open partial laryngectomies led to the preservation of many larynxes around the world while reporting adequate oncological and functional outcomes (voice, breathing and swallowing). Although promising/beneficial for the patient, these approaches have some limitations. First, they require a transient tracheostomy and the use of feeding tubes and are associated with long hospital stays. The voice and swallowing rehabilitation program is long and requires patient motivation. Moreover, the surgery is associated with aesthetic sequelae, such as cervical scars.

In the past thirty years, major modifications in the way we treat LSCC, due to the decreasing incidence of tobacco-related LSCC in the West, as well as advances in technology (Transoral Laser Microsurgery, Transoral Robotic Surgery) and medical oncology, have led to a decline in the use of partial laryngectomy as a first-line treatment of LSCC.

7. In Tribute

This paper is a tribute to Professor Henri Laccourreye, Head of the ENT and Head and Neck Surgery Department at Laënnec Hospital from 1978 to 1992; we also thank Associate Professor Ollivier Laccourreye and Madeleine Ménard.

This paper is also a tribute to Professor Daniel Brasnu, Head of ENT and Head and Neck Surgery at Hôpital Laënnec from 1992 to 2000, and then Head of ENT and Head and Neck Surgery at Hôpital Européen Georges Pompidou from 2000 to 2015.

Author Contributions: Conceptualization, validation, resources, review and editing: J.R.L., S.H. and R.B.; methodology: F.C., M.P.C., L.C.-B. and Q.L. All authors have read and agreed to the published version of the manuscript.

Funding: This research received no external funding.

Institutional Review Board Statement: Not applicable.

Informed Consent Statement: Not applicable.

Data Availability Statement: The study did not report any data.

Conflicts of Interest: The authors declare no conflict of interest.

References

1. Global Burden of Disease Cancer Collaboration. Global, Regional, and National Cancer Incidence, Mortality, Years of Life Lost, Years Lived with Disability, and Disability-Adjusted Life-Years for 29 Cancer Groups, 1990 to 2017: A Systematic Analysis for the Global Burden of Disease Study. *JAMA Oncol.* **2019**, *5*, 1749–1768.
2. Bradley, P.J. Laryngeal cancer in nondrinker nonsmoker young patients: A distinct pathological entity? *Curr. Opin. Otolaryngol. Head Neck Surg.* **2016**, *24*, 140–147. [CrossRef] [PubMed]
3. Aupérin, A. Epidemiology of head and neck cancers: An update. *Curr. Opin. Oncol.* **2020**, *32*, 178–186. [CrossRef] [PubMed]
4. Succo, G.; Peretti, G.; Piazza, C.; Remacle, M.; Eckel, H.E.; Chevalier, D.; Simo, R.; Hantzakos, A.G.; Rizzotto, G.; Lucioni, M.; et al. Open partial horizontal laryngectomies: A proposal for classification by the working committee on nomenclature of the European Laryngological Society. *Eur. Arch. Otorhinolaryngol.* **2014**, *271*, 2489–2496. [CrossRef]
5. Silver, C.E. *Survey for Cancer of the Larynx and Related Structures*; Churchill Livingstone: New York, NY, USA, 1981.
6. Sands, H.B. Case of cancer of the larynx, successfully removed by laryngotomy; With an analysis of 50 cases of tumors of the larynx, treated by operation. *N. Y. Med. J.* **1865**, *1*, 110–126.
7. Solis-Cohen, J. Modern procedures in excision of intrinsic malignant growths of the larynx. *Laryngoscope* **1907**, *17*, 365.
8. Moure, E.J. *Maladies du Larynx*; Octave Doin: Paris, France, 1890.
9. Kirchner, J.A. A historical and histological view of partial laryngectomy. *Bull. N. Y. Acad. Med.* **1986**, *62*, 808–817.
10. Pack, G.T.; Campbelle, R. Historical case records of cancer: Laryngeal cancer of Frederick III of Germany. *Ann. Med. Hist.* **1940**, *2*, 151–170.
11. Laurenson, R.D. The Emporor who smoked a pipe. *J. Laryngol. Otol.* **1995**, *109*, 1–4. [CrossRef]
12. Germain, H.H. Laryngectomy for cancer. *JAMA* **1904**, *42*, 954–955. [CrossRef]
13. Sendziak, J. *The Malignant Laryngeal Tumours Carcinomata, Sarcomata; Their Diagnosis and Treatment*; Bergmann: Wiesbaden, Germany, 1897; Volume 3.
14. Lombard, E. *Indications et Techniques de Laryngectomie pour Cancer*; Rapport de la Société Française d'Oto-rhino-laryngologie; Société Française d'Oto-rhino-laryngologie: Paris, France, 1914.
15. Hajek, J. Anatomische untersuchungen uber das larynxo edem. *Arch. Klin. Chir.* **1891**, *42*, 46–93.
16. Laccourreye, H. Evolution of surgical treatment for cancer of the larynx in the 20th century. *Ann. Otolaryngol. Chir. Cervicofac.* **2000**, *117*, 237–247. [PubMed]
17. Kirchner, J.A. Two hundred laryngeal cancers: Patterns of growth and spread as seen in serial section. *Laryngoscope* **2015**, *125*, 281. [CrossRef]
18. Garcia, M. Physiological observations on the human voice. *Proc. Roy. Soc.* **1855**, *7*, 399–410.
19. Reinhard, M.; Eberhardt, E. Alfred Kirstein (1863–1922)—Pioneer in direct laryngoscopy. *Anasthesiol. Intensivmed. Notfallmed. Schmerzther.* **1995**, *30*, 240–246. [CrossRef]
20. Berteşteanu, S.V.; Popescu, C.R.; Grigore, R.; Popescu, B. Pharyngoesophageal junction neoplasia—Therapeutic management. *Chirurgia* **2012**, *107*, 33–38.
21. Zeitels, S.M. Chevalier Jackson's contributions to direct laryngoscopy. *J. Voice* **1998**, *12*, 1–6. [CrossRef]
22. Leroux-Robert, J. *Les Epitheliomas Intra-Laryngés. Etudes Comparées Cliniques, Radiographiques et Anatomo-Topographiques*; Doin: Paris, France, 1936; 172p.
23. Leroux-Robert, J. A statistical study of 620 laryngeal carcinomas of the glottic region personally operated upon more than five years ago. *Laryngoscope* **1975**, *85*, 1440–1452. [CrossRef]
24. Biacabe, B.; Crevier-Buchman, L.; Hans, S.; Laccourreye, O.; Brasnu, D. Phonatory mechanisms after vertical partial laryngectomy with glottic reconstruction by false vocal fold flap. *Ann. Otol. Rhinol. Laryngol.* **2001**, *110*, 935–940. [CrossRef]
25. Aubry, M. *Chirurgie de L'oreille, du Nez, du Pharynx et du Larynx*; Masson: Paris, France, 1949.
26. Brasnu, D.; Laccourreye, H.; Dulmet, E.; Jaubert, F. Mobility of the vocal cord and arytenoid in squamous cell carcinoma of the larynx and hypopharynx: An anatomical and clinical comparative study. *Ear Nose Throat J.* **1990**, *69*, 324–330.
27. Biller, H.F.; Lawson, W. Partial laryngectomy for vocal cord cancer with marked limitation or fixation of the vocal cord. *Laryngoscope* **1986**, *96*, 61–64. [CrossRef]
28. Rouviere, H. *Anatomy of the Human Lymphatic System*; Edwards: Ann Arbor, MI, USA, 1938.
29. Baclesse, F. Carcinoma of the larynx. *Br. J. Radiol.* **1949**, *3*, 1–62.
30. Trotter, W. The principles and techniques of the operative treatment of malignant disease of the mouth and pharynx. *Lancet* **1913**, *1*, 1147–1152.
31. Alonso, J.M. Conservation surgery of cancer of the larynx. *Trans. Am. Acad. Ophthalmol. Otolaryngol.* **1947**, *51*, 633–642.
32. Bocca, E. Supraglottic laryngectomy and functional neck dissection. *J. Laryngol. Otol.* **1966**, *80*, 831–838. [CrossRef]
33. Laccourreye, H.; Brasnu, D.F.; Beutter, P. Carcinoma of the laryngeal margin. *Head Neck Surg.* **1983**, *5*, 500–507. [CrossRef]
34. Tucker, H.H.; Wood, B.G.; Levine, H.; Katz, R. Glottic reconstruction after near total laryngectomy. *Laryngoscope* **1979**, *89*, 609–618. [CrossRef]
35. Majer, E.H.; Rieder, W. Technic of laryngectomy permitting the conservation of respiratory permeability (cricohyoidopexy). *Ann. Otolaryngol.* **1959**, *76*, 677–681.
36. Piquet, J.J.; Desaulty, A.; Decroix, G. Crico-hyoido-epiglotto-pexy. Surgical technic and functional results. *Ann. Otolaryngol. Chir. Cervicofac.* **1974**, *91*, 681–686.

37. Laccourreye, H.; Laccourreye, O.; Weinstein, G.S.; Menard, M.; Brasnu, D. Supracricoid laryngectomy with cricohyoidoepiglottopexy: A partial laryngeal procedure for glottic carcinomas. *Ann. Otol. Rhinol. Laryngol.* **1999**, *99*, 421–426. [CrossRef]
38. Bocca, E.; Oreste Pignataro Piña, J.P. Conservative horizontal-vertical laryngectomy ventricular cancer. *Acta Otorinolaryngol. Iber. Am.* **1971**, *22*, 117–127. [PubMed]
39. Dedo, H.H. A technique for verticle hemilaryngectomy to prevent stenosis and aspiration. *Laryngoscope* **1975**, *85*, 978–984. [CrossRef] [PubMed]
40. Labayle, J.; Bismuth, R. Total laryngectomy with reconstitution. *Ann. Otolaryngol. Chir. Cervicofac.* **1971**, *88*, 219–328. [PubMed]
41. Laccourreye, H.; Laccourreye, O.; Weinstein, G.S.; Menard, M.; Brasnu, D. supracricoid laryngectomy with cricohyoidopexy: A partial laryngeal procedure for selected supraglottic and transglottic carcinomas. *Laryngoscope* **1990**, *100*, 735–741. [CrossRef]
42. Lefebvre, J.L. What is the role of primary surgery in the treatment of laryngeal and hypopharyngeal cancer? *Hayes Martin Lecture. Arch. Otolaryngol. Head Neck Surg.* **2000**, *126*, 285–288. [CrossRef]
43. Biacabe, B.; Crevier-Buchman, L.; Hans, S.; Laccourreye, O.; Brasnu, D. Vocal function after vertical partial laryngectomy with glottic reconstruction by false vocal fold flap: Durational and frequency measures. *Laryngoscope* **1999**, *109*, 698–704. [CrossRef]
44. Crevier-Buchman, L.; Laccourreye, O.; Wuyts, F.L.; Monfrais-Pfauwadel, M.C.; Pillot, C.; Brasnu, D. Comparison and evolution of perceptual and acoustic characteristics of voice after supracricoid partial laryngectomy with cricohyoidoepiglottopexy. *Acta Otolaryngol.* **1998**, *118*, 594–599. [CrossRef]
45. Crevier-Buchman, L.; Laccourreye, O.; Weinstein, G.; Garcia, D.; Jouffre, V.; Brasnu, D. Evolution of speech and voice following supracricoid partial laryngectomy. *J. Laryngol. Otol.* **1995**, *109*, 410–413. [CrossRef]
46. Miyamaru, S.; Minoda, R.; Kodama, N. Long-term changes in vocal function after supracricoid partial laryngectomy with cricohyoidoepiglottopexy for laryngeal cancer. *Head Neck.* **2019**, *41*, 139–145. [CrossRef]
47. Silver, C.E.; Beitler, J.J.; Shaha, A.R.; Rinaldo, A.; Ferlito, A. Current trends in initial management of laryngeal cancer: The declining use of open surgery. *Eur. Arch. Otorhinolaryngol.* **2009**, *266*, 1333–1352. [CrossRef]
48. Hartl, D.M.; Brasnu, D.F.; Shah, J.P.; Hinni, M.L.; Takes, R.P.; Olsen, K.D.; Kowalski, L.P.; Rodrigo, J.P.; Strojan, P.; Wolf, G.T.; et al. Is open surgery for head and neck cancers truly declining? *Eur. Arch. Otorhinolaryngol.* **2013**, *270*, 2793–2802. [CrossRef]
49. Ferlito, A.; Takes, R.P.; Silver, C.E.; Strojan, P.; Haigentz, M., Jr.; Robbins, K.T.; Genden, E.M.; Hartl, D.M.; Shaha, A.R.; Rinaldo, A.; et al. The changing role of surgery in the current era of head and neck oncology. *Eur. Arch. Otorhinolaryngol.* **2013**, *270*, 1971–1973. [CrossRef]
50. Laccourreye, O.; Weinstein, G.; Naudo, P.; Cauchois, R.; Laccourreye, H.; Brasnu, D. Supracricoid partial laryngectomy after failed laryngeal radiation therapy. *Laryngoscope* **1996**, *106*, 495–498. [CrossRef]
51. De Virgilio, A.; Pellini, R.; Mercante, G.; Cristalli, G.; Manciocco, V.; Giannarelli, D.; Spriano, G. Supracricoid partial laryngectomy for radiorecurrent laryngeal cancer: A systematic review of the literature and meta-analysis. *Eur. Arch. Otorhinolaryngol.* **2018**, *275*, 1671–1680. [CrossRef]

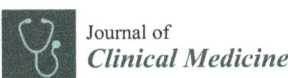

Article

Salvage Partial Laryngectomy after Failed Radiotherapy: Oncological and Functional Outcomes

Mélanie Gigot [1], Antoine Digonnet [2], Alexandra Rodriguez [1,†] and Jerome R. Lechien [1,3,4,5,*,†]

1. Department of Otorhinolaryngology and Head and Neck Surgery, CHU Saint-Pierre, 1000 Brussels, Belgium
2. Department of Surgery, Bordet Institute, Brussel Free University, 1050 Brussels, Belgium
3. Department of Otolaryngology, Polyclinic of Poitiers, Elsan, 86000 Poitiers, France
4. Department of Human Anatomy and Experimental Oncology, Faculty of Medicine, UMONS Research Institute for Health Sciences and Technology, University of Mons, 7000 Mons, Belgium
5. Department of Otolaryngology-Head & Neck Surgery, Foch Hospital, School of Medicine, UFR Simone Veil, Université Versailles Saint-Quentin-en-Yvelines, 92150 Paris, France
* Correspondence: jerome.lechien@umons.ac.be
† These authors contributed equally to this work.

Abstract: Objective: To investigate oncological and functional outcomes in patients treated with salvage partial laryngectomy (SPL) after failed radio/chemotherapy. Study design: Retrospective multicenter chart review. Methods: Medical records of patients treated with SPL from January 1998 to January 2018 in two University Medical centers were retrieved. The SPL included horizontal supraglottic laryngectomy, hemi-laryngectomy and crico-hyoido-epiglottopexy. The following outcomes were investigated: histopathological features; overall survival (OS); recurrence-free survival (RFS) local and regional controls; post-operative speech recovery; and the oral diet restart and decannulation. Results: The data of 20 patients with cT1–cT3 laryngeal cancer were collected. The mean follow-up of patients was 69.7 months. The mean hospital stay was 43.0 days (16–111). The following complications occurred in the immediate post-operative follow-up: neck fistula (N = 6), aspiration pneumonia (N = 5), and chondronecrosis (N = 2). Early or late total laryngectomy was carried out over the follow-up period for the following reasons: positive margins and local recurrence/progression (N = 7), chondronecrosis (N = 2) and non-functional larynx (N = 1). The restart of the oral diet was carried out in 12/15 (80%) SPL patients (five patients being excluded for totalization). All patients recovered speech, and decannulation was performed in 14 patients (93%). The 5-year OS and RFS were 50% and 56%, respectively. The 5-year local and regional control rates were 56% and 56%, respectively. Conclusions: Partial laryngectomy is an alternative therapeutic approach to total laryngectomy in patients with a history of failed radiation.

Keywords: otolaryngology; head neck surgery; laryngectomy; partial; cancer; oncological; survival; voice; swallowing

Citation: Gigot, M.; Digonnet, A.; Rodriguez, A.; Lechien, J.R. Salvage Partial Laryngectomy after Failed Radiotherapy: Oncological and Functional Outcomes. *J. Clin. Med.* **2022**, *11*, 5411. https://doi.org/10.3390/jcm11185411

Academic Editor: Matteo Fermi

Received: 3 August 2022
Accepted: 3 September 2022
Published: 15 September 2022

Publisher's Note: MDPI stays neutral with regard to jurisdictional claims in published maps and institutional affiliations.

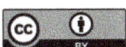

Copyright: © 2022 by the authors. Licensee MDPI, Basel, Switzerland. This article is an open access article distributed under the terms and conditions of the Creative Commons Attribution (CC BY) license (https://creativecommons.org/licenses/by/4.0/).

1. Introduction

Head and neck squamous cell carcinoma (HNSCC) is the 6th most common adult malignancy worldwide, accounting for 5.3% of all cancers [1]. Laryngeal squamous cell carcinoma (LSCC) is the second most prevalent HNSCC, corresponding to 211,000 new cases and 126,000 deaths per year worldwide [2,3]. According to the stage and location of tumor, the main therapeutic options include surgery, radiotherapy or concurrent chemoradiotherapy. Radiotherapy may achieve local control rates of 77% to 100% of cT1, 62% to 83% of cT2, and 50% to 76% of cT3 supraglottic SCCs [4]. In cases of local failure, the most common therapeutic option remains total laryngectomy, which may be associated with complications and poor quality of life outcomes [5]. However, a recent systematic review of the literature suggested that the realization of salvage partial laryngectomy (SPL) in place of total laryngectomy may be an option in selected cases of glottic or supraglottic SCC recurrence or post-radiotherapy failure, reporting adequate local control and survival outcomes [6].

In this study, we retrospectively reviewed the oncological, histopathological and functional outcomes of patients who benefited from SPL after failed radiotherapy.

2. Materials and Methods

The data of patients treated with post-radiotherapy SPL for glottic or supraglottic SCC from 1998 to 2021 were retrieved. Patients were recruited and treated in two University medical centers (CHU Saint-Pierre and Jules Bordet Institute, Brussels, Belgium). The SCCs were located in glottic or supraglottic region. The SPL indication was based on cTNM tumor (cT1–cT3), medical history of patients, the MRI/CT-scan findings and swallowing tests. All patients underwent diagnostic preoperative workup with laryngeal fibroscopy, in-suspension laryngoscopy (biopsy) and injected tomodensitometry or Pet-CT. The SPL was considered as a therapeutic option if it was possible to preserve one cricoarytenoid unit after the surgery. The SPL was not recommended for the following patient/tumor outcomes: cricoid invasion; large invasion of laryngeal posterior commissure or thyroid cartilage; and pharyngeal or prevertebral invasion (cT4). The SPL decision was approved by the multidisciplinary oncological board. The local institutional review boards of both centers approved the study design (CE171211 et CE2849).

2.1. Procedures

Surgeries were performed under general anesthesia. According to the European Laryngological Society classification [7], the following SPL were considered: open partial horizontal supraglottic (hemi) laryngectomy (type I), supracricoid laryngectomy with cricohyoidoepiglottopexy (type IIa) or cricohyoidopexy (type IIb; Appendix A). Note that in all procedures, surgeons performed extemporaneous analyses. In the case of positive margins, the surgeon completed the surgery with recut of the positive tissue section. We did not extend the resection from one type of open partial laryngectomy to another. Only the definitive margin analyses were considered for the follow-up decisions. The surgical techniques were described in previous studies [7]. According to the tomodensitometry findings, unilateral or bilateral selective neck dissection(s) of levels II-IV were carried out in cT3 and selected cT2 patients.

Patients had tracheostomies and feeding tubes. All patients benefited from post-operative speech therapy (3- to 5 sessions weekly), which was started 7 days after the surgery. All patients received 7-day antibiotics and 1-month proton pump inhibitors. An oral diet was restarted from 7 days post-SPL depending on the speech therapist and oto-laryngologist's agreement. Regarding the evolution of swallowing, speech and breathing, patients were decannulated and discharged as soon as possible after a fiberoptic endoscopic evaluation of swallowing.

The total laryngectomy was considered in patients with (i) positive margins at the post-SPL histopathological analysis, (ii) post-operative chondronecrosis or non-functional larynx, or (iii) for local recurrence. If the salvage total laryngectomy was performed in the 6-month post-SPL follow-up, the total laryngectomy was considered as an early procedure, while when the surgeon carried out the total laryngectomy after 6 months of follow-up, the salvage laryngectomy was considered as late. Note that positive margins (R1) were followed before the decision of total laryngectomy according to the difficulties to have reliable histopathological findings in radiation tissues.

The neck dissection was proposed by the multidisciplinary oncological team in patients with suspicion of positive nodes at the tomodensitometry even if the cTNM classification reported cN0 (<1 cm diameter). Unilateral neck dissection was proposed for suspicion of unilateral node(s), while bilateral neck dissection was proposed for suspected bilateral nodes.

2.2. Outcomes

The following postoperative outcomes were retrieved: infectious complications; fistula; chondronecrosis; aspiration pneumonia; death. The functional outcomes included the postoperative speech recovery; restart of an oral diet; and the removal of the tracheostomy tube. Post-operative speech recovery was defined as the ability of the patient to be understood by other people without repetition. The usual voice and speech clinical tools (e.g., speech rate; GRBASI, voice handicap index) were not used because they are inappropriate for post-partial laryngectomy voice and speech evaluations and there was no systematic use of clinical voice/speech tools in our centers. The following oncological outcomes were considered: 3- and 5-year overall survival (OS); recurrence-free survival (RFS); and local and regional control rates.

3. Results

3.1. Setting and Patients

Twenty patients underwent SPL after failed radiotherapy (N = 17) or concurrent chemoradiotherapy (N = 3), including supracricoid laryngectomy with cricohyoidoepiglottopexy (type 2a, N = 11); open partial horizontal supraglottic laryngectomy (type 1, N = 6), and open partial horizontal hemi-laryngectomy (type 1, N = 3). The flow chart of the study is described in Figure 1.

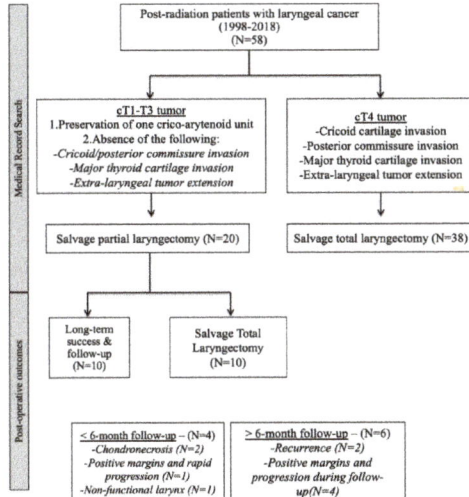

Figure 1. Flow chart.

There were 14 males and the mean age was 54.0 years old. Eighteen patients (90%) reported a history of tobacco consumption prior to the initial radiation treatment, while 14/16 (88%) had a history of chronic alcohol consumption (>3 IU/day). The radiotherapy doses of initial treatment are reported in Appendix A. Two patients had chemoradiation prior to salvage surgery (cisplatin). The surgeons performed six unilateral and five bilateral neck dissections. There were 7, 10, and 3 cT1, cT2, and cT3N0M0 glottic or supraglottic SCC, respectively (Table 1).

Synchronous cancer was detected in two patients (esophagus and lung cancer).

The histopathological findings are reported in Table 1. Frozen sections were positive in 7 cases, leading to preoperative revision. Among them, four definitive histopathological examinations reported R1, which led to a follow-up approach and total laryngectomy for recurrence (Appendix A). Three of eleven neck dissections were positive. Among them, two patients had extra-capsular node invasion; which led to post-operative chemo-radiotherapy and palliative chemotherapy, respectively. As described in Appendix A, the initial cTNM assessment was lower than the pTNM for five patients with two with pT4 cancer at the histopathological examination.

Table 1. Epidemiological, clinical and surgical features.

Outcomes	Mean/N
Age (mean, range)	54 (40–69)
Gender (F/M)	6/14
Tumor features	
Second location (N, mean month delay)	4 (52.5)
Recurrence (N, mean month delay)	16 (34.8)
Locations	
Supraglottic	7 (35)
Glottic	10 (50)
Laryngopharyngeal	3 (15)
Stages	
cT1N0M0	7 (35)
cT2N0M0	10 (50)
cT3N0M0	3 (15)
Surgeries	
Cricohyoidoepiglottopexy	11 (55)
Horizontal supraglottic laryngectomy	6 (30)
Horizontal hemi-laryngectomy	3 (15)
Tracheostomy	20 (100)
Feeding tube	20 (100)
Histopathological Findings	**N (%)**
Margins	
R0	13 (65)
R1	7 (35)
Management of R1	
Re-intervention	5 (71)
Total laryngectomy	2 (29)
Neck dissection	
pN+	3 (27)
pN0	8 (73)
Management of N+	
Follow-up	1 (33)
Chemoradiotherapy	1 (33)
Palliative chemotherapy	1 (33)
Functional Outcomes	**N (%)**
Early total laryngectomy	5 (25)
Chondronecrosis	2 (10)
Positive margins	2 (10)
Non-functional larynx	1 (5)
Late total laryngectomy	5 (25)
Positive margins	2 (10)
Recurrences	3 (15)
Oral diet rehabilitation	
Success of restart	12 (80)
Definitive gastrostomy	3 (20)
Delay (mean, days)	49.0
Cricohyoidoepiglottopexy	34.3
Horizontal supraglottic laryngectomy	163.0
Horizontal hemi-laryngectomy	58.5
Speech rehabilitation	
Success	15 (100)
Delay (mean, days)	60.7
Cricohyoidoepiglottopexy	52.8
Horizontal supraglottic laryngectomy	90.0
Horizontal hemi-laryngectomy	56.6
Tracheostomy	
Decannulation	14/15 (93)
Delay (mean, days)	11.2
Cricohyoidoepiglottopexy	10.4
Horizontal supraglottic laryngectomy	13.8
Horizontal hemi-laryngectomy	7.6

Abbreviations: F/M = female/male; R = margin status; N = number of cases.

The mean hospital stay was 43.0 days (16–111). The following complications occurred in the immediate post-operative follow-up: neck fistula (N = 6), aspiration pneumonia (N = 5), and chondronecrosis (N = 2). There was no local infection (abscess) or death during the post-operative course. Three patients with fistula required re-intervention and the following flaps were used: pectoral (N = 1), supraclavicular (N = 1) and temporal (N = 1) flap. Two patients with chondronecrosis, one patient with positive margins and rapid (<6-month) progression (R1) and one patient with non-functional larynx were treated with an early total laryngectomy (<6-month post-SPL). Late total laryngectomy (>6 months of follow-up) was carried out in six patients (Figure 1). Two had positive margins but refused the total laryngectomy and three had late recurrences. Finally, total laryngectomy was carried out in 10 patients (50%) for the following reasons: positive margins and follow-up recurrence/progression (N = 7); chondronecrosis (N = 2); and non-functional larynx (N = 1; Appendix A).

3.2. Functional Outcomes

The functional outcomes are summarized in Table 1. The restart of an oral diet was carried out in 12/15 (80%) SLP patients without early total laryngectomy with a mean delay of 49.0 days. Three patients did not restart an oral diet because of severe aspiration (N = 2) or malnutrition related to synchronous chest cancer. These patients benefited from permanent gastrostomy. The speech rehabilitation was successfully completed in all patients with a mean delay of 60.7 days (mean of speech session: three times weekly). Decannulation was carried out in 14 patients (93%) with a mean delay of 11.2 days. The restart of oral diet, speech rehabilitation and decannulation delays varied between surgeries (Table 1).

3.3. Oncological Outcomes

The mean follow-up of patients was 69.7 months (6–178). The 3- and 5-year OS were 50.0% and 50.0%, respectively. The 3- and 5-year local control rates were 55.5% and 55.5%, respectively. The 3- and 5-year RFS were 55.5% and 55.5%, respectively. At the end of the follow-up, five patients were alive and five were lost of follow-up (after the 5-year initial follow-up). The causes of death of the 10 remaining patients were local recurrence or distant metastasis (N = 5); non-oncological origin (N = 3); and metachronous non-head and neck cancer (N = 2). Note that 3/6 patients who underwent salvage total laryngectomy were alive at the end of the follow-up period (five patients were lost of follow-up). In the SPL group, 5/10 patients were alive at the end of the follow-up period (Appendix A).

4. Discussion

Residual or recurrent LSCC after failed radiotherapy is a challenging issue. The salvage total laryngectomy was the main option for post-radiation LSCC and only a few case series with a low number of patients investigated the oncological and functional outcomes of SLP [6].

The primary finding of the present study was the demonstration of adequate functional post-operative outcomes, including decannulation, speech rehabilitation and oral diet restart. All patients with SPL were successfully decannulated after 60 days. Our decannulation rate was slightly above that of those found in the literature despite a longer delay of decannulation in the present study [8–12]. The oral restart was possible in 80% of patients with a mean delay of 49 days. Kim et al. reported oral restart rates of 100% versus 74.2% in patients who underwent salvage supraglottic laryngectomy or TL, respectively [12]. The mean removal time of the feeding tube was 25 days in the study of Kim et al., which was, however, substantially shorter than our delay [12]. In the study of Philippe et al., 15/20 (75%) patients treated with SPL for LSCC after failed radiotherapy were able to restart an oral diet in the post-operative few months [11]. Others reported similar rates of the restart of an oral diet with delays ranging from 15 to 74 days [6,8–10,12,13]. Our study reports an adequate post-operative speech rehabilitation rate despite longer delays than those of some studies in which authors started speech exercises 3 days after the SLP [6,10]. The functional outcome in comparison with other studies is still limited regarding the heterogeneity across studies about the types of SPL, the patient comorbidities, and the TNM features. Moreover, as supported by Paleri et al., the differences between world regions in speech therapy access and program may support different speech rehabilitation outcomes [14].

The complications after salvage partial laryngectomy depend on the type of surgery and the features of the population (comorbidities), and include most commonly fistula, hemorrhage, wound infection, aspiration pneumonia and dysphagia [10–17]. In this case series, aspiration pneumonia (25%), fistula (15%) and chondronecrosis (10%) were the main complications. The rate of fistula in SPL patients after failed radiotherapy ranged from 2% to 81% [15–18] and was influenced by the radiotherapy doses rather than the type of surgery [15]. The tobacco and the reflux histories are additional contributing factors to fistula [19]. In these case series, Philippe et al. carried out total laryngectomy in two patients (10%) with a non-functional larynx and recurrent aspiration pneumonia, which corroborates our rate of a non-functional larynx [11]. Aspiration pneumonia occurred in 20% of our patients. The literature rate of aspirations ranges from 3% to 40% [8,11,20,21].

In the present study, the 5-year OS and RFS were 50% and 55%, respectively. The OS and RFS data in the literature substantially vary from one study to another. Overall, both OS and RFS ranged from 52% to 95% but depend on the features of patients (comorbidities), tumor stage and treatment [10,11,16,17,21–23]. According to Kim et al., the OS and DFR were non-significantly higher in the salvage SPL than in the salvage TL [12]. Authors reported 5-year OS and RFS of 87.5% and 41.9% in their SPL patients, which were significantly higher for OS than our rate. Interestingly, they highlighted the importance of margin status in survival and recurrence outcomes, which supports the need for a close follow-up in patients with post-SLP positive margins or re-intervention. In the study of Makaieff et al., the 5-year OS was 69% [20], while Philippe et al. reported a 3-year OS of 66% [11]. As for other studies of the literature [9,10,15], the main cohort difference between our case series and these studies was the inclusion of cT3 LSCC in the present study, which is known to be associated with poorer OS and RFS data [15]. Interestingly, our study reported that the initial cTNM assessment may be biased according to the radiation history. Indeed, for six patients, the pTNM was higher than the cTNM, both having a T4 LSCC at the histopathological examination. The tissue fibrosis related to radiation may influence the clinical and imaging staging leading to the inclusion of patients with more advanced disease. This point is an additional factor supporting the low but literature-comparable OS and RFS rates.

The main limitations of the present study were the retrospective design and the low number of patients. However, the SPL after failed radiotherapy remains a rare surgical approach because the current trend in head and neck oncology is to propose salvage total laryngectomy for patients with such LSCC. However, since the possible risk of conversion in total laryngectomy exists, appropriate information about the patient is a mainstay in this therapeutic approach.

5. Conclusions

The salvage partial laryngectomy after radiotherapy failure is an alternative therapeutic option to total laryngectomy for patients with cT1-T3 LSCC. Otolaryngologists had to be careful about the risk of preoperative mis-staging. Aspiration and fistula were the most common complications occurring in 15% to 20% of cases.

Author Contributions: Conceptualization, A.D., M.G., A.R. and J.R.L.; methodology, A.D., M.G., A.R. and J.R.L.; formal analysis, and investigation, A.D., M.G., A.R. and J.R.L.; writing—original draft preparation, M.G. and J.R.L.; writing—review and editing, A.D. and A.R. All authors have read and agreed to the published version of the manuscript.

Funding: This research received no external funding.

Institutional Review Board Statement: The local institutional review board approved the study design (CHU Saint-Pierre, number CE171211, 12 January 2018).

Informed Consent Statement: Not applicable.

Data Availability Statement: Data are available on request.

Acknowledgments: Gilbert Chantrain (retained) for the supervision of the work.

Conflicts of Interest: The authors declare no conflict of interest.

Appendix A

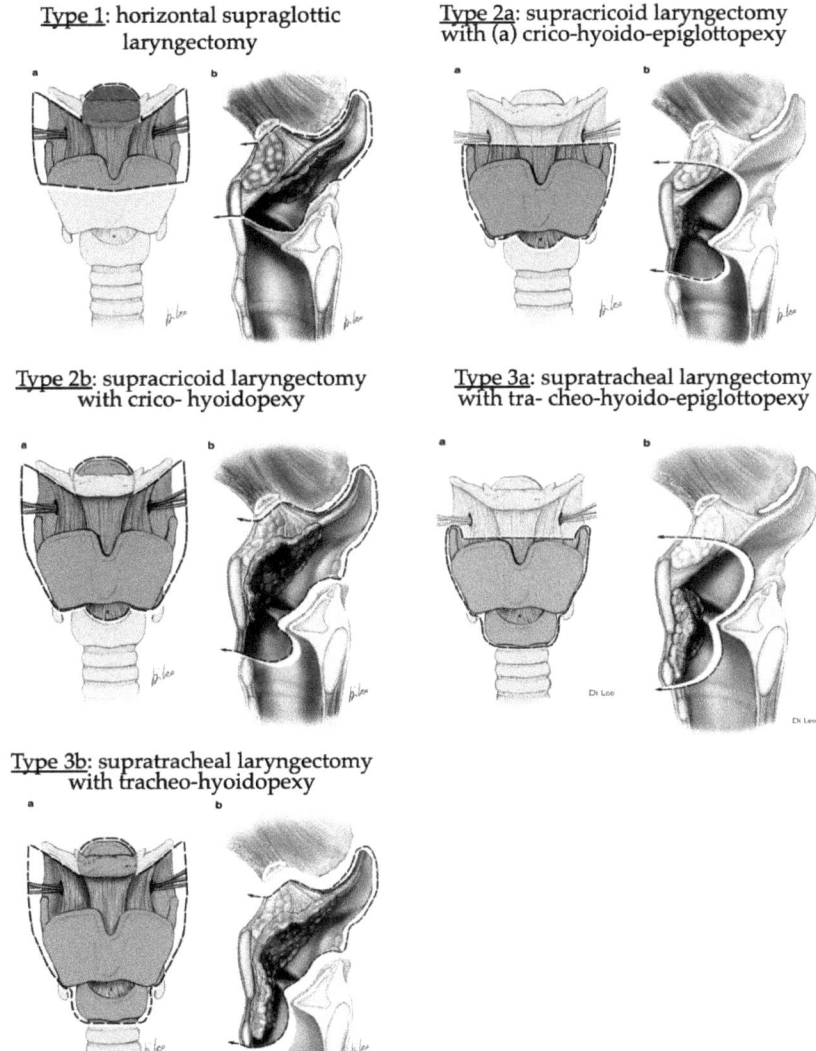

Figure A1. European Laryngological Society Classification of Partial Laryngectomy. a = coronal plan, b = saggital plan.

Table A1. Patient Features.

N	Tob.	Alcohol	Surgery	RT (Gy)	CT	ND	cTNM	pTNM*	EHE m	DHE m	Adj.T.	2d Cancer	Complications	Flap	TL	Cause	PG	Death
1	+	-	CHEP	70	-	-	cT2N0	T2N0	R1	R1	-	-	-	-	-	-	-	Lost
2	+	+	CHEP	70	-	-	cT1N0	T1N0	R0	R0	-	-	Chondronecrosis, fistula	Yes	Late	R1	-	Yes
3	+	+	HL	63	-	+	cT1N0	T1N2+	R0	R0	-	-	Fistula	Yes	Early	CN	Yes	Yes
4	+	+	CHEP	70	-	+	cT2N0	T4N0	R1	R0	-	-	Chondronecrosis	-	-	-	-	No
5	+	+	CHEP	70	-	+	cT2N0	T4N1	R1	R1	CRT	-	-	-	Early	CN	-	Yes
6	+	N.A.	HL	70	-	-	cT2N0	T2N0	R0	R0	-	Esophagus	-	-	Late	R1	-	No
7	+	+	CHEP	70	-	-	cT2N0	T1N0	R0	R0	-	-	-	-	-	-	-	No
8	+	+	HSGL	70	-	+	cT2N0	T2N0	R1	R1	-	-	Aspiration P.	-	-	-	-	Lost
9	+	N.A.	HL	70	+	+	cT2N0	T2N2+	R0	R0	C	Lung	-	-	Late	R1	Yes	Yes
10	+	N.A.	CHEP	70	-	+	cT3N0	T3N0	R0	R0	-	-	Fistula	-	-	-	-	Yes
11	+	+	CHEP	70	-	+	cT2N0	T2N0	R0	R0	-	-	Aspiration P., fistula	Yes	-	-	-	No
12	+	+	CHEP	70	-	-	cT2N0	T2N0	R0	R0	-	-	Aspiration P., fistula	-	-	-	-	No
13	+	+	CHEP	65	-	+	cT3N0	T3N0	R1	R0	-	-	Fistula	-	Early	R1	-	Lost
14	-	+	CHEP	70	-	+	cT3N0	T3N0	R0	R0	-	-	-	-	Late	Recurrence	-	Yes
15	+	+	HSGL	70	+	-	cT2N0	T3N0	R0	R0	-	-	-	-	-	-	-	No
16	+	+	CHEP	70	-	+	cT1N0	T1N0	R0	R0	-	-	Aspiration P.	-	Late	Recurrence	-	Yes
17	+	-	HSGL	70	-	+	cT1N0	T1N0	R0	R0	-	-	-	-	-	-	Yes	Yes
18	+	+	HSGL	63	-	-	cT1N0	T2N0M1	R1	R1	-	-	-	-	Late	R1	-	Lost
19	-	+	HSGL	63	-	-	cT1N0	T2N0	R0	R0	-	-	Aspiration P.	-	-	-	Yes	Yes
20	+	N.A.	HSGL	70	+	+	cT1N0	T2N0	R0	R0	-	-	Non-functional larynx	-	Early	Functional	-	Lost

* The pTNM classification was based on the 6th TNM classification. Abbreviations: Adj.T. = immediate adjuvant treatment; CN=chondronecrosis; CT = chemotherapy associated with radiotherapy in the initial treatment; C/CRT = chemo/chemoradiotherapy; CHEP = crico-hyoido-epiglottopexy (type 2a); D/EHH m = definitive/extemporaneous histopathological examination margins; Gy = Gray; HL = hemi-laryngectomy (type 1); HSGL = horizontal sugraglottic laryngectomy (type 1); N = number; ND = neck dissection; P. = pneumopathy; PG = permanent gastrostomy; RT = radiation doses priori to surgery (initial radiotherapy); TL = total laryngectomy; Tob = tobacco consumption history prior to surgery.
NA = not available.

References

1. Global Burden of Disease Cancer Collaboration. Global, Regional, and National Cancer Incidence, Mortality, Years of Life Lost, Years Lived With Disability, and Disability-Adjusted Life-Years for 29 Cancer Groups, 1990 to 2017: A Systematic Analysis for the Global Burden of Disease Study. *JAMA Oncol.* **2019**, *5*, 1749–1768. [CrossRef] [PubMed]
2. Bradley, P.J. Laryngeal cancer in nondrinker nonsmoker young patients: A distinct pathological entity? *Curr. Opin. Otolaryngol. Head Neck Surg.* **2016**, *24*, 140–147. [CrossRef] [PubMed]
3. Aupérin, A. Epidemiology of head and neck cancers: An update. *Curr. Opin. Oncol.* **2020**, *32*, 178–186. [CrossRef]
4. Ambrosch, P. The role of laser microsurgery in the treat- ment of laryngeal cancer. *Curr. Opin. Otolaryngol. Head Neck Surg.* **2007**, *15*, 82–88. [CrossRef]
5. Locatello, L.G.; Licci, G.; Maggiore, G.; Gallo, O. Non-Surgical Strategies for Assisting Closure of Pharyngocutaneous Fistula after Total Laryngectomy: A Systematic Review of the Literature. *J. Clin. Med.* **2021**, *11*, 100. [CrossRef]
6. Shapira, U.; Warshavsky, A.; Muhanna, N.; Oestreicher-Kedem, Y.; Nachalon, Y.; Ungar, O.J.; Safadi, A.; Carmel Neiderman, N.N.; Horowitz, G. Laryngectomy-free survival after salvage partial laryngectomy: A systematic review and meta-analysis. *Eur. Arch. Otorhinolaryngol.* **2022**, *279*, 3021–3027. [CrossRef]
7. Succo, G.; Peretti, G.; Piazza, C.; Remacle, M.; Eckel, H.E.; Chevalier, D.; Simo, R.; Hantzakos, A.G.; Rizzotto, G.; Lucioni, M.; et al. Open partial horizontal laryngectomies: A proposal for classification by the working committee on nomenclature of the European LaryngologicalSociety. *Eur. Arch. Otorhinolaryngol.* **2014**, *271*, 2489–2496. [CrossRef]
8. Bertolin, A.; Lionello, M.; Ghizzo, M.; Cena, I.; Leone, F.; Valerini, S.; Mattioli, F.; Crosetti, E.; Presutti, L.; Succo, G.; et al. Salvage open partial horizontal laryngectomy after failed radiotherapy: A multicentric study. *Laryngoscope* **2020**, *130*, 431–436. [CrossRef]
9. Sperry, S.M.; Rassekh, C.H.; Laccourreye, O.; Weinstein, G.S. Supracricoid partial laryngectomy for primary and recurrent laryngeal cancer. *JAMA Otolaryngol. Head Neck Surg.* **2013**, *139*, 1226–1235. [CrossRef]
10. Rodríguez-Cuevas, S.; Labastida, S.; Gonzalez, D.; Briseño, N.; Cortes, H. Partial laryngectomy as salvage surgery for radiation failures in T1-T2 laryngeal cancer. *Head Neck.* **1998**, *20*, 630–633. [CrossRef]
11. Philippe, Y.; Espitalier, F.; Durand, N.; Ferron, C.; Bardet, E.; Malard, O. Partial laryngectomy as salvage surgery after radiotherapy: Oncological and functional outcomes and impact on quality of life. A retrospective study of 20 cases. *Eur. Ann. Otorhinolaryngol. Head Neck Dis.* **2014**, *131*, 15–19. [CrossRef] [PubMed]
12. Kim, J.H.; Kim, W.S.; Koh, Y.W.; Kim, S.H.; Byeon, H.K.; Choi, E.C. Oncologic and functional outcomes of salvage supracricoid partial laryngectomy. *Acta Otolaryngol.* **2018**, *138*, 1117–1122. [CrossRef] [PubMed]
13. Spriano, G.; Pellini, R.; Romano, G.; Muscatello, L.; Roselli, R. Supracricoid partial laryngectomy as salvage surgery after radiation failure. *Head Neck.* **2002**, *24*, 759–765. [CrossRef]
14. Paleri, V.; Thomas, L.; Basavaiah, N.; Drinnan, M.; Mehanna, H.; Jones, T. Oncologic outcomes of open conservation laryngectomy for radiorecurrent laryngeal carcinoma: A systematic review and meta-analysis of english-language literature. *Cancer* **2011**, *117*, 2668–2676. [CrossRef] [PubMed]
15. Ganly, I.; Patel, S.G.; Matsuo, J.; Singh, B.; Kraus, D.H.; Boyle, J.O.; Wong, R.J.; Shaha, A.R.; Lee, N.; Shah, J.P. Results of surgical salvage after failure of definitive radiation therapy for early-stage squamous cell carcinoma of the glottic larynx. *Arch. Otolaryngol. Head Neck Surg.* **2006**, *132*, 59–66. [CrossRef]
16. Toma, M.; Nibu, K.-I.; Nakao, K.; Matsuzaki, M.; Mochiki, M.; Yuge, T.; Pazzaia, A.; Laudadio, P.; Piazza, C.; Peretti, G.; et al. Partial laryngectomy to treat early glottic cancer after failure of radiation therapy. *Arch. Otolaryngol. Head Neck Surg.* **2002**, *128*, 909–912. [CrossRef]
17. Pellini, R.; Pichi, B.; Ruscito, P.; Ceroni, A.R.; Caliceti, U.; Rizzotto, G.; Pazzaia, A.; Laudadio, P.; Piazza, C.; Peretti, G.; et al. Supracricoid partial laryngectomies after radiation failure: A multi-institutional series. *Head Neck.* **2008**, *30*, 372–379. [CrossRef]
18. Deganello, A.; Gallo, O.; De Cesare, J.M.; Ninu, M.B.; Gitti, G.; de' Campora, L.; Radici, M.; de' Campora, E. Supracricoid partial laryngectomy as salvage surgery for radiation therapy failure. *Head Neck.* **2008**, *30*, 1064–1071. [CrossRef]
19. Seikaly, H.; Park, P. Gastroesophageal reflux prophylaxis decreases the incidence of pharyngocutaneous fistula after total laryngectomy. *Laryngoscope* **1995**, *105*, 1220–1222. [CrossRef]
20. Hong, J.C.; Kim, S.W.; Lee, H.S.; Han, Y.J.; Park, H.S.; Lee, K.D. Salvage transoral laser supraglottic laryngectomy after radiation failure: A report of seven cases. *Ann. Otol. Rhinol. Laryngol.* **2013**, *122*, 85–90. [CrossRef]
21. Makeieff, M.; Venegoni, D.; Mercante, G.; Crampette, L.; Guerrier, B. Supracricoid partial laryngectomies after failure of radiation therapy. *Laryngoscope* **2005**, *115*, 353–357. [CrossRef] [PubMed]
22. Yiotakis, J.; Stavroulaki, P.; Nikolopoulos, T.; Manolopoulos, L.; Kandiloros, D.; Ferekidis, E.; Adamopoulos, G. Partial Laryngectomy after Irradiation Failure. *Otolaryngol.-Head Neck Surg.* **2003**, *128*, 200–209. [CrossRef] [PubMed]
23. Schwaab, G.; Mamelle, G.; Lartigau, E.; Parise, O.; Wibault, P.; Luboinski, B. Surgical salvage treatment of T1/T2 glottic carcinoma after failure of radiotherapy. *Am. J. Surg.* **1994**, *168*, 474–475. [CrossRef]

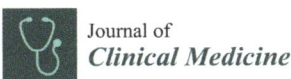

Article

A New Animal Model of Laryngeal Transplantation

Pierre Philouze [1,*], Olivier Malard [2], Sébastien Albert [3], Lionel Badet [4], Bertrand Baujat [5], Frédéric Faure [6], Carine Fuchsmann [1], Franck Jegoux [7], Jean Lacau-St-Guily [5], Jean-Paul Marie [8], Antoine Ramade [1], Sebastien Vergez [9], Philippe Ceruse [1] and Olivier J. Gauthier [10]

1. Département d'ORL et Chirurgie Cervico-Faciale, Croix-Rousse Hospital, Université Lyon 1, 69004 Lyon, France
2. Service d'ORL, Hôtel-Dieu, Université Nantes, 44093 Nantes, France
3. Service d'ORL, Hôpital Bichat, University Paris VII, AP-HP, 75018 Paris, France
4. Service de Chirurgie de la Transplantation et d'Urologie, Hôpital Edouard-Herriot, Université Lyon 1, 69347 Lyon, France
5. Service d'ORL et Chirurgie Cervico-Faciale, Hôpital Tenon, APHP, Sorbonne Université, 75013 Paris, France
6. Département d'ORL et Chirurgie Cervico-Faciale, Hôpital Edouard Herriot, Université Lyon 1, 69100 Lyon, France
7. Service d'ORL et Chirurgie Maxillo-Faciale, CHU Pontchaillou, Université Rennes, 35033 Rennes, France
8. Service ORL et Chirurgie Cervico-Faciale, Hôpital Charles-Nicolle, CHU Rouen, Université Rouen Normandie, UR 3830 GRHVN, 76000 Rouen, France
9. Service ORL et Chirurgie Cervicofaciale, CHU Toulouse Rangueil-Larrey, Université Toulouse, 31059 Toulouse, France
10. Department of Small Animal Surgery and Anesthesia, Nantes-Atlantic College of Veterinary Medicine, Food Science and Engineering (ONIRIS), 44307 Nantes, France
* Correspondence: pierre.philouze@chu-lyon.fr

Abstract: Only three laryngeal transplants have been described in the literature to date, and none of the techniques has enabled a completely satisfactory functional result to be obtained. This article presents a new model of laryngeal transplantation, with quality of revascularisation of the transplant being the principal objective and optimisation of the various steps of the procedure, with the integration of a new reinnervation technique as a secondary objective. We present a preclinical animal study. Three pig larynges removed in vivo underwent allotransplantation according to the same protocol. The quality of the revascularisation was examined immediately after the surgery as well as by endoscopy for one animal on the fourth day after the operation. The mean time of cold ischaemia was 3 h 15 min. The anaesthetic tolerance of the pigs was excellent. Revascularisation was achieved and judged to be excellent for the three transplants immediately after the operation and the endoscopy performed for one pig on the fourth day after the operation confirmed this result. The anatomical similarities also enabled the application and integration of an innovative technique of laryngeal reinnervation into the various phases of the operation. We describe a reliable and reproducible animal model for laryngeal transplantation. Its application in humans can be envisaged.

Keywords: larynx; allotransplantation; model; preclinical; laryngeal transplantation; allograft

1. Introduction

Since the 1960s, much progress has been made in the field of organ transplantation, which enables transplants to be performed today in the treatment of handicaps; hand and face transplants, for example, enter into this field of application [1,2]. Despite this progress, there are scarce data concerning laryngeal transplantation and, to our knowledge, only few cases have been published in the English language literature [3,4].

The first larynx allotransplant dates to 1969 and was performed by Kluyskens on a patient who had had a total laryngectomy due to epidermoid carcinoma [5]. The patient no longer required tracheotomy and survived eight months until relapse of the carcinoma. This first surgery cannot really be considered as a vascularised allotransplant but more as a graft of allogenic tissue. There was no true vascular anastomosis, with the larynx only being "nursed". It was in 1998 that Strome [6] performed the first true larynx allotransplant, but the patient's tracheotomy tube was never removed, and the larynx had to be removed 14 years later due to chronic rejection of the graft [7]. The second published larynx allotransplant is more recent, but in this case as well the patient was still tracheotomised four years after the operation [8]. These positive results prove the feasibility of allotransplantation, but the procedure needs to be optimised to render it functional, as none of the three transplanted larynx has regained normal or subnormal mobility and the patients remained tracheotomised in the latter two cases.

The complexity of the vascularisation and innervation of this organ is responsible in part for the difficulties encountered in obtaining a reliable model for laryngeal transplantation.

Nevertheless, there is a unique and very interesting experiment that has passed completely unnoticed in the field of laryngeal transplantation, as it was only published indirectly: the article concerns the management of 13 larynx or trachea donors [9]. This Colombian team describe a reliable and reproducible model of laryngeal removal and transplantation that enables one of the major difficulties concerning the problem of vascularisation.

The second difficulty concerns the reinnervation of the larynx, and the Colombian model does not allow an intrinsic mobility of the larynx. We have therefore conceived of a model of laryngeal transplantation combining the Colombian model and the laryngeal reinnervation model described by J.P. Marie et al. in the rehabilitation of laryngeal diplegia [10].

Thus, herein, an animal model is presented, using pigs, the animal which presents the closest anatomical similarity with the human larynx.

2. Materials and Methods

Six female Land Race × Large White crossed pigs, 35 kg in weight, three months of age, were used for this study with the authorisation of the Animal Welfare Committee of Nantes Veterinary School pursuant to European Directive 86/609/EEC regarding the protection of animals used for experimental and other scientific purposes.

Three laryngeal allografts were carried out with a standardised anaesthetic protocol: premedication with midazolam (0.2 mg/kg i.m.), ketamine (5 mg/kg i.m.), and medetomidine (20 µg/kg i.m.); induction with propofol (6–8 mg/kg i.v.) and analgesia with morphine (1 mg/kg i.v.); CRI fentanyl 10 µg/kg/h + ketamine 0.5 mg/kg/h and meloxicam 0.4 mg/kg.

2.1. Removal of the Graft

After a U-shaped (bilateral curved) cervical incision, prolonged vertically along the presternal midline, the dissection started with bilateral identification of the vasculo-nervous elements: vagus and superior laryngeal nerves, the ligature of the internal jugular vein, as well as the internal carotid artery and the branches of the external carotid artery beyond the superior laryngeal artery.

Vascular dissection continued lower down, after sternotomy, until the ascending aorta and the superior vena cava were identified. The recurrent nerves were also dissected. The ascending aorta was then canulated and the piece perfused and flushed with organ perfusion and flushing solution (Custodiol®, Methapharm Inc, Brantford, ON, Canada). The transplant was then completely freed by performing the equivalent of a total circular pharyngolaryngectomy, including approximately 10 trachea rings and the entire visceral, vascular, and nervous axis in the piece (Figure 1).

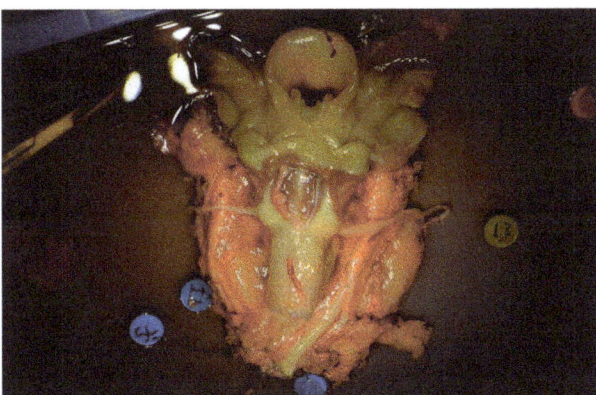

Figure 1. The transplant was completely harvested by performing the equivalent of a total circular pharyngolaryngectomy, including about 10 trachea rings and the entire visceral, vascular and nervous axis.

2.2. Preparation of the Graft

The graft was then prepared in ice for transplantation. First, the vessels were chosen with opening of the brachiocephalic arterial trunk so as to identify the origin of the common carotid arteries: the trunk was retained for 1 cm below the origin of the carotid arteries so as to be able to perform an arterial anastomosis of reasonable diameter. The technique was similar for the venous axes.

The infrahyoid muscles were then resected and the hypopharyngeal mucosa prepared: section of the oesophagus, respecting the recurrent nerves, then opening of the hypopharynx respecting the mucosa of the piriform sinuses as far as possible, were carried out. The retrocricoid mucosa was then partially resected so as to cover the arytenoids and the nervous graft on the posterior cricoarytenoid muscles.

The neurological step then began, with bilateral neurotisation of the posterior cricoarytenoid muscles using a Y-shaped graft of large auricular nerve taken from the donor (Figure 2).

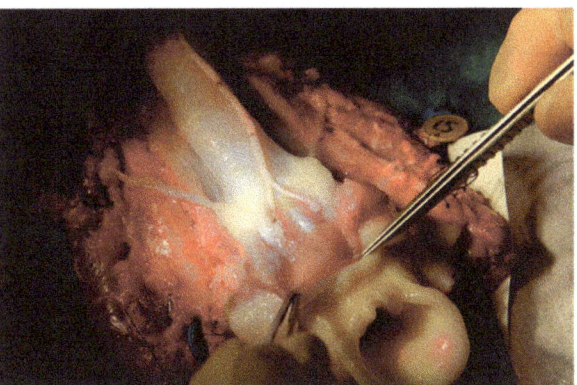

Figure 2. The neurological step with bilateral neurotisation of the posterior cricoarytenoid muscles using a Y-shaped graft of large auricular nerve taken from the donor.

2.3. Preparation of the Recipient

At the same time as the removal of the graft, the recipient animal was prepared for transplantation. The incision was midline at the cervical level: this was preferred to a

U-shaped incision that would lead to skin necrosis in an animal. The entire arterial and venous axes were bilaterally dissected.

During the neurological step, the hypoglossal nerve and its thyrohyoid branch, the vagus nerve, and the superior laryngeal nerve were identified. The phrenic nerve was dissected higher up so as to locate the roots and anastomoses with C5.

Once all the vascular nervous elements had been identified and marked, a total laryngectomy with preservation of the hyoid bone and as much laryngeal mucosa as possible was carried out.

2.4. Transplantation

The posterior face of the trachea was first fixed in order to correctly fix the transplant. Then lateral sutures of the mucosae were made. The vascular phase then began by adapting the technique to the anatomy of the pig, which is variable and different to that of the human. For this study, the anastomosis performed were: for the arteries, the brachiocephalic trunk (including the two common carotid arteries) terminolaterally with the left subclavicular artery of the recipient, and for the veins, on the right and on the left, the subclavicular vein terminoterminally with the external jugular vein of the recipient.

After reperfusion of the graft, the reinnervation step began. The superior laryngeal nerves of the donor and of the recipient were anastomosed, as was the Y-shaped nerve transplant with the left phrenic nerve of the recipient. Finally, the recurrent nerves of the donor were anastomosed with the thyroid branch of the hypoglossal nerve on the right and on the left (Figure 3).

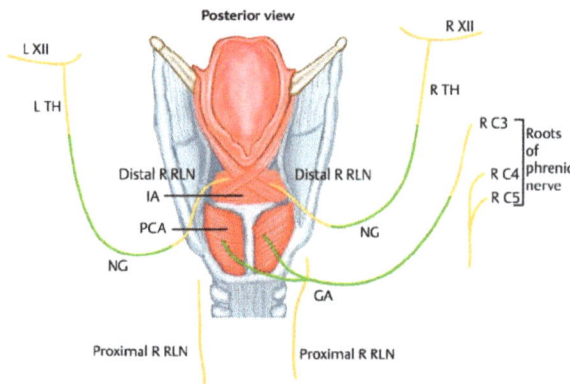

Figure 3. Reinnervation technique: R XII: right XII nerve; R TH: right thyro hyoid branch; NG: nerve graft; R RLN: right recurrent laryngeal nerve; PCA: posterior crico arytenoid muscle; IA: interarytenoid muscle.

The suture of the hypopharyngeal mucosa, the trachea, and an inferior tracheotomy were performed at the end.

2.5. Post-Operative Progress

The donor animals were euthanised once the removal had been carried out (pentobarbital sodium 364.4 g i.v.).

The first two recipient animals were monitored for a few hours to verify the revascularisation, and then euthanised.

The third recipient pig was kept in monitoring for four days, awake and with a tracheotomy tube. Pharyngolaryngeal endoscopy was performed immediately after the operation and on the fourth post-operative day.

An immunosuppressant protocol (tacrolimus 0.3 mg/kg/d and prednisolone 2 mg/kg/d) and prophylactic antibiotic treatment with amoxicillin/clavulanic acid and metronidazole were administered intravenously.

3. Results

The mean time of intervention, including removal, preparation of the recipient and of the graft and transplantation, was 10 h 30 min (minimum 9 h 30 min, maximum 11 h 40 min).

The cold ischaemia time (time between flushing and the start of anastomoses) of the graft was 2 h on average, and the warm ischaemia time (time between the start of vascular anastomoses and the clamping) was 1 h 5 min. Results are shown in Table 1.

Table 1. Operative time, ischemia times, tolerance and post-operative revascularisation assessment for the three transplantations.

	Transplantation 1	Transplantation 2	Transplantation 3	Mean Time
Operative time	570 min	620 min	700 min	630 min
Cold ischemia	140 min	115 min	105 min	120 min
Warm ischemia	60	65	70	65 min
Anesthesia tolerance	Excellent	Excellent	Excellent	
Post operative revascularisation assesment	none	none	Endoscopic at day 0 and day 4	

The tolerance of anaesthesia was excellent for the six pigs, both donors and recipients.

The different phases of the transplantation could be respected in all cases, and adaptation to the inter-individual anatomical variability did not constitute an obstacle. The transplantation protocol was correctly and reproducibly followed in the three operations.

Once the anastomoses had been carried out, the vessels were de-clamped and perfect in vivo revascularisation of the transplant could be observed after a few minutes (Figure 4).

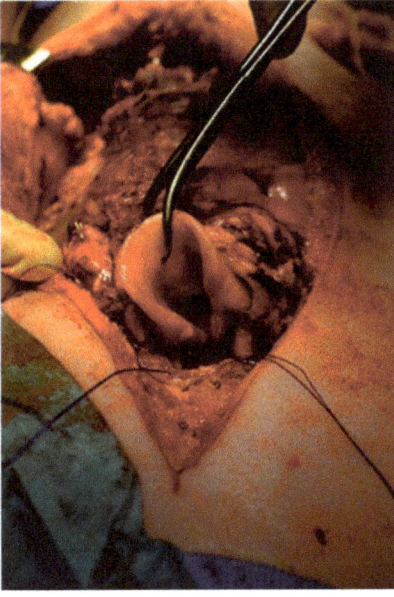

Figure 4. Once the anastomoses had been carried out, the vessels were de-clamped and perfect in vivo revascularisation of the transplant could be observed after a few minutes.

An endoscopy was immediately performed after the surgery in the third recipient animal and confirmed the correct revascularisation of the transplant (Figure 5).

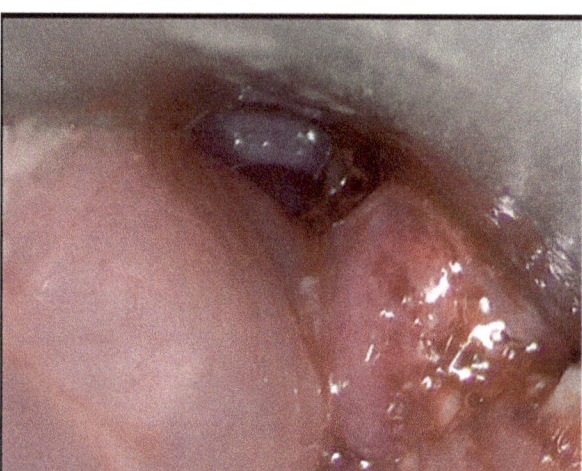

Figure 5. Endoscopy immediately performed after the surgery in the third recipient animal confirmed the correct revascularisation of the transplant.

The animal was monitored for four days with no significant problems. Endoscopy on the fourth day confirmed the viability of the transplant. The animal died on the fifth day after the operation, and the autopsy revealed massive mesenteric infarction.

4. Discussion

The complexity of the laryngeal vascularisation and innervation is probably one of the reasons explaining the small number of larynx transplants published to date. Furthermore, to our knowledge, there is no real description of larynx removal that would allow the results that have been published to date to be reproduced [4,6]. It seemed important to us to obtain a reproducible model of larynx transplant before undertaking a transplantation program in humans.

The pig model seemed the most appropriate to us; it has also been chosen in particular by Birchall et al., who also showed its reliability [11]. In comparison with the rat [12], the anatomical elements of the pig are closely comparable to those of humans, which also allows the reinnervation technique to be studied [13–15]. The dog has also been chosen, especially in the earliest work on allotransplantation, but the morbi-mortality of this model was high [16–18] and its current use in animal experimentation is limited for ethical reasons.

Furthermore, even if our objective was to evaluate the feasibility and reproducibility of the technique that we have developed, the good tolerance to immunosuppression in pigs allows immunological studies, as shown by studies for the transplantation of other organs, in particular bronchi and trachea [19,20].

In our experience, the choice of the pig as an animal model enables the transplantation model to be as close as possible to humans, thanks to the close anatomical similarities. The variations, particularly in the vascular network, did not hinder the revascularisation of the transplant, in part due to the single-block removal up to the ascending aorta and the vena cava. This animal model shows the feasibility and reproducibility, in terms of vascularisation, of this laryngeal removal and transplantation technique. We were able to obtain three transplanted vascularised larynges, to at one hour after the operation and the third at four days after the operation. Preferring large vessels for the vascular anastomoses enables a perfect viability of the transplant to be ensured.

The principal objective of this work was not concerned with the reinnervation because the first results, either in terms of reinnervation or respiration to be able to envisage removal of the tracheotomy tube, would only be visible after several months. This period seemed to us to be technically, ethically, and financially incompatible with keeping a transplanted and tracheotomised animal alive. Nevertheless, the anatomical similarities between the pig model and humans enabled us to carry out the nervous anastomoses, which is important in the progress of the different steps of a transplantation. This allowed us to model a complete transplantation in both vascular and neurological terms and so to precisely determine the order of the different operative steps.

This original technique of laryngeal reinnervation was inspired by the work of J.P. Marie et al. on laryngeal diplegia [21,22]. Marie et al. propose a neurotisation of the posterior cricoarytenoid muscles by a Y-shaped graft of the large auricular nerve. This graft is then unilaterally micro-anastomosed with the superior root of the phrenic nerve without significantly affecting diaphragm function and without respiratory impact. In this way, the dilator muscles of the glottis are stimulated on inhalation. At the same time the adductor muscles are re-innervated by the thyrohyoid branch of the hypoglossal nerve, for contraction on swallowing, in a bilateral fashion so as to avoid erroneous reinnervation of these adductor muscles by branches of the phrenic nerve. The identification of the thyrohyoid branch is difficult and requires a certain amount of practice.

This technique, which has shown its utility in the treatment of laryngeal diplegia [23], seems applicable to laryngeal transplantation in our model. It constitutes one of the innovative elements, compared to techniques previously described in the literature, aiming to obtain a functional larynx. This allows us to envisage the possibility of larynx transplant with a mobile larynx and patients without a tracheotomy tube, something which, to our knowledge, has never been carried out to date. The studies of reinnervation for bilateral recurrent paralysis have shown that the selective reinnervation via the phrenic nerve allows sufficient laryngeal opening to envisage the removal of the tracheotomy tube and even preservation of the quality of the voice [8]. This technique is therefore an alternative to the arytenoidopexy performed by the Colombian team (unpublished results).

5. Conclusions

With the technique of removal in a single block and anastomoses with large vessels, we can consider that this animal model of laryngeal transplantation is reliable and reproducible with regard to revascularisation. These results encourage us to continue this work in order to consider offering this technique to humans in the near future.

Author Contributions: Conceptualization, O.M., S.A., L.B., B.B., F.F., C.F., F.J., J.L.-S.-G., J.-P.M., A.R., S.V., P.C. and O.J.G.; data curation, O.J.G.; formal analysis, P.C.; funding acquisition, P.C.; investigation, P.P., O.M., S.A., L.B., B.B., F.F., C.F., F.J., J.L.-S.-G., J.-P.M., A.R., S.V., P.C. and O.J.G.; methodology, P.P., P.C. and O.J.G.; project administration, O.J.G.; resources, P.P.; supervision, P.C. and O.J.G.; validation, P.C.; writing—original draft, P.P.; writing—review & editing, P.P., O.M., S.A., L.B., B.B., F.F., C.F., F.J., J.L.-S.-G., J.-P.M., A.R., S.V. and P.C. All authors have read and agreed to the published version of the manuscript.

Funding: This research received no external funding.

Institutional Review Board Statement: Authorisation of the Animal Welfare Committee of Nantes Veterinary School pursuant to European Directive 86/609/EEC regarding the protection of animals used for experimental and other scientific purposes.

Conflicts of Interest: The authors declare no conflict of interest.

References

1. Petruzzo, P.; Testelin, S.; Kanitakis, J.; Badet, L.; Lengelé, B.; Girbon, J.P.; Parmentier, H.; Malcus, C.; Morelon, E.; Devauchelle, B.; et al. First human face transplantation: 5 years outcomes. *Transplantation* **2012**, *93*, 236–240. [CrossRef] [PubMed]
2. Dubernard, J.M.; Owen, E.; Herzberg, G.; Lanzetta, M.; Martin, X.; Kapila, H.; Dawahra, M.; Hakim, N.S. Human hand allograft: Report on first 6 months. *Lancet* **1999**, *353*, 1315–1320. [CrossRef]

3. Bewley, A.F.; Farwell, D.G. Laryngeal Transplantation. In *Advances in Oto-Rhino-Laryngology*; Karger: Basel, Switzerland, 2020; pp. 125–132.
4. Krishnan, G.; Du, C.; Fishman, J.M.; Foreman, A.; Lott, D.G.; Farwell, G.; Belafsky, P.; Krishnan, S.; Birchall, M.A. The current status of human laryngeal transplantation in 2017: A state of the field review. *Laryngoscope* 2017, *127*, 1861–1868. [CrossRef] [PubMed]
5. Kluyskens, P.; Boedts, D.; Dhont, G.; Weghe, J.P.V.; Vandenhove, P.; Van Clooster, R.; Bilo, F.; Ringoir, S.; Daneels, R. Preliminary note on the transplantation of larynx. *Acta Oto-Rhino-Laryngol. Belg.* 1969, *23*, 5–8.
6. Strome, M.; Stein, J.; Esclamado, R.; Hicks, D.; Lorenz, R.R.; Braun, W.; Yetman, R.; Eliachar, I.; Mayes, J. Laryngeal Transplantation and 40-Month Follow-up. *N. Engl. J. Med.* 2001, *344*, 1676–1679. [CrossRef]
7. Lorenz, R.R.; Strome, M. Total laryngeal transplant explanted: 14 years of lessons learned. *Otolaryngol. Head Neck Surg.* 2014, *150*, 509–511. [CrossRef]
8. Farwell, D.G.; Birchall, M.A.; Macchiarini, P.; Luu, Q.C.; De Mattos, A.M.; Gallay, B.J.; Perez, R.V.; Grow, M.P.; Ramsamooj, R.; Salgado, M.D.; et al. Laryngotracheal transplantation: Technical modifications and functional outcomes. *Laryngoscope* 2013, *123*, 2502–2508. [CrossRef]
9. Duque, E.; Duque, J.; Nieves, M.; Mejía, G.; López, B.; Tintinago, L. Management of larynx and trachea donors. *Transplant. Proc.* 2007, *39*, 2076–2078. [CrossRef]
10. Marina, M.B.; Marie, J.-P.; Birchall, M.A. Laryngeal reinnervation for bilateral vocal fold paralysis. *Curr. Opin. Otolaryngol. Head Neck Surg.* 2011, *19*, 434–438. [CrossRef]
11. Gorti, G.K.; Birchall, M.A.; Haverson, K.; Macchiarini, P.; Bailey, M. A preclinical model for laryngeal transplantation: Anatomy and mucosal immunology of the porcine larynx. *Transplantation* 1999, *68*, 1638–1642. [CrossRef]
12. Birchall, M.A.; Ayling, S.M.; Harley, R.; Murison, P.J.; Burt, R.; Mitchard, L.; Jones, A.; Macchiarini, P.; Stokes, C.R.; Bailey, M. Laryngeal transplantation in minipigs: Early immunological outcomes. *Clin. Exp. Immunol.* 2011, *167*, 556–564. [CrossRef] [PubMed]
13. Birchall, M.A.; Kingham, P.J.; Murison, P.J.; Ayling, S.M.; Burt, R.; Mitchard, L.; Jones, A.; Lear, P.; Stokes, C.R.; Terenghi, G.; et al. Laryngeal transplantation in minipigs: Vascular, myologic and functional outcomes. *Eur. Arch. Oto-Rhino-Laryngol.* 2011, *268*, 405–414. [CrossRef] [PubMed]
14. Strome, S.; Sloman-Moll, E.; Samonte, B.R.; Wu, J.; Strome, M. Rat model for a vascularized laryngeal allograft. *Ann. Otol. Rhinol. Laryngol.* 1992, *101*, 950–953. [CrossRef] [PubMed]
15. Knight, M.; Birchall, M. 29 A neuroanatomical study of the porcine larynx: Establishing a model for reinnervation studies. *J. Anat.* 2002, *201*, 425. [PubMed]
16. Stavroulaki, P.; Birchall, M. Comparative study of the laryngeal innervation in humans and animals employed in laryngeal transplantation research. *J. Laryngol. Otol.* 2001, *115*, 257–266. [CrossRef] [PubMed]
17. Mounier-Kuhn, P.; Haguenauer, J.P. Autotransplantation of the larynx in the dog. *Arch. Ital. Otol. Rinol. Laringol. Patol. Cervicofacc.* 1970, *81*, 341–352. [PubMed]
18. Anthony, J.P.; Allen, D.B.; Trabulsy, P.P.; Mahdavian, M.; Mathes, S.J. Canine laryngeal transplantation: Preliminary studies and a new heterotopic allotransplantation model. *Eur. Arch. Oto-Rhino-Laryngol.* 1995, *252*, 197–205. [CrossRef]
19. Macchiarini, P.; Lenot, B.; de Montpreville, V.; Dulmet, E.; Mazmanian, G.-M.; Fattal, M.; Guiard, F.; Chapelier, A.; Dartevelle, P. Heterotopic pig model for direct revascularization and venous drainage of tracheal allografts. *J. Thorac. Cardiovasc. Surg.* 1994, *108*, 1066–1075. [CrossRef]
20. Alessiani, M.; Spada, M.; Dionigi, P.; Arbustini, E.; Regazzi, M.; Fossati, G.S.; Zonta, A. Combined immunosuppressive therapy with tacrolimus and mycophenolate mofetil for small bowel transplantation in pigs. *Transplantation* 1996, *62*, 563–567. [CrossRef]
21. Marie, J.P.; Tardif, C.; Lerosey, Y.; Gibon, J.; Hellot, M.; Tadié, M.; Andrieu-Guitrancourt, J.; Dehesdin, D.; Pasquis, P. Selective resection of the phrenic nerve roots in rabbits: Part II: Respiratory effects. *Respir. Physiol.* 1997, *109*, 139–148. [CrossRef]
22. Marie, J.-P.; Lacoume, Y.; Laquerrière, A.; Tardif, C.; Fallu, J.; Bonmarchand, G.; Vérin, E. Diaphragmatic effects of selective resection of the upper phrenic nerve root in dogs. *Respir. Physiol. Neurobiol.* 2006, *154*, 419–430. [CrossRef] [PubMed]
23. Marie, J.-P. Reinnervation, new frontiers. *Diagn. Treat. Voice Disord.* 2014, *4*, 855–870.

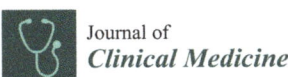

Review

Narrative Review of Classification Systems Describing Laryngeal Vascularity Using Advanced Endoscopic Imaging

Peter Kántor [1,2,*], Lucia Staníková [1,2], Anna Švejdová [3], Karol Zeleník [1,2] and Pavel Komínek [1,2]

1. Department of Otorhinolaryngology and Head and Neck Surgery, University Hospital Ostrava, 708 52 Ostrava, Czech Republic
2. Department of Craniofacial Surgery, Faculty of Medicine, University of Ostrava, 701 03 Ostrava, Czech Republic
3. Department of Otorhinolaryngology and Head and Neck Surgery, University Hospital Hradec Králové, Faculty of Medicine in Hradec Králové, Charles University, 500 03 Hradec Králové, Czech Republic
* Correspondence: peter.kantor@fno.cz; Tel.: +420-722-437-109

Abstract: Endoscopic methods are critical in the early diagnosis of mucosal lesions of the head and neck. In recent years, new examination methods and classification systems have been developed and introduced into clinical practice. All of these new techniques target the notion of optical biopsy, which tries to assess the nature of the lesion before histology examination. Many methods suffer from interpretation issues due to subjective interpretation of the findings. Therefore, multiple classification systems have been developed to assist the proper interpretation of mucosal findings and reduce the error rate. They provide various perspectives on the assessment and interpretation of mucosa changes. This article provides a comprehensive and critical view of the available classification systems as well as their advantages and disadvantages.

Keywords: enhanced contact endoscopy; narrow-band imaging; Storz Professional Image Enhancement System; leukoplakia; larynx; laryngeal cancer

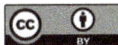

1. Introduction

Endoscopy of the upper aerodigestive tract has become a common practice in otolaryngology and remains an inseparable part of in-office diagnostics of head and neck cancer. Nowadays, laryngeal squamous cell carcinoma is the most common form of head and neck cancer [1]. Unfortunately, the mucosal changes caused by a malignant tumor in the early stages are usually small and similar to non-neoplastic lesions. Therefore, differentiating between neoplastic and non-neoplastic tissue changes remains a diagnostic challenge even for experienced clinicians. Moreover, every surgical intervention in the larynx may lead to the deterioration of the voice after surgery due to the scarring of the vocal cords [2]. If a malignant tumor is present, then a resection margin of the healthy tissue is often required to successfully remove the lesion [3]. Therefore, advanced endoscopy methods are needed to identify patients who can be treated with less aggressive surgery or who can even be managed without surgical intervention. Attempting to differentiate between malignant and benign changes with naked eye or regular white light endoscopy is very difficult and histology examination remains the gold standard for the identification of cancerous changes [4]. Thus, many new endoscopy techniques have been developed. These techniques strive towards the concept of pre-histology diagnosis, which tries to determine the lesion histology before the biopsy.

Most methods try to utilize metabolic or morphological tissue changes induced by the lesion. The most popular methods are Narrow Band Imaging® (NBI, Olympus, Tokyo, Japan) or IMAGE 1S® (Karl Storz, Tuttingen, Germany). These methods utilize morphological changes of mucosa vascularization. Changes are caused by the capability of malignant tumors to induce neoangiogenesis. When the tumor is very small, nutrients are supplied to it by simple diffusion from the surrounding extracellular fluid [5]. If the tumor continues to grow, then diffusion becomes insufficient in providing enough nutrients for further cell growth; the tumor thus begins to experience ischemia [5]. Tissue ischemia triggers neoangiogenesis growth factors such as vascular endothelial growth factor (VEGF) [5]. When VEGF comes into contact with endothelial cells, it triggers a signaling cascade initiating the process of neoangiogenesis [5]. The result of this process is the formation of pathological vascularization [5].

Advanced endoscopy imaging methods enhance mucosa vascularization. According to these changes, we can determine with a certain probability if the observed lesion is benign or malignant. A meta-analysis performed by Zhui et al. pooled 25 studies and reported a sensitivity of 88.5% and a specificity 95.6% [6]. Unfortunately, interpretations of the results of the examinations are subjective and therefore may be prone to interpretation errors. One of the possibilities to achieve relative objectivity is to use a classification system. Multiple classification systems have been developed and can be used to determine the character of the laryngeal lesions. They provide interpretation guidelines, which are very useful for the proper assessment of the lesion character. Unfortunately, these classification systems are not uniform, and each has advantages and drawbacks. Thus, the aim of the paper is to provide a complex and critical overview of available classification systems for mucosal laryngeal lesions.

2. Materials and Methods

PubMed, the Cochrane Library, and Google Scholar databases were searched using the term "endoscopy", "head and neck cancer", "larynx", and "classification" to identify articles published on the topic within the period 2000–2022. The search was conducted by two independent authors during November 2022. All articles were reviewed and only those written in the English language, dealing with adult patients, and describing a classification system of laryngeal lesions were retained for analysis. All duplicates were removed. Identification of the relevant studies was conducted according to the PRISMA guidelines. The selection process of relevant articles can be seen on the Preferred Reporting Items for Systematic Reviews and Meta-Analyses (PRISMA) flow diagram (Figure 1) [7].

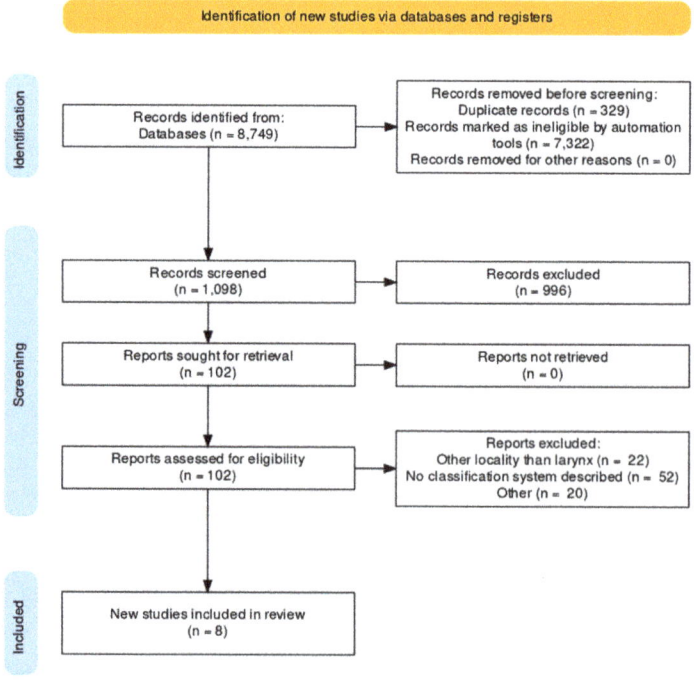

Figure 1. PRISMA flow diagram of the selection process of the relevant articles.

3. Results

3.1. Current Classification Systems Used in the Description of Laryngeal Mucosal Vascularization

- **Classification according to Ni et al. (2011) [2]**

The first available classification system was described by Ni et al. This classification is widely used by many ENT clinicians and was originally designed to be used with the NBI technology. This classification can be used with other technologies such as IMAGE 1S (Karl Storz) with similar results [3].

This system classifies endoscopy findings according to the changes of intrapapillary capillary loops (IPCLs) into five categories [2]. Lesions in category I–IV are considered to be benign (Figure 2) [2]. Category V lesions are considered malignant lesions and are divided into three subcategories: Va, Vb, and Vc (Figure 3) [2]. Ni et al. reported a cancer lesion detection sensitivity of 88.9% and a specificity of 93.2% [2]. Many subsequent studies and meta-analyses have confirmed the diagnostic value of this classification system [4–6,8]. The overview of this classification can be seen in Table 1.

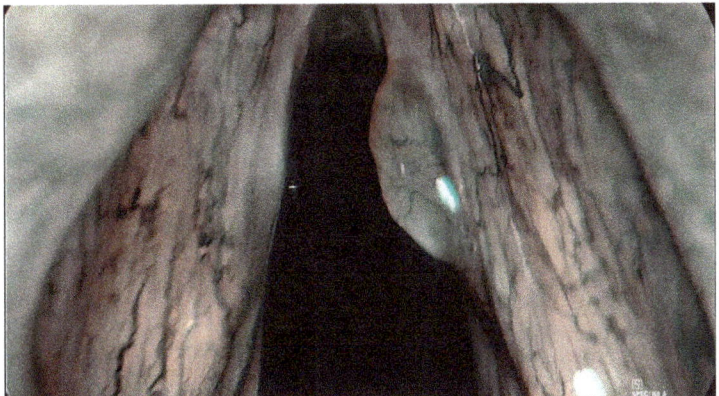

Figure 2. Histologically verified polyp of the right vocal cord, Ni type II of the mucosal vascularization, ELS classification—longitudinal type of vascularization.

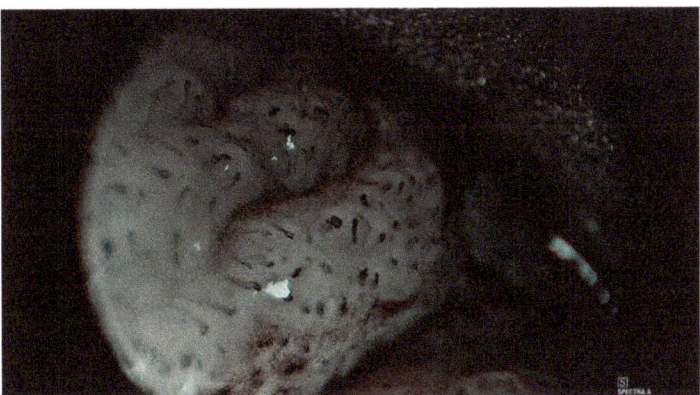

Figure 3. Histologically verified supraglottic squamous cell carcinoma. Ni type Vb of the mucosal vascularization, ELS classification—perpendicular type of vascularization.

Table 1. Narrow-band imaging endoscopic classification of the laryngeal lesions according to Ni et al. (2011) [2].

Endoscopic Pattern	Morphology of Vessels	IPCLs
Type I	Small, oblique, and arborescent	Not visible
Type II	Enlarged, oblique, and arborescent	Not visible
Type III	Obscured or seen indistinctly by white mucosa	Not visible
Type IV	Oblique and arborescent vessels not visible	Small and dark brown spots
Type Va	Oblique and arborescent vessels not visible	Dilated, solid, or hollow, with a brownish, speckled pattern, and various shapes
Type Vb	Oblique and arborescent vessels not visible	Tortuous, irregular, with a snake, earthworm, tadpole, or branch-like shapes
Type Vc	Oblique and arborescent vessels not visible	Tortuous or brownish speckles with irregular distribution

Abbreviation: IPCLs—intrapapillary capillary loops.

- **Classification proposed by the European Laryngological Society (2016) [9]**

  This classification system was published by Arens et al. in 2016 [9]. It separates lesions according to their vascular architecture into two categories: longitudinal or perpendicular [9]. Longitudinal vascularization passes parallel to the mucosa and is associated with benign lesions (Figure 2) [9]. Perpendicular vascularization runs upright in the mucosa and is interpreted as suspicious (Figure 3) [9]. Perpendicular vascularization is specific for papilloma, high-grade dysplastic lesions, carcinoma in situ, and invasive carcinoma [9].

  The high diagnostic yield of the classification has been confirmed by other authors [10,11]. Šifrer et al. studied 104 patients and described perpendicular vascularization in only 9.3% of benign lesions [10]. Histologically verified papillomatosis and malignant lesions showed perpendicular vascularization in 96.2% of subjects [10]. Table 2 overviews this classification.

Table 2. Classification according to the European Laryngological Society by Arens et al. (2016) [9].

Endoscopic Pattern	Morphology of Vessels	
Longitudinal vascular changes	Ectasia	Dilated vessels
	Meander	Meandering, tortuous vessels
	Varicose	Advanced meandering and dilated vessels
	Convolute	Organized coil/tangle of vessels
	Number of vessels	Increased vessels number
	Branches of vessels	Increased branches of vessels
	Change of direction	Abrupt change of vessels direction
Perpendicular vascular changes	Enlarged vessel loops	Abnormal IPCLs with wide-angled turning points
	Dot-like vessel loops	Abnormal IPCLs with narrow-angled turning points
	A Worm-like vessels	Abnormal vessels with spiral morphology and bizarre course

Abbreviation: IPCLs—intraepithelial capillary loops.

- **Classification according to Puxxedu et al. (2016) [12]**

  This classification system was designed exclusively for enhanced contact endoscopy [12]. This technology combines enhanced endoscopy imaging (such as NBI or IMAGE 1S) and a special magnifying endoscope with a magnification up to 150x. Magnification of the observed tissue allows precise description of the changes in vascular microarchitecture. This technology is suitable only for use under general anesthesia due to the lack of flexible magnifying endoscopes.

  The classification separates mucosal findings into types 0-IV, where 0 means normal mucosa, type I is interpreted as an inflammatory lesion, and type II is hyperplasia or papillomatosis if the capillary loop is encased by mucosal papilloma (Figure 4) [12]. Type III implies mild to moderate dysplasia [12]. Type IV should be interpreted as either high-grade dysplasia, carcinoma in situ, or invasive carcinoma (Figure 5) [12]. The results provided by Puxxedu et al. are promising and suggest that the sensitivity and specificity of the method in differentiating normal tissue vs. histological alterations is 100% [12]. The same sensitivity and specificity were achieved for differentiation of normal and inflammatory lesions vs. invasive carcinoma [12]. To differentiate between normal tissue and hyperplasia vs. dysplasia and invasive carcinoma, Puxxedu found a sensitivity and specificity of 97.6% [12]. We could not find other studies that confirm or contradict the results of this study. The overview of this classification can be seen in Table 3.

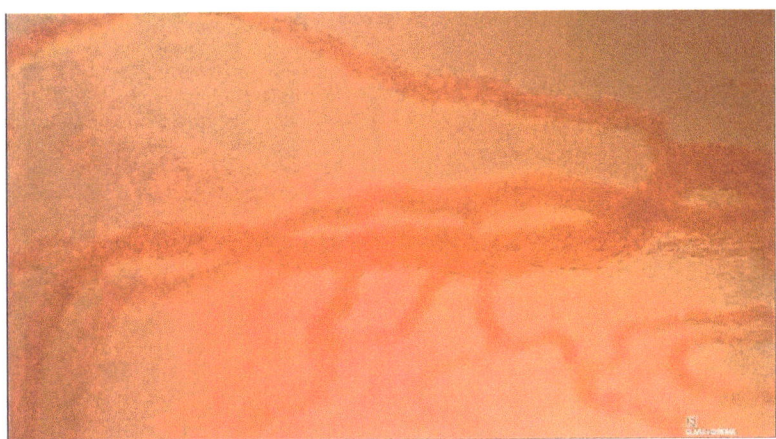

Figure 4. Histologically verified polyp of the left vocal cord. Puxxedu classification type I.

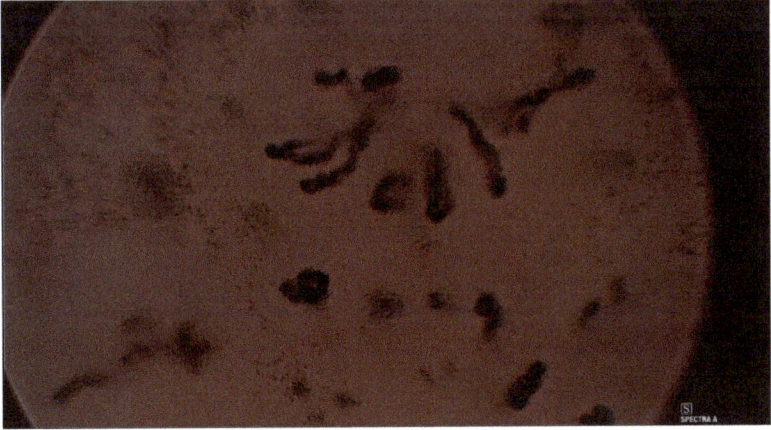

Figure 5. Histologically verified supraglottic squamous cell carcinoma. Puxxedu classification type IV.

Table 3. Classification according to Puxxedu et al. (2016) [12].

Vascular Pattern	Diagnosis	Description
Type 0	Normal mucosa	Thin-end regular subepithelial vessels connecting with a thicker and deeper arborescent vascular network running parallel to the epithelium.
Type I	Inflammation	The subepithelial vessels are increased in number and size with irregular and sometimes crossing directions.
Type II	Hyperplasia	Intra-CLs are visible running toward the surface when the hyperplasia is at the initial stage. In this phase, CLs are generally still very thin and short, arising from the underlying inflammatory vasculature with a scattered distribution. In the case of mature hyperplasia, the deeper inflammatory vascular network is not visible, and only the elongated CLs can be easily seen. In the case of vegetating keratosis, the deeper inflammatory vascular network is often not visible, and the elongated CLs are difficult to see. A particular type of "bobby-pin" can be seen in laryngeal papillomatosis. The typical papilla encases the "bobby-pin" inside the papilloma.
Type III	Mild–moderate dysplasia	Vascular changes become progressively more consistent with elongated small vessels in the typical "bobby-pin" shape, but some arborescence appears at the end of the CLs.
Type IV	High-grade dysplasia/carcinoma in situ/invasive carcinoma	The vascularity of the chorion is more evident and CLs appear significantly dilated with various shapes and a wide range of vascular architectural changes such as corkscrews or tree-like patterns.

Abbreviation: CLs—capillary loops.

3.2. Classification Systems Used in Examination of Leukoplakia

Leukoplakia represents a specific diagnostic and therapeutic problem, and thus particular classification systems for describing this distinct pathology have been developed. Leukoplakia is a descriptive term used to name white patch-like lesions present on the mucosa [13]. Leukoplakia of the larynx can be mostly observed on the vocal cords. It is caused by extensive irritation of the laryngeal mucosa by alcohol, smoking, voice overuse, or laryngopharyngeal reflux [13]. The irritation causes formation of a keratin layer. Another cause of laryngeal leukoplakia is the use of inhalation corticosteroids [14]. Even though the term leukoplakia has been used for decades, it is descriptive but not clinically useful because it does not provide the risk stratification of the lesion. Histologically, the lesions can vary from hyperkeratosis to invasive cancer [15]. Therefore, early identification of the character of the lesion is crucial for a good prognosis and outcome of the treatment.

The pre-histological diagnosis of leukoplakia is difficult. Even though as much as 50% of the samples return as non-dysplastic lesions from the histopathology exam, a diagnosis of invasive cancer is made in 6–22% of the samples [16–18]. Therefore, lesion biopsy under general anesthesia remains common practice.

A few classification systems have been developed, and some of them can be used with white light endoscopy while others require enhanced imagining such as NBI. However, the proper NBI examination is difficult and sometimes impossible due to the "umbrella effect" [13]. This phenomenon causes the reflection of the light emitted from the light source. Therefore, the emitted light does not reach the IPCLs in the mucosa, which limits examination [13]. Nevertheless, vascularization around the leukoplakia can be observed and can yield important information about the observed lesion. It can be classified according to one of the available classifications. According to multiple authors, changes in the vascular architecture surrounding the primary lesion yield valuable information about the features of the lesion [13,19]. Stanikova et al. reported that perpendicular vascularization surrounding the leukoplakia was associated with malignant lesions (carcinoma in situ or invasive carcinoma). This was histologically confirmed in 84.6% of cases [19]. Leukoplakia surrounded by longitudinal type of vascularization was histologically benign (hyperkeratosis or low-grade dysplasia) in 83.8% of cases [19]. The authors also suggest that leukoplakia with favorable surrounding findings in NBI endoscopy can be followed conservatively without surgical intervention [19].

- **Clinical scoring of leukoplakia according to Young et al. (2014) [20]**

Young et al. proposed a scoring system of vocal cord leukoplakia based on their macroscopical appearance during white light endoscopy [20]. His classification stratifies leukoplakia by seven macroscopical features: color, texture, size, hyperemia, thickness, symmetry, and oedema [20]. Color, texture, size, and hyperemia significantly correlated with final histopathology and therefore were proposed as one of the possible ways to select high-risk patients. Interrater reliability of the classification was found to be from 68 to 79% [20]. Lesions with lower scores had very high probability to be less aggressive and should be managed conservatively [20]. Unfortunately, the study did not provide an optimal cut-off point that could be used to differentiate between low-risk and high-risk lesions. The overview of this classification can be seen in Table 4.

Table 4. Clinical scoring of leukoplakia according to Young et al. (2014) [20].

Factors	Categories	Score	Definitions of the Vocal Cord Leukoplakia
Color	Homogenous	0	The color is distributed evenly.
	Non-homogeneous	1	The color is not distributed evenly.
Texture	Regular	0	The surface is smooth and flat.
	Irregular	1	The surface showed granular appearance.
Size	Small	0	The sum of all vocal cord leukoplakia is less than half a length of one true vocal cord.
	Large	1	The sum of all vocal cord leukoplakia exceeds half a length of one true vocal cord.
Hyperemia	Absence	0	The vocal cord leukoplakia is without peripheral erythema or increased vascularity.
	Presence	1	The vocal cord leukoplakia is associated with peripheral erythema or increased vascularity.
Thickness	Thin	0	The lesion is thin and blood vessels beneath the lesion are visible.
	Thick	1	The lesion is thick and blood vessels beneath the lesion are invisible.
Symmetry	Symmetric	0	Lesions are distributed at similar sites of bilateral vocal cords.
	Asymmetric	1	Lesions are located at one or unopposed sites.
Edema	Exist	0	Existence of vocal edema.
	Absence	1	Absence of vocal edema.

- **Clinical scoring of leukoplakia by Fang et al. (2016) [21]**

Fang et al. continued the previous research and removed one of the criteria (edema) from the Young et al. scoring system. Therefore, a six-tier system was established. Observed morphological features of the leukoplakia were useful in differentiation between malignant and benign lesions [21]. The morphological features were color, texture, size, hyperemia, thickness, and symmetry. The scoring system achieved good sensitivity (80.4%) and specificity (81.5%) with good interrater reliability [21]. Unfortunately, this study did not provide a specific cut-off that could be used to differentiate between benign and malignant lesion. Rather, the authors advised clinicians to set the cut-off point for each institution individually [21]. The overview of this classification can be seen in Table 5.

Table 5. Clinical scoring of leukoplakia according to Fang et al. (2016) [21].

	Factors	Score	Definitions
Color	Homogenous	0	The color of vocal cord leukoplakia is distributed evenly.
	Heterogeneous	1	The color of vocal cord leukoplakia is not distributed evenly.
Texture	Regular	0	The surface of vocal cord leukoplakia is smooth and flat.
	Irregular	1	The surface of vocal cord leukoplakia showed granular appearance.
Size	Small	0	The sum of all vocal cord leukoplakia is less than half length of one true vocal cord.
	Large	1	The sum of all vocal cord leukoplakia exceeds the half length of one true vocal cord.
Hyperemia	Absence	0	The vocal cord leukoplakia is without peripheral erythema or increased vascularity.
	Presence	1	The vocal cord leukoplakia is associated with peripheral erythema or increased vascularity.
Thickness	Thin	0	The lesion is thin and blood vessels beneath the lesion are visible.
	Thick	1	The lesion is thick and blood vessels beneath the lesion are invisible.
Symmetry	Symmetric	0	Lesions are distributed at similar sites of the bilateral cords.
	Asymmetric	1	Lesions are located at one or unopposed sites.

- **Laryngoscopic classification of vocal cord leukoplakia by Zhang et al. (2017)** [17]

Zhang et al. tried to simplify classifications mentioned before by stratifying vocal cord leukoplakia into three subtypes: type I—flat and smooth; type II—bulged and smooth; and type III—bulged and rough [17]. According to the results, type I is mostly histologically interpreted as keratinization or hyperplasia without dysplastic changes (Figure 6) [17]. In type II, the dominant histology was mild to moderate dysplasia [17]. Type III presented the highest incidence of cancerous lesion (carcinoma in situ or invasive carcinoma), while incidence of non-cancerous lesions (keratosis or hyperplasia) was the lowest from all types (Figure 7) [17]. The authors further proposed conservative treatment in type I leukoplakia and surgical resection in type III leukoplakia [17]. Type II remains a grey zone, but the authors stated that leukoplakia in this stage is irreversible and may contain moderate or severe dysplasia [17]. The overview of this classification can be seen in Table 6.

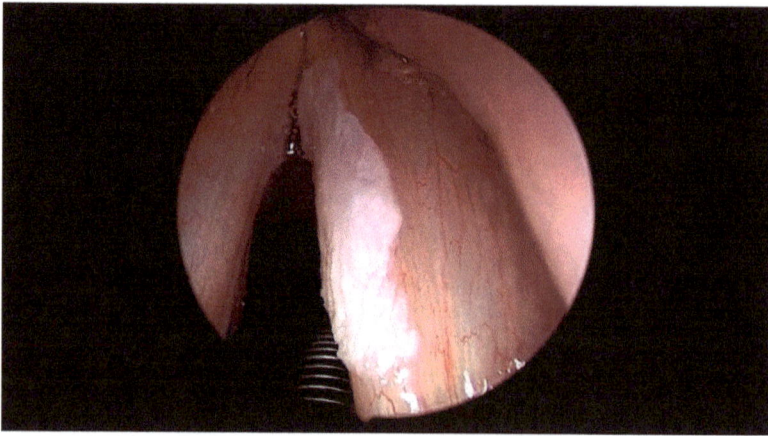

Figure 6. Histologically-verified parakeratosis of the right vocal cord presenting as leukoplakia. Young scoring system—3 points, Fang scoring system—3 points, Zhang type I—flat and smooth.

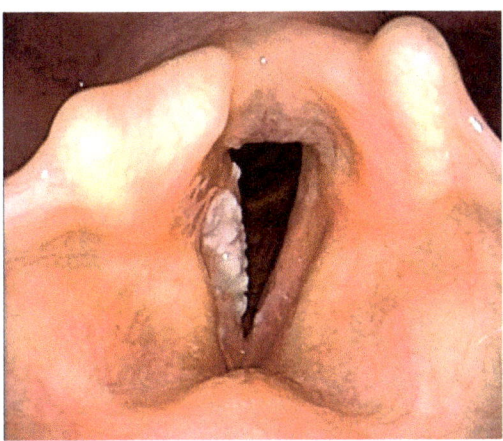

Figure 7. Histologically-verified squamous cell carcinoma of the right vocal cord presenting as leukoplakia. Young scoring system—5 points, Fang scoring system—5 points, Zhang type III—bulge and rough.

Table 6. Laryngoscopic classification of vocal cord leukoplakia by Zhang et al. (2017) [17].

Type of Lesion		Description
Type I	flat and smooth	Localized white plaque lesion having a uniform thin smooth homogeneous surface or white patch is raised slightly, but the edge of the white patch is continuous with the surrounding mucosa.
Type II	bulge and smooth	White plaque lesion is homogeneous and significantly bulged with a constant texture throughout. It is higher than the mucosa around the plaque. The edge of the white patch is discontinuous with the surrounding mucosa.
Type III	bulge and rough	Grayish-white, nodular, verrucous, granular, non-homogeneous, and (or) exophytic lesions with irregular blunt or sharp projections. They have an irregular surface associated with erosion or ulceration that is higher than the mucosa around the plaque.

A similar classification system was also proposed by Chen et al. [22]. This classification also used a three-tier classification system with similar categories: flat and smooth, elevated and smooth, and rough leukoplakia [22]. This study included 375 patients treated for vocal cord leukoplakia and confirmed that the morphology of the leukoplakia correlates significantly with the final histology examination [22].

- **Narrow-Band Imaging endoscopic classification of laryngeal leukoplakia according to Ni et al. (2019) [23]**

Attempts to introduce advanced endoscopic methods used the modified Ni et al. classification. This classification stratifies leukoplakia into six types. Types 1–3 indicate benign leukoplakia (Figure 8) and types 4–6 suggest possibility of malignancy (Figure 9) [23]. The accuracy of the classification in judging the pathological nature of the leukoplakia was 90.8% [23]. The overview of this classification can be seen in Table 7.

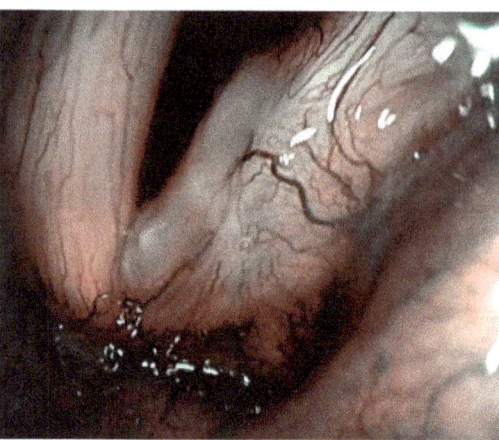

Figure 8. Histologically-verified low-grade dysplasia presenting as leukoplakia of the left vocal cord. Ni classification of laryngeal leukoplakia—type I.

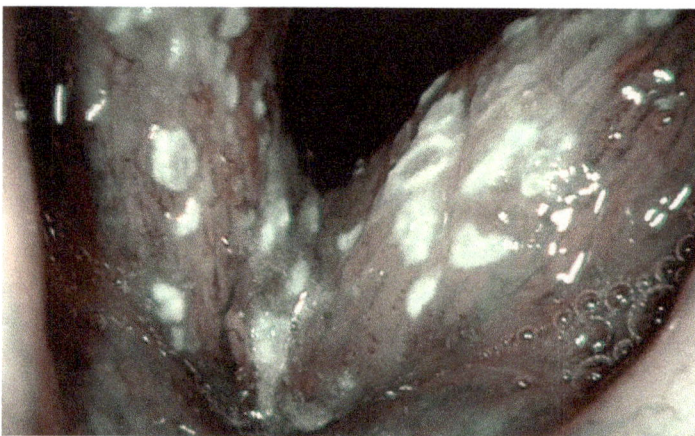

Figure 9. Histologically-verified squamous cell carcinoma presenting as leukoplakia of both vocal cords. IPCLs can be seen around leukoplakia. Ni classification of laryngeal leukoplakia—type III–IV.

An examination that can provide additional information about the lesion is laryngeal videostroboscopy. According to Rzepakowska et al., non-invasive leukoplakia (parakeratosis, low-grade dysplasia, etc.) tends to preserve the mucosal wave of the vocal cord [24]. On the other hand, the mucosal wave tends to diminish in the case of an invasive form of leukoplakia (high-grade dysplasia, invasive carcinoma, etc.) [24]. As stated by El-Demerdash, the overall accuracy of laryngeal videostroboscopy versus histology was 95% [25]. Those results were further confirmed by studies by other authors [25–27].

Table 7. Narrow-band imaging endoscopic classification of laryngeal leukoplakia according to Ni et al. (2019) [23].

Type	Interpretation	Description
Type I	Benign leukoplakia	There are no IPCLs but white plaque can be observed on the vocal cord with obliquely running vessels and branching vessels indistinctly present under the white plaque.
Type II	Benign leukoplakia	There are white patches on the vocal cord but neither IPCLs nor obliquely running vessels or branching vessels can be found.
Type III	Benign leukoplakia	IPCLs can be seen at the surface of the vocal cord mucosa where the epithelium is not covered by the leukoplakia, thus showing small brown spots with a relatively regular arrangement without clear boundaries. No obliquely running vessels or branching vessel were seen.
Type IV	Malignant leukoplakia	IPCLs can be observed on the vocal cord, showing large brown spots embedded at the surface of white plaque.
Type V	Malignant leukoplakia	IPCLs on the vocal cord can be seen with large brown spots that appear at the surface of the vocal cord mucosa outside the leukoplakia with obvious boundaries.
Type VI	Malignant leukoplakia	IPCLs are visible at the surface of the vocal cord and are characterized by large brown spots or twisted earthworm-like vessels distributed at the surface of the leukoplakia as well as on the surface of the vocal cord epithelium outside the leukoplakia.

Abbreviation: IPCLs—intrapapillary capillary loops.

4. Discussion

Every classification system carries certain advantages and disadvantages. One of the major advantages of ELS classification is its simplicity. This two-stage system allows the examinator to classify mucosal vasculature findings as either perpendicular or longitudinal. Mehlum et al. found low interrater variability and suitability of the classification for inexperienced examiners [28]. A major disadvantage of this system is that it does not try to specify what the lesion is histologically according to endoscopy findings. The question is if specification of the histology of the lesion pre-operatively is required.

Ni classification provides ample information about the nature of the lesion. It also tries to state its histological character according to endoscopy findings. Unfortunately, the Ni classification has a few disadvantages. The major problem is the blurry cut-off line between malignant and benign lesions. According to the classification, Ni IV IPCLs have the appearance of small and dark brown spots, and should be interpreted as benign lesions [2]. Unfortunately, this appearance of IPCLs would be interpreted as perpendicular and therefore suspect according to ELS classification [9]. Therefore, a study determining whether Ni IV should be interpreted as a benign or suspect lesion is required. Another problem that affects multiple classification systems is the use of the old classification of laryngeal dysplasia. The terms "mild", "moderate", and "severe dysplasia" should no longer be used according to the new World Health Organization (WHO) revision of laryngeal dysplasia terms [29]. These terms should be replaced and reclassified to low-grade dysplasia and high-grade dysplasia according to the WHO [29].

The Puxxedu classification for ECE yields interesting data—it provides histological specifications of the examined lesion, and very high sensitivity and specificity are stated in the original work. Unfortunately, the sensitivity and specificity are calculated in a sub-optimal way in the original paper. Puxxedu stated his sensitivity and specificity rates according to healthy tissue vs. malignant tumors or inflammation changes vs malignant tumors [12]. These changes are usually very well pronounced and easy to differentiate even without ECE; therefore, the results may be biased. A study that compares sensitivity and specificity calculated according to the Puxxedu classification vs. final histology examination is therefore required. Also, the Puxxedu classification still uses the old classification of laryngeal dysplasia and should be modified to fit the new WHO recommendations.

Moreover, the situation is even more difficult if the patient has undergone radiotherapy. The vasculature is influenced by radiation and it is difficult to interpret vascular character properly. This makes differentiating between recurrence of the malignant tumors and post-radiation changes very difficult. The experience of the examiner comes into play more significantly. On the other hand, according to Zabrodsky et al., NBI is a good tool for follow-up of patients after radiotherapy for laryngeal and hypopharyngeal cancer with sensitivity of 92%, specificity of 76%, and overall accuracy of 88% [30].

Management of vocal cord leukoplakia remains a challenging topic in modern otolaryngology. Biopsy under general anesthesia and histological verification of the leukoplakia remains a common practice. Fortunately, clinicians have started to stratify the risk of malignancy of the leukoplakia using various classification systems as mentioned above to properly assess the risk of malignancy. A management algorithm combining the morphology of the leukoplakia, laryngeal videostroboscopy, and assessment of IPCLs around the lesion should be used to assess the risk of malignancy. If it remains low, then conservative treatment is suggested by some authors [19,20,22,31,32]. However, when managing the leukoplakia conservatively, clinicians should be very cautious and in case of any doubt examination under general anesthesia with histology examination of the leukoplakia should be performed.

Isenberg et al. provided a systematic review of 2188 biopsies of leukoplakia and showed that mild to moderate dysplasia was found in 33.5% of cases, and high-grade dysplasia or carcinoma in situ was found in 15.2% of cases [16]. According to Weller et al., laryngeal dysplasia carries a significant risk of malignant transformation [33]. The risk triples with increasing severity of dysplasia [33]. Therefore, clinicians should be aware of the possibility of malignant transformation of the vocal cord leukoplakia and patients should be tightly observed. Early discharge of patients with vocal cord leukoplakia should not be a common practice.

Unfortunately, we are still far from the concept of optical biopsy and pre-histology diagnosis. None of the advanced endoscopy methods can overcome histological verification of the lesion. The important point is that examinators should not assess laryngeal lesions solely according to their vasculature changes, appearance, or preservation of the mucosa wave. All available examinations should be performed to gather as much information as possible. Only complex and detailed examination allows the highest accuracy and diagnostic yield.

The future in differential diagnosis of laryngeal lesions is probably artificial intelligence (AI) and machine learning. These systems will probably be able to eliminate the problems with the subjective evaluation of the mentioned endoscopic classifications. Żurek et al. analyzed 11 studies that used AI in the early diagnosis of laryngeal lesions. Although various AI models were used, the overall accuracy was very high—from 80.6% to 99.7% [34]. The pooled sensitivity and specificity for differentiation between benign and malignant lesions were also very high: 91% and 94%, respectively [34].

5. Conclusions

ENT endoscopy remains a rapidly evolving and dynamic field of medicine, but the concept of optical biopsy and pre-histology diagnosis remains a challenging problem. The available classification systems provide very good sensitivity and specificity. However, the non-coherence of the classification systems remains an issue, and therefore a unified classification system is needed. Further research is needed to determine whether the Ni IV should be interpreted as a benign or a suspicious lesion. Also, research on the field of leukoplakia risk assessment is required. Artificial intelligence will probably be a valuable assistant in laryngeal examination in the future.

Author Contributions: Conceptualization, P.K. (Peter Kántor) and A.Š.; methodology, L.S.; validation, K.Z. and P.K. (Pavel Komínek); formal analysis, L.S.; investigation, P.K. (Peter Kántor); resources, L.S.; data curation, A.Š.; writing—original draft preparation, P.K. (Peter Kántor); writing—review and editing, L.S., K.Z. and P.K. (Pavel Komínek); supervision, P.K. (Pavel Komínek); project administration, K.Z.; funding acquisition, P.K. (Peter Kántor). All authors have read and agreed to the published version of the manuscript.

Funding: This research was funded by University of Ostrava, grant number SGS08/LF/2022.

Institutional Review Board Statement: The study was conducted in accordance with the Declaration of Helsinki, and approved by the Ethics Committee of University hospital Ostrava (protocol code 08/LF/2022, date of approval 31 March 2022) for studies involving humans.

Informed Consent Statement: Patient consent was waived due to the review nature of the study.

Data Availability Statement: Data sharing not applicable.

Conflicts of Interest: The authors declare no conflict of interest.

References

1. Tsetsos, N.; Poutoglidis, A.; Vlachtsis, K.; Stavrakas, M.; Nikolaou, A.; Fyrmpas, G. Twenty-Year Experience with Salvage Total Laryngectomy: Lessons Learned. *J. Laryngol. Otol.* **2021**, *135*, 729–736. [CrossRef] [PubMed]
2. Ni, X.-G.; He, S.; Xu, Z.-G.; Gao, L.; Lu, N.; Yuan, Z.; Lai, S.-Q.; Zhang, Y.-M.; Yi, J.-L.; Wang, X.-L.; et al. Endoscopic Diagnosis of Laryngeal Cancer and Precancerous Lesions by Narrow Band Imaging. *J. Laryngol. Otol.* **2011**, *125*, 288–296. [CrossRef] [PubMed]
3. Abdullah, B.; Rasid, N.S.A.; Lazim, N.M.; Volgger, V.; Betz, C.S.; Mohammad, Z.W.; Hassan, N.F.H.N. Ni Endoscopic Classification for Storz Professional Image Enhancement System (SPIES) Endoscopy in the Detection of Upper Aerodigestive Tract (UADT) Tumours. *Sci. Rep.* **2020**, *10*, 6341. [CrossRef] [PubMed]
4. Zhou, H.; Zhang, J.; Guo, L.; Nie, J.; Zhu, C.; Ma, X. The Value of Narrow Band Imaging in Diagnosis of Head and Neck Cancer: A Meta-Analysis. *Sci. Rep.* **2018**, *8*, 515. [CrossRef] [PubMed]
5. Bertino, G.; Cacciola, S.; Fernandes, W.B.; Fernandes, C.M.; Occhini, A.; Tinelli, C.; Benazzo, M. Effectiveness of Narrow Band Imaging in the Detection of Premalignant and Malignant Lesions of the Larynx: Validation of a New Endoscopic Clinical Classification: Validation of a New Endoscopic Clinical Classification. *Head Neck* **2015**, *37*, 215–222. [CrossRef] [PubMed]
6. Sun, C.; Han, X.; Li, X.; Zhang, Y.; Du, X. Diagnostic Performance of Narrow Band Imaging for Laryngeal Cancer: A Systematic Review and Meta-Analysis. *Otolaryngol. Neck Surg.* **2017**, *156*, 589–597. [CrossRef]
7. Page, M.J.; McKenzie, J.E.; Bossuyt, P.M.; Boutron, I.; Hoffmann, T.C.; Mulrow, C.D.; Shamseer, L.; Tetzlaff, J.M.; Akl, E.A.; Brennan, S.E.; et al. The PRISMA 2020 Statement: An Updated Guideline for Reporting Systematic Reviews. *BMJ* **2021**, *10*, 89. [CrossRef]
8. Ahmadzada, S.; Tseros, E.; Sritharan, N.; Singh, N.; Smith, M.; Palme, C.E.; Riffat, F. The Value of Narrowband Imaging Using the Ni Classification in the Diagnosis of Laryngeal Cancer. *Laryngoscope Investig. Otolaryngol.* **2020**, *5*, 665–671. [CrossRef]
9. Arens, C.; Piazza, C.; Andrea, M.; Dikkers, F.G.; Tjon Pian Gi, R.E.A.; Voigt-Zimmermann, S.; Peretti, G. Proposal for a Descriptive Guideline of Vascular Changes in Lesions of the Vocal Folds by the Committee on Endoscopic Laryngeal Imaging of the European Laryngological Society. *Eur. Arch. Otorhinolaryngol.* **2016**, *273*, 1207–1214. [CrossRef]
10. Šifrer, R.; Rijken, J.A.; Leemans, C.R.; Eerenstein, S.E.J.; van Weert, S.; Hendrickx, J.-J.; Bloemena, E.; Heuveling, D.A.; Rinkel, R.N.P.M. Evaluation of Vascular Features of Vocal Cords Proposed by the European Laryngological Society. *Eur. Arch. Otorhinolaryngol.* **2018**, *275*, 147–151. [CrossRef]
11. Missale, F.; Taboni, S.; Carobbio, A.L.C.; Mazzola, F.; Berretti, G.; Iandelli, A.; Fragale, M.; Mora, F.; Paderno, A.; Del Bon, F.; et al. Validation of the European Laryngological Society Classification of Glottic Vascular Changes as Seen by Narrow Band Imaging in the Optical Biopsy Setting. *Eur. Arch. Otorhinolaryngol.* **2021**, *278*, 2397–2409. [CrossRef] [PubMed]
12. Puxeddu, R.; Sionis, S.; Gerosa, C.; Carta, F. Enhanced Contact Endoscopy for the Detection of Neoangiogenesis in Tumors of the Larynx and Hypopharynx: ECE for Detection of Neoangiogenesis. *Laryngoscope* **2015**, *125*, 1600–1606. [CrossRef] [PubMed]
13. Klimza, H.; Jackowska, J.; Tokarski, M.; Piersiala, K.; Wierzbicka, M. Narrow-Band Imaging (NBI) for Improving the Assessment of Vocal Fold Leukoplakia and Overcoming the Umbrella Effect. *PLoS ONE* **2017**, *12*, e0180590. [CrossRef]
14. Mirza, N.; Kasper Schwartz, S.; Antin-Ozerkis, D. Laryngeal Findings in Users of Combination Corticosteroid and Bronchodilator Therapy. *Laryngoscope* **2004**, *114*, 1566–1569. [CrossRef]
15. Kostev, K.; Jacob, L.; Kalder, M.; Sesterhenn, A.; Seidel, D. Association of Laryngeal Cancer with Vocal Cord Leukoplakia and Associated Risk Factors in 1,184 Patients Diagnosed in Otorhinolaryngology Practices in Germany. *Mol. Clin. Oncol.* **2018**, *8*, 689–693. [CrossRef] [PubMed]
16. Isenberg, J.S.; Crozier, D.L.; Dailey, S.H. Institutional and Comprehensive Review of Laryngeal Leukoplakia. *Ann. Otol. Rhinol. Laryngol.* **2008**, *117*, 74–79. [CrossRef] [PubMed]
17. Zhang, N.; Cheng, L.; Chen, M.; Chen, J.; Yang, Y.; Xie, M.; Li, C.; Chen, X.-L.; Zhou, L.; Wu, H.-T. Relationship between Laryngoscopic and Pathological Characteristics of Vocal Cords Leukoplakia. *Acta Otolaryngol.* **2017**, *137*, 1199–1203. [CrossRef] [PubMed]
18. Ricci, G.; Molini, E.; Faralli, M.; Simoncelli, C. Retrospective Study on Precancerous Laryngeal Lesions: Long-Term Follow-Up. *Acta Otorhinolaryngol. Ital.* **2003**, *23*, 362–367.
19. Staníková, L.; Šatanková, J.; Kučová, H.; Walderová, R.; Zeleník, K.; Komínek, P. The Role of Narrow-Band Imaging (NBI) Endoscopy in Optical Biopsy of Vocal Cord Leukoplakia. *Eur. Arch. Oto-Rhino-Laryngol.* **2017**, *274*, 355–359. [CrossRef]

20. Young, C.-K.; Lin, W.-N.; Lee, L.-Y.; Lee, L.-A.; Hsin, L.-J.; Liao, C.-T.; Li, H.-Y.; Chen, I.-H.; Fang, T.-J. Laryngoscopic Characteristics in Vocal Leukoplakia: Inter-Rater Reliability and Correlation with Histology Grading: Characteristics in Vocal Leukoplakia. *Laryngoscope* **2015**, *125*, E62–E66. [CrossRef]
21. Fang, T.-J.; Lin, W.-N.; Lee, L.-Y.; Young, C.-K.; Lee, L.-A.; Chang, K.-P.; Liao, C.-T.; Li, H.-Y.; Yen, T.-C. Classification of Vocal Fold Leukoplakia by Clinical Scoring: Clinical Predictors in Vocal Leukoplakia. *Head Neck* **2016**, *38*, E1998–E2003. [CrossRef] [PubMed]
22. Chen, M.; Li, C.; Yang, Y.; Cheng, L.; Wu, H. A Morphological Classification for Vocal Fold Leukoplakia. *Braz. J. Otorhinolaryngol.* **2019**, *85*, 588–596. [CrossRef] [PubMed]
23. Ni, X.-G.; Zhu, J.-Q.; Zhang, Q.-Q.; Zhang, B.-G.; Wang, G.-Q. Diagnosis of Vocal Cord Leukoplakia: The Role of a Novel Narrow Band Imaging Endoscopic Classification: NBI for Diagnosis of Vocal Cord Leukoplakia. *Laryngoscope* **2019**, *129*, 429–434. [CrossRef] [PubMed]
24. Rzepakowska, A.; Sobol, M.; Sielska-Badurek, E.; Niemczyk, K.; Osuch-Wójcikiewicz, E. Morphology, Vibratory Function, and Vascular Pattern for Predicting Malignancy in Vocal Fold Leukoplakia. *J. Voice* **2020**, *34*, 812.e9–812.e15. [CrossRef] [PubMed]
25. El-Demerdash, A.; Fawaz, S.A.; Sabri, S.M.; Sweed, A.; Rabie, H. Sensitivity and Specificity of Stroboscopy in Preoperative Differentiation of Dysplasia from Early Invasive Glottic Carcinoma. *Eur. Arch. Otorhinolaryngol.* **2015**, *272*, 1189–1193. [CrossRef]
26. Cui, W.; Xu, W.; Yang, Q.; Hu, R. Clinicopathological Parameters Associated with Histological Background and Recurrence after Surgical Intervention of Vocal Cord Leukoplakia. *Medicine* **2017**, *96*, e7033. [CrossRef]
27. Gugatschka, M.; Kiesler, K.; Beham, A.; Rechenmacher, J.; Friedrich, G. Hyperplastic Epithelial Lesions of the Vocal Folds: Combined Use of Exfoliative Cytology and Laryngostroboscopy in Differential Diagnosis. *Eur. Arch. Otorhinolaryngol.* **2008**, *265*, 797–801. [CrossRef]
28. Mehlum, C.S.; Døssing, H.; Davaris, N.; Giers, A.; Grøntved, Å.M.; Kjaergaard, T.; Möller, S.; Godballe, C.; Arens, C. Interrater Variation of Vascular Classifications Used in Enhanced Laryngeal Contact Endoscopy. *Eur. Arch. Otorhinolaryngol.* **2020**, *277*, 2485–2492. [CrossRef]
29. El-Naggar, A.K.; Chan, J.K.C.; Takata, T.; Grandis, J.R.; Slootweg, P.J. The Fourth Edition of the Head and Neck World Health Organization Blue Book: Editors' Perspectives. *Hum. Pathol.* **2017**, *66*, 10–12. [CrossRef]
30. Zabrodsky, M.; Lukes, P.; Lukesova, E.; Boucek, J.; Plzak, J. The Role of Narrow Band Imaging in the Detection of Recurrent Laryngeal and Hypopharyngeal Cancer after Curative Radiotherapy. *BioMed Res. Int.* **2014**, *2014*, 175398. [CrossRef]
31. Chen, M.; Cheng, L.; Li, C.; Chen, J.; Shu, Y.; Wu, H. Nonsurgical Treatment for Vocal Fold Leukoplakia: An Analysis of 178 Cases. *BioMed Res. Int.* **2017**, *2017*, 6958250. [CrossRef] [PubMed]
32. Staníková, L.; Kučová, H.; Walderová, R.; Zeleník, K.; Komínek, P. Úloha Narrow Band Imaging (NBI) v Hodnocení Leukoplakií Hrtanu. *Otorinolaryngol. Foniatr.* **2015**, *64*, 186–190.
33. Weller, M.D.; Nankivell, P.C.; McConkey, C.; Paleri, V.; Mehanna, H.M. The Risk and Interval to Malignancy of Patients with Laryngeal Dysplasia; a Systematic Review of Case Series and Meta-Analysis: Risk and Interval to Malignancy of Patients with Laryngeal Dysplasia. *Clin. Otolaryngol.* **2010**, *35*, 364–372. [CrossRef] [PubMed]
34. Żurek, M.; Jasak, K.; Niemczyk, K.; Rzepakowska, A. Artificial Intelligence in Laryngeal Endoscopy: Systematic Review and Meta-Analysis. *J. Clin. Med.* **2022**, *11*, 2752. [CrossRef] [PubMed]

Disclaimer/Publisher's Note: The statements, opinions and data contained in all publications are solely those of the individual author(s) and contributor(s) and not of MDPI and/or the editor(s). MDPI and/or the editor(s) disclaim responsibility for any injury to people or property resulting from any ideas, methods, instructions or products referred to in the content.

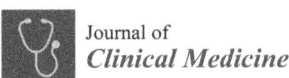

Article

Results of Primary Treatment and Salvage Treatment in the Management of Patients with Non-Squamous Cell Malignant Tumors of the Sinonasal Region: Single Institution Experience

Urszula Kacorzyk [1], Marek Kentnowski [1], Cezary Szymczyk [2], Ewa Chmielik [3], Barbara Bobek-Billewicz [4], Krzysztof Składowski [1] and Tomasz Wojciech Rutkowski [1,*]

[1] I Radiation and Clinical Oncology Department, Maria Sklodowska-Curie National Research Institute of Oncology Gliwice Branch, Wybrzeże Armii Krajowej 15, 44-101 Gliwice, Poland
[2] Department of Oncological and Reconstructive Surgery, Maria Sklodowska-Curie National Research Institute of Oncology Gliwice Branch, Wybrzeże Armii Krajowej 15, 44-101 Gliwice, Poland
[3] Tumor Pathology Department, Maria Sklodowska-Curie National Research Institute of Oncology Gliwice Branch, Wybrzeże Armii Krajowej 15, 44-101 Gliwice, Poland
[4] Department of Radiodiagnostics, Maria Sklodowska-Curie National Research Institute of Oncology Gliwice Branch, Wybrzeże Armii Krajowej 15, 44-101 Gliwice, Poland
* Correspondence: tomasz.rutkowski@io.gliwice.pl; Tel./Fax: +48-32-2788328

Abstract: Non-squamous cell carcinoma-related malignant sinonasal tract tumors (non-SCC MSTT) are rare and diverse malignancies. In this study, we report our experience in the management of this group of patients. The treatment outcome has been presented, involving both primary treatment and salvage approaches. Data from 61 patients treated radically due to non-SCC MSTT between 2000 and 2016 at the National Cancer Research Institute, Gliwice branch, were analyzed. The group consisted of the following pathological subtypes of MSTT: adenoid cystic carcinoma (ACC), undifferentiated sinonasal carcinoma (USC), sarcoma, olfactory neuroblastoma (ONB), adenocarcinoma, small cell neuroendocrine carcinoma (SNC), mucoepidermic carcinoma (MEC), and acinic cell carcinoma, which were found in nineteen (31%), seventeen (28%), seven (11.5%), seven (11.5%), five (8%), three (5%), two (3%) and one (2%) of patients, respectively. There were 28 (46%) males and 33 (54%) females at the median age of 51 years. Maxilla was the primary tumor localization followed by the nasal cavity and ethmoid sinus in thirty-one (51%), twenty (32.5%), and seven (11.5%) patients, respectively. In 46 (74%) patients, an advanced tumor stage (T3 or T4) was diagnosed. Primary nodal involvement (N) was found in three (5%) cases, and all patients underwent radical treatment. The combined treatment consisted of surgery and radiotherapy (RT) and was given to 52 (85%) patients. The probabilities of overall survival (OS), locoregional control (LRC), metastases-free survival (MFS), and disease-free survival (DFS) were assessed in pathological subtypes and grouped together, along with the ratio and effectiveness of salvage. Locoregional treatment failure was seen in 21 (34%) patients. Salvage treatment was performed in fifteen (71%) patients and was effective in nine (60%) cases. There was a significant difference in OS between patients who underwent salvage and those who did not (median: 40 months vs. 7 months, $p = 0.01$). In the group of patients who underwent salvage, OS was significantly longer when the procedure was effective (median: 80.5 months) than if it failed (median: 20.5 months), $p < 0.0001$. OS in patients after effective salvage was the same as in patients who were primary cured (median: 80.5 months vs. 88 months, $p = 0.8$). Distant metastases developed in ten (16%) patients. Five and ten year LRC, MFS, DFS, and OS were 69%, 83%, 60%, 70%, and 58%, 83%, 47%, 49%, respectively. The best treatment results were observed for patients with adenocarcinoma and sarcoma, while USC gave the poorest results in our set of patients. In this study, we indicate that salvage is possible in most patients with non-SCC MSTT with locoregional failure and that it may significantly prolong their overall survival.

Keywords: sinonasal carcinoma; salvage; radiotherapy; surgery

Citation: Kacorzyk, U.; Kentnowski, M.; Szymczyk, C.; Chmielik, E.; Bobek-Billewicz, B.; Składowski, K.; Rutkowski, T.W. Results of Primary Treatment and Salvage Treatment in the Management of Patients with Non-Squamous Cell Malignant Tumors of the Sinonasal Region: Single Institution Experience. *J. Clin. Med.* **2023**, *12*, 1953. https://doi.org/10.3390/jcm12051953

Academic Editors: Oreste Gallo and Luca Giovanni Locatello

Received: 9 February 2023
Revised: 23 February 2023
Accepted: 24 February 2023
Published: 1 March 2023

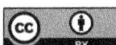

Copyright: © 2023 by the authors. Licensee MDPI, Basel, Switzerland. This article is an open access article distributed under the terms and conditions of the Creative Commons Attribution (CC BY) license (https://creativecommons.org/licenses/by/4.0/).

1. Introduction and Aim of the Study

Malignant sinonasal tract tumors (MSTT) are rare neoplasms that account for only 3% of head and neck carcinomas (HNC) and about 0.5% of all malignant diseases [1–3]. In contrast to other head and neck malignances, which are in the overwhelming majority squamous cell carcinomas, the pathology of MSTT is complex and diverse. Although the distribution of histological types varies in reported series, generally squamous cell carcinoma (SCC) accounts for about half of all MSTT and is followed by adenocarcinoma (10–27%), lymphoma (3–15%), adenoid cystic carcinoma (ACC), olfactory neuroblastoma (ONB), sarcoma, and mucosal melanoma, respectively, in 10%, 3%, 3%, and 2% [4–11]. Other, even more rare pathological types involve undifferentiated sinonasal carcinoma (USC), mucoepidermic carcinoma (MEC), small cell neuroendocrine carcinoma (SNC), and acinic cell carcinoma. The other reason for heterogeneity is a few tumor sites with various topography in the upper part of the head where MSTT may arise. Some correlation between tumor site and pathology type could be observed, like the fact that ethmoid tumors are mostly adenocarcinomas, or ONB, while SCC prevails in the maxillary sinus [5,8]. Latent and asymptomatic tumor growth or symptoms imitating sinusitis at the beginning of the disease usually turn into a late diagnosis and an advanced stage of the disease (stages T3–T4) when the tumor already infiltrates adjacent structures [3,9,12,13]. Numerous data indicate that less than 20% of primary-diagnosed MSTT are early-stage tumors [5,8,9,14–17]. Due to the above-mentioned rarity, heterogeneity, and challenging diagnosis, prospective studies on treatment efficacy have never been performed, and most treatment recommendations are based on one institution's reports, usually with a limited number of cases. In this study, we report our experience with the management of patients with non-SCC MSTT. Treatment outcomes involving both primary treatment and a salvage approach are presented.

2. Material and Methods

A review of retrospective clinical data of 233 consecutive patients with MSTT treated between 2000 and 2016 at the National Cancer Research Institute, Gliwice branch, was performed. The study was conducted according to the guidelines of the Declaration of Helsinki and approved by the Ethics Committee of the Maria Skłodowska-Curie National Research Institute of Oncology, Gliwice Branch (decision code: KB/430-73/21; date of approval: 10 May 2021). As many as 81 patients underwent a palliative approach, and 12 patients with benign tumors were excluded. Additionally, 79 cases with SCC were excluded. Finally, the analyzed group consisted of 28 (46%) males and 33 (54%) females with a median age of 51 years. Thirty-six patients (59%) had never smoked, and 25 (41%) were smokers. The median duration of symptoms before diagnosis was 10 months. Maxilla was the primary tumor localization, followed by the nasal cavity and ethmoid sinus in 31 (51%), 20 (32.5%), and 7 (11.5%) patients, respectively. The 8th edition of the American Joint Committee on Cancer (AJCC) staging was used for pretreatment staging [18]. In 46 (74%) patients, an advanced tumor stage (T3 or T4) was diagnosed. Primary nodal involvement (N) was found in only 3 (5%) cases. The choice of the sequence of treatment methods depended mostly on the stage of the disease and tumor pathology. All patients underwent radical treatment. The combined treatment consisted of surgery and radiotherapy (RT) and was given to 52 (85%) patients. Among them postoperative RT alone was given to 43 patients, and RT combined with chemotherapy (chemotherapy—CHT, RT combined with CHT—CHRT) in 9 cases. RT alone was given to 2 patients. Induction chemotherapy was followed by RT alone in 2 patients and by CHRT in 3 patients. CHRT was given to 1 patient. Surgery alone was applied to one patient. All chemotherapy sessions were platinum-based. Monochemotherapy was used as concomitant therapy during RT. Platinum combined with either 5FU as PF or taxanes as TPF were used as induction agents. An RT dose in the range of 66–70 Gy was used to eradicate macroscopic tumor infiltration with RT alone or if surgery was R2. For eradication of microscopic extension of disease (surgery: R1) at least 66 Gy was used. For elective RT, the dose prescribed was in the range of 50–60 Gy.

Persistent disease was defined as either a local or regional tumor that did not disappear after treatment or recurred within 6 months of treatment completion. Recurrence was defined as either a local or regional tumor that recurred later than 6 months after treatment completion or that recurred anytime in patients who underwent postoperative treatment.

Salvage treatment was defined as an attempt to apply the radical management of a persistent tumor or recurrence after the completion of primary radical therapy. Successful (effective) salvage was reported when the treated tumor was either no longer observed for at least 3 months or remained stable for at least 6 months after the salvage procedure. Following the previous salvage, a subsequent recurrence was defined as either a recurrence or progression.

The analysis of the treatment outcome was based on follow-up data. Patients were seen 1–2 months after treatment completion, then every 3 months for the first year, every 6 months for another year, and then annually. At each follow-up visit, a physical examination, including palpation of the neck, was performed. Routine imaging was done with MRI, CT, or positron emission tomography scans every 6 months or at the physician's discretion based on physical examination findings.

Both cumulative survival and tumor control rates were calculated using the Kaplan–Meier product-limited (actuarial) method. A p value of < 0.05 was considered statistically significant. A detailed analysis of the time and site of the primary treatment failure was performed. The ratio and effects of salvage were analyzed. The probabilities of overall survival (OS), locoregional control (LRC), metastases-free survival (MFS), and disease-free survival (DFS) were estimated from the end of primary treatment using the Kaplan–Meier product limit estimate and were compared using the log-rank test.

3. Results

3.1. Treatment Results in All Groups

The median follow-up in all groups was 86 months (range: 1–305 months). In general, locoregional treatment failure was seen in 21 (34%) patients. Persistent disease was found in four (6.5%) patients, and in all cases, it was localized in the primary site of the tumor. In one case, the persistent disease was concomitantly localized in the neck nodes. Recurrence appeared in 17 (28%) cases involving local, regional, or concomitantly locoregional sites in eleven, one, and five patients, respectively. The median time to recurrence was 21.5 months (range: 2–96 months). Distant metastases developed in ten (16%) patients, but only in six cases was this the sole reason for disease progression. The median time to metastases was 17 months (range: 3–60 months). In the remaining four patients, metastases appeared in patients with persistent disease (one case) or in patients with recurrence (three cases). Five and ten years LRC, MFS, DFS, and OS were 69%, 83%, 60%, 70% and 58%, 83%, 47%, 49%, respectively. Despite locoregional failure, six (29%) patients have not been admitted to salvage procedures due to: (a) quickly progressing persistent tumor after primary treatment (two cases); (b) advanced stage of recurrent disease (two cases); (c) lack of pathologically proven recurrence despite radiological progression (one case); and (d) persistent tumor without progression for about 7 years. Salvage treatment was given to the remaining fifteen (71%) patients and was effective in nine (60%) cases. In the group with effective salvage, surgery was undertaken as the first treatment modality in eight patients, and in one patient, it was RT. In five patients from the group, recurrence occurred more than once. In these cases, the salvage approach (surgery or RT) was given from two to five times. There was a significant difference in OS between patients who underwent salvage and those who did not (median: 40 months vs. 7 months, p = 0.01). In the group of patients who underwent salvage, OS was significantly longer when the procedure was effective (median: 80.5 months) than if it failed (median: 20.5 months), p < 0.0001. What is interesting is that OS in patients after effective salvage was the same as in patients who were primary cured (median: 80.5 months vs. 88 months, p = 0.8). (Figure 1). A detailed distribution of patients' characteristics according to individual pathologies is presented in Table 1. The results of primary treatment, the salvage ratio, and its effects distributed according to pathological type and in all groups are presented in Table 2.

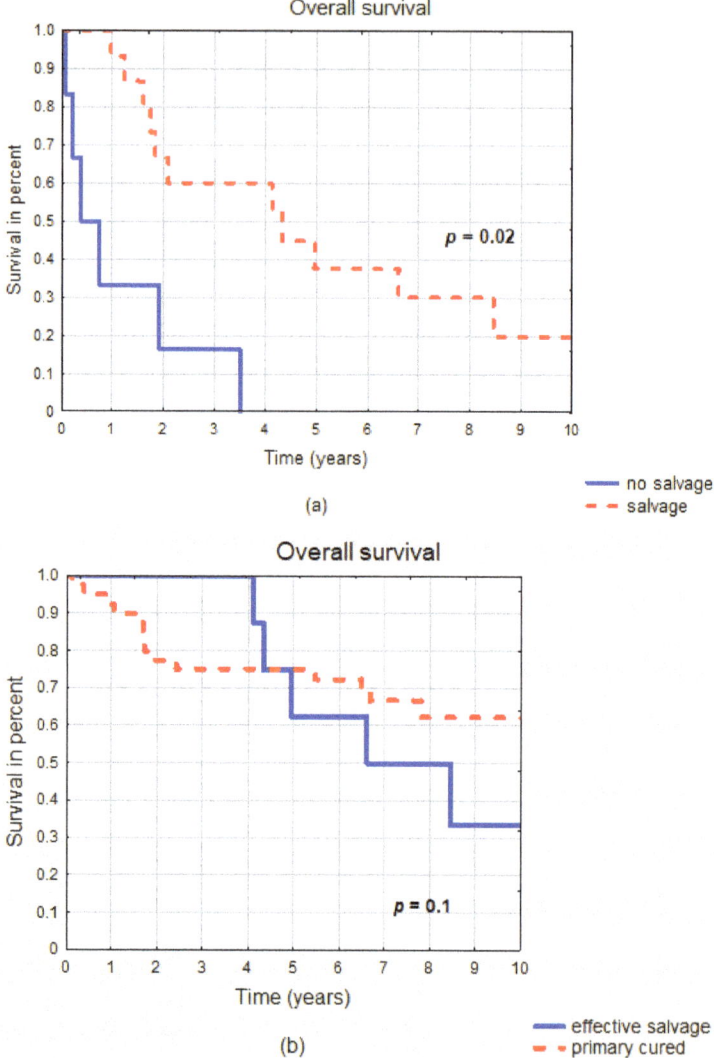

Figure 1. Overall survival considering salvage after primary treatment failure. (**a**) Patients with treatment failure: salvage vs. no salvage. (**b**) Patients cured primarily vs. cured after salvage.

Table 1. Patients' characteristics according to histopathological types and in all groups. ACC—adenoid-cystic carcinoma, USC—undifferentiated sinonasal carcinoma, ENB—olfactory neuroblastoma, MEC—mucoepidermic carcinoma, and SNC—small cell neuroendocrine carcinoma. CHRT—radiochemotherapy.

Pathology	No/%	Age (Median)	Man/Woman	Maxilla	Nasal Cavity	Ethmoid Sinus	Other	Surgery + pRT/CHRT	Surgery Alone	RT/CHRT Alone	RT Dose (Gy) 66–70/50–60
ACC	19/31	52	6/13	13	4	1	orbit	17/1	1	1/0	10/8
USC	17/28	54	6/11	7	7	2	frontal sin.	11/3	0	0/3	8/9
Sarcoma	7/11.5	44	3/4	3	3	0	frontal sin.	6/0	0	1/0	2/5
ENB	7/11.5	39	4/3	0	3	4	-	4/1	0	2/0	2/5
Adenocarcinoma	5/8	56.5	2/3	4	1	0	-	5/0	0	0/0	1/4
SNC	3/5	53	1/2	2	1	0	-	1/1	0	0/1	2/1
MEC	2/3	46.5	1/1	2	0	0	-	1/1	0	0/0	0/2
Acinic cell carcinoma	1/2	59	0/1	0	1	0	-	1/0	0	0	0/1
All groups	61/100	51	23/38	31	20	7	3	46/7	1	4/4	25/35

Table 2. Primary treatment results and results of salvage according to histopathological types and in all groups. Rec—recurrence, L—local, N—nodal, LN—local and nodal, ND—no data, ACC—adenoid-cystic carcinoma, USC—undifferentiated sinonasal carcinoma, ENB—olfactory neuroblastoma, MEC—mucoepidermic carcinoma, LRC—locoregional control, SNC—small cell neuroendocrine carcinoma. MFS—metastases-free survival, OS—overall survival.

Pathology	No/%	Persistant Tumor	Rec L	Rec N	Rec LN	Rec %	Met %	5 Year LRC (%)	5 Year MFS (%)	5 Year OS (%)	10 Year OS (%)	Salvage No/%	Effective Salvage No/%
ACC	19/31	0	6	0	1	37	26	77	82	74	38	4/57	2/50
USC	17/28	2	3	0	2	41	23.5	55	78	64	25	6/88	2/33
Sarcoma	7/11.5	1	0	0	0	14	0	83	83	71	71	1/100	1/100
ENB	7/11.5	1	1	0	2	28	14	57	85	71	57	2/50	2/100
Adenocarcinoma	5/8	0	0	1	0	20	0	80	100	100	100	1/100	1/100
SNC	3/5	0	0	0	0	0	33	100	63	33	33	0/0	0/0
MEC	2/3	0	0	0	0	0	0	100	100	50	50	0/0	0/0
Acinic cell carcinoma	1/2	0	1	0	0	100	0	0	100	100	100	1/100	1/100
All groups	61/100	4	11	1	5	31	16	69	83	70	49	15/24.5	9/60

3.2. Adenoid Cystic Carcinoma

Our group consisted of 19 (31%) patients with ACC. The maxillary sinus (68%) and nasal cavity (21%) were the most common sites of primary ACC tumors. The median age in this group was 56 years, and the women/men ratio was 13/6. In all but one patient, surgery was the primary treatment, which was followed by RT. Only one patient did not receive postoperative RT due to the lack of patient agreement. Additionally, due to an unresectable primary tumor, one patient received RT alone following induction CHT. The median time between surgery and RT was 4 months. In 10 cases 66–70 Gy was administered due to a residual macroscopic tumor. In the remaining eight patients 57.6–60 Gy was administered to eradicate the microscopic disease. In seven (37%) cases, local recurrence of the disease was found at the median time of 43 months (range: 2–96 months) after primary treatment completion. In one case from this group, 5 months after a local recurrence, a regional one appeared, and in the next 10 months, a distant spread developed. Distant metastases appeared in three more patients from this group in a median time of 35 months. There were also three other primary malignant tumors that appeared in patients 25, 7, and 209 months after primary treatment completion. Salvage was provided to four (57%) of the seven patients with locoregional failure. In three patients, it was surgery for the first failure and RT for the subsequent ones. In one case, RT alone was provided. In two patients, salvage was 50% effective. Five and ten years LRC, MFS, DFS, and OS were 77%, 82%, 62%, 74% and 46%, 82%, 30%, 38%, respectively.

4. Undifferentiated Sinonasal Carcinoma

Our group consists of 17 (28%) patients with USC pathology. The nasal cavity and maxillary sinus were the most common sites of primary tumors in this group, accounting for 41% each. The median age was 55 years, with a female/male ratio of 6/11. Additionally, in this group, in most cases, primary surgery followed by RT/CHRT was the main approach and was carried out in 14 (82%) patients. In three patients from this group CHRT was used. In three patients, no surgery was performed due to the advanced stage of the disease. In two patients from this group, induction chemotherapy was given with either RT or CHRT, and in one case, CHRT alone was given. The median time between surgery and RT was 2.5 months. After treatment completion, persistent tumors were found in two cases. In five patients recurrence appeared in a median time of 16 months. From this group, in three cases, local recurrence alone was found. In the next two patients, there was also nodal recurrence that preceded local recurrence in one case and followed it in the second one. Metastatic disease was found in four cases, but only in one patient was it the only reason for failure. Out of seven patients with locoregional failure, salvage was provided to six (85.5%). Surgery was used on three patients, and on the three others, RT was used as salvage. In two (33%) patients, salvage was effective; both cases had surgery. Five and 10 years LRC, MFS, DFS, and OS were 55%, 78%, 51%, 64% and 55%, 78%, 51%, 25%, respectively.

4.1. Sarcoma

Our group consisted of seven (11.5%) patients with sarcoma. The nasal cavity and maxillary sinus were the most common sites of the primary tumor in this group, accounting for 43% each. The median age in this group was 44 years, and the man/woman ratio was 3/4. In all but one patient, surgery was the primary treatment, which was followed by RT. In one patient, RT alone was applied due to an advanced tumor, and RT was not completed because the patient was lost to therapy after the dose of 28 Gy. Additionally, in one patient, postoperative RT was preceded with induction chemotherapy due to progression shortly after surgery. The median time between surgery and RT was 3 months. In one patient from this group, treatment failure was found as a persistent tumor. Salvage surgery was performed, followed by RT, but only the subsequent salvage and stereotactic RT were successful, and the patient was eventually cured. Five and 10 years LRC, MFS, DFS, and OS were 83%, 83%, 68%, 71% and 83%, 83%, 68%, 71%, respectively.

4.2. Olfactory Neuroblastoma

There were seven (11.5%) patients with ONB in our group. The ethmoid sinus (57%) and nasal cavity (43%) were the most common sites of the primary tumor in this group. The median age was 39 years, and the male/female ratio was 4/3 in this series. Additionally, in this group, in most cases, primary surgery followed by RT was the main approach and was carried out on five patients. In two patients, no surgery was performed due to the advanced stage. Concomitant CHRT was used in one patient from this group, and RT alone was used in another. The median time between surgery and RT was 2.8 months. In five cases, 60 Gy was given to eradicate microscopic diseases. In two cases, 66–68 Gy were given due to the macroscopic tumor. There were four treatment failures: a residual tumor in one case and recurrence in three cases. A patient who had a persistent tumor had a distant spread of the disease. Salvage was given to two (50%) patients from this group, and in both cases, it consisted of surgery, RT, and systemic treatment repeated a few times. This effort was successful for both patients. Five and 10 years LRC, MFS, DFS, and OS were 57%, 85%, 57%, 71% and 43%, 85%, 43%, 57%, respectively.

4.3. Adenocarcinoma

Our group consisted of five (8%) patients with this pathology. The maxillary sinus (80%) and nasal cavity (20%) were the most common primary sites of this malignancy. The median age was 56.6 years, and the male/female ratio was 2/3. In all cases, primary surgery followed by RT was the main treatment approach. The median time between surgery and RT was 2.3 months. In four cases, 60 Gy was given to eradicate the microscopic disease. In one case, 66 Gy was given due to a residual macroscopic tumor. The results of primary treatment were excellent; in only one patient, nodal recurrence appeared 21 months after primary treatment completion. Surgical salvage was successful in this case. Five and ten years LRC, MFS, DFS, and OS were 80%, 100%, 80%, 100% and 80%, 100%, 80%, 100%, respectively.

4.4. Small Cell Neuroendocrine Carcinoma

There were three (5%) patients with a small cell neuroendocrine carcinoma in this group. It was localized in the nasal cavity and maxillary sinus in two and one case, respectively. There were two women and one man, with a median age of 53 years. In two patients, primary surgery followed by RT was carried out, and in another patient, CHRT was used. The median time between surgery and RT was 3.2 months. All patients were cured, and only in one case did a distant spread to the lung appear about a year after the completion of primary treatment. CHT was not effective, and the patient died about 2 months later.

4.5. Mucoepidermic Carcinoma

There were two (3%) patients with mucoepidermic carcinoma in this group, and both cases had a primary tumor localized in the maxillary sinus. They were a man and a woman, ages 30 and 63, respectively. In both patients' surgeries, primary treatment was followed by RT with elective doses. The median time between surgery and RT was 2.9 months. Both patients were cured, but one of them died 21 months later due to another reason.

4.6. Acinic Cell Carcinoma

There was one (2%) patient with this rare pathology in our group. The tumor in the 59-year-old woman was localized in the nasal cavity. The patient underwent surgery, which was followed by RT 2.5 months after surgery at a dose of 60 Gy. After 4 years of follow-up, a local recurrence was found, and the patient underwent stereotactic RT. After the next 4 years, the patient underwent endoscopic surgery due to a subsequent recurrence. There was another stereotactic RT in the next 4 years due to the next recurrence and four cycles of palliative CHT in the next 2 years due to a subsequent recurrence. The patient died in the next 1.5 years due to the progression of local infiltration of the cancer.

5. Discussion

The rarity of MSTT, which is even more sparse due to diverse pathology, means that reports considering this type of cancer are usually from one institution and usually with a limited number of cases. In this study, we described the results of the radical treatment of 61 patients who suffered from MSTT, taking into account the follow-up period and the results of a salvage approach. To refer to as many clinical outcomes as possible, we presented the results of an entire group first and subsequently the results in each pathological cohort. All patients were treated at a single cancer center, the National Cancer Research Institute, Gliwice branch, Poland. The patient's distribution was generally consistent with other series, with the majority of patients having advanced stages (T3, T4), and only 5% of them having involved regional lymph nodes [19,20]. There were more women in our group, probably due to a relatively large subgroup of patients with ACC and USC. Females dominating in these groups were also found in other series [21,22]. The predominating primary site of the MSTT differs slightly between our cohort and other reported groups. We found most cases with primary infiltration in the maxilla, followed by the nasal cavity, whereas Hafstrom et al. reported an inverse distribution, and Dirix et al. pointed to the ethmoid sinus as the most frequent primary site of MSTT [20,21]. Contrary to other authors' reports listing adenocarcinoma as the second most common malignancy in this region [23], ACC and USC were predominating in our group.

A five year OS rate of 70% established in our group is comparable to the survival rate reported by other authors (38–69%) [6,7,14,21,24–28]. Due to the relatively long follow-up period, we were also able to assess the 10 year OS, which was 49%. Other authors reported a 10 year OS rate in the range of 35–48% [21,24,25].

Five and 10 years of DFS were at 60% and 47% in our group, which is comparable to 42–63% and 54–59%, respectively, reported by other authors [21,24,25]. In our group, only four (6.5%) patients were never in remission after primary treatment. The ratio of persistent disease after primary treatment was between 6% and 14%, which was also reported by other authors [21,28]. In patients with a persistent tumor, salvage was performed in two patients (50%) and was finally successful in both cases. Mirghani et al. reported effective salvage in only two patients (9%) out of twenty-two with a persistent tumor after primary treatment [28].

In our group, locoregional failure was seen in 38% of cases but isolated local ones in 18%. In one of the largest series aiming to report recurrences during follow-up in MSTT patients performed by Zochi et al., at least one recurrence during follow-up was shown in 28% of patients, and in almost 75% it developed in the first three years after primary treatment [29]. In that study, the median time to first relapse was 17 months [29]. Mattaveli et al. assessed the median time to recurrence as 18 months, which is shorter than the 21 months assessed in our study [25]. According to Mattavelli et al., over 60% of all recurrences in the group were local, which is similar to our group, where 65% of patients with recurrences developed it in a primary site [25]. Additionally, other authors show local recurrence as the most common site of relapse in MSTT patients in the range of 15–73% and an average of 30–40% [1,7,14,19,20,25,28,30–32]. However, the most commonly cited factors increasing the risk of local recurrence, such as T-staging and pathology, as well as primary treatment performed outside referral centers, could also be an adverse factor [1,25,29]. Due to the high risk of local failure, post-treatment surveillance seems essential for early detection of failure. It is, however, challenging due to lack of both surveillance recommendations (how often and what diagnostic procedure is optimal) and evidence of its influence on survival prolongation [33]. Despite other benefits of surveillance like comprehensive nutritional assessment, rehabilitation after surgery, and RT [10], the evidence of an effective salvage may support the significance of early detection of treatment failure [34]. Most of the data concerning the role of salvage for MSTT patients refers to SCC as the most common pathology. For this malignancy, salvage is possible in 30–70% of patients [34–36]. It has been shown that even patients in whom salvage was not effective presented an improved OS compared with those with failure but no salvage at all. Moreover, effective salvage appeared to compensate for failure, giving the same ultimate OS as in primarily cured patients [34]. In non-SCC patients, the relevance of salvage is more difficult to assess due to the pathological diversity in this group. For such patients, Kaplan et al. proposed a therapeutic algorithm that considered, among other things, pathology and the site of recurrence. Based on the series of 49 patients with recurrence, surgery was strongly recommended for low-grade tumors, while a rather palliative approach was recommended for high-grade lesions with orbital or skull-base invasions [2]. Mattaveli et al. also suggested a multiparametrical score defining groups A, B, and C with excellent survival estimation, intermediate prognosis, and poor estimated survival comparable to those of metastatic head and neck cancer, respectively. The authors concluded that, similarly to primary tumors, in the recurrent setting, histology and tumor biology are critical, strongly influencing final results. In cases of unfavorable pathology, SNC has been included, while ONB and USC presented the best survival estimates in this analysis [25]. Contrary to this observation, USC malignancies gave the poorest results in our set of patients, with the highest ratio of recurrence and relatively low salvage success. Additionally, according to other authors, the prognosis of patients with USC remains poor [21,37]. We obtained the best primary treatment results for patients with adenocarcinoma and sarcoma. Despite a relatively higher ratio of locoregional failure, due to effective salvage, patients with ACC and ENB could be considered good predictors. Additionally, according to Hafstrom et al., adenocarcinoma and ENB have a relatively good prognosis [21].

Not much data concerning the results of salvage for patients with the presented pathological types are available. Mirghani et al. found salvage to be an effective treatment in 20% of isolated local recurrences and in 16% of cases with both local and nodal failure [28]. In our series, time to recurrence did not significantly influence salvage effectiveness and was similar in those who experienced effective or ineffective salvage. Our data suggest that salvage was possible in over 70% of recurrent patients and was effective in 60% of those who underwent this procedure. The results of salvage assessed in this group of patients are consistent with those obtained for SCC patients [34]. We were able to confirm that salvage is an effective procedure and may significantly prolong OS, reducing the adverse effect of recurrence for patients with non-SCC MSTT.

Isolated regional relapse usually is rare. In most series, it does not exceed 10%, usually being in the range of 4–6%. We found recurrent disease in regional nodes in 4% of our patients. Mirghani et al. described the issue of regional failure in detail, and pointed out that nodal recurrence appeared in 10% of patients in all groups, but 6.5% while considering patients without local failure, and 4% of those with initially cN0 [28]. Despite generally rare regional relapse pathological types like SCC or USC without prophylactic neck treatment may develop more nodal recurrences than ACC or MEC [38]. Other risk factors include T-stage in the context of local invasiveness, especially at sites with a rich lymphatic network [20,39,40]. Recommendations for elective nodal treatment to prevent regional recurrence are not well defined and vary between authors, usually due to the heterogeneity of the groups and a limited number of neck relapses [28]. For patients with an isolated nodal recurrence, salvage remains a good option. In our group, only one patient presented with an isolated nodal relapse and underwent effective salvage. In two patients in whom a nodal recurrence developed prior to or simultaneously with a local one, surgical salvage was effective in both cases. In the remaining three cases, local recurrences appeared prior to a nodal one. The median preceding time was 5 months, which may suggest a rather nodal progression from local recurrence than metastatic failure after primary treatment. Such a scenario has also been suggested by Mirghani et al., who stressed the separation between isolated neck recurrence and that associated with local failure. Such misinterpretation may lead, according to this author, to an overstated indication for prophylactic neck management [28]. In addition, successful nodal salvage has been reported by other authors. Cantu et al., in a group of 399 patients with maxillary sinus cancer, found 281 recurrences and 31 isolated nodal ones among them. Due to effective salvage, only two of them died of nodal-only metastases [41]. Dirix et al. found an isolated nodal recurrence in six patients in a group of one hundred and twenty-seven patients with MTSS. All of them underwent salvage neck dissection, followed by postoperative RT (no elective RT was given during primary treatment), which was effective, and none of them died due to nodal relapse [20].

5.1. Adenoid Cystic Carcinoma

ACC is a relatively slow-growing tumor characterized by perineural invasion and a high rate of local recurrence. In the distribution of histological types of MSTT, ACC usually accounts for about 10% [8], but in our series, it was the most common type (SCC was excluded from this analysis). In our group, females were dominant (sex ratio: 2.0). Atallach et al. also found more females in their group (sex ratio: 1.5) [42]. The five to ten years local recurrence rate is 30% to 75% [43]. In our group, locoregional recurrence was found in 37% of patients, and in 57% of them, salvage was performed. It was successful in 50% of patients who underwent this procedure. It resulted in a 5 and 10 years OS ratio of 74% and 38%, respectively. Other authors report 5 and 10 years of OS at 68–85% [42,44]

and 52–67%, respectively [42,44,45]. Long-term survival in ACC is usually affected by a high risk of distant metastases (40–50%), but we found it only in 15% [42,44].

5.2. Undifferentiated Sinonasal Carcinoma

Sinonasal undifferentiated carcinoma is a rare and aggressive tumor. This malignancy was second as to the number of subgroup cases in our study, with almost two times more females in the group, which is in contrast with other data [46]. Over 80% of our patients undergo surgery followed by RT or CHRT. Kuo et al. showed that surgery, RT, and CHT as a combined modality are the most effective treatment, with a 5 year survival rate of 41.5% [47]. Other authors showed 5 years of OS after surgery combined with RT in the range of 36–39%, indicating that RT is a critical component in the treatment [46]. Additionally, CHT is almost always included as part of the therapy regimen, and the role of induction CHT has been raised [48]. In general, the overall 5 year survival rate for this malignancy is less favorable than for other MSTT malignancies. It was also confirmed in our results. Despite that, locoregional failure was found in 41% of our patients, and salvage was performed in all but one case. It was effective in one-third of patients.

5.3. Sarcoma

Sarcomas are extremely rare, accounting for only ~1% of all the malignancies in the head and neck region. Moreover, the nasal cavity and paranasal sinus location represents only about 5% of all head and neck sarcomas. Malignant peripheral nerve sheath tumor (MPNST) was diagnosed in three cases in our group, while in the literature, not more than 25 cases have been reported so far [49]. In our group, five out of seven cases underwent surgery followed by RT. Such management seems to be optimal for these type of malignances. Although preoperative RT is well tolerated and provides a high rate of local control [50], RT is most commonly followed by definitive surgery [51]. Treatment results in our group were good and 5 and 10 years OS was 71%. In one case, recurrence salvage was performed and appeared to be effective. Five years of OS and the local control ratio reported by other authors are in the range of 56–82% and 41–83%, respectively [50,52]. One should remember, however, that pathological subtype, site of primary tumor, histological grade, and percentage of gross total resections, among others, may significantly impact the outcome.

5.4. Olfactory Neuroblastoma

Olfactory neuroblastoma is a rare tumor arising from the olfactory neuroepithelium in the sinonasal cavity. ENB presents a bimodal age distribution with peaks in the second and sixth decades [10]. It was the youngest subgroup in our study, with a median age of 39 years. In general, the combination of surgery and RT is the most frequently used treatment and was associated with the best average survival results (65%) in the meta-analysis performed by Dulguerov et al. The 5 year and 10 year OS rates in our group were 71% and 57%, respectively, which is better than in other reports. The mean overall survival and disease-free survival at 5 years was 45% (range: 0–86%), and the average OS at 10 years was 52% [53]. Despite the main roles of surgery and RT, CHT has been increasingly used by Thawani [10]. There was a local failure of 57% in our group, which is higher than the 29% reported by Dulguerov et al. Salvage was possible in 50% of our patients, which is consistent with others, indicating possible salvage in 33–50% of patients with a local recurrence [54]. A salvage approach in our group was multimodal according to subsequent recurrences in these patients and turned into additional years of overall survival.

5.5. Adenocarcinoma

Contrary to other data, which indicate this type as the second most common malignancy, we found it only in 8% in our group (Castelnuovo and Arnold) [23,24]. We found the maxilla most often as the primary site of this tumor, while others pointed out the nasal cavity and ethmoid sinus (Bhayani) [54]. We noticed excellent results from surgery followed by RT. A successful salvage neck dissection due to reginal recurrence was performed, resulting in a 5 years OS of 100%. Arnold et al. in a group of 21 cases reported 53% of 5 and 10 years OS. (Arnold) [24]. In fact, the 5 year overall survival (OS) rates in this group vary widely among studies, ranging from 36% to 86% (Maccariello) [55].

5.6. Small Cell Neuroendocrine Carcinoma

A rare cancer arising mostly in the ethmoid sinus [56]. There were three patients with this tumor in our group, and the primary localization was the maxilla in two of them. According to the literature, surgery followed by RT remains the main treatment approach, although some data indicate that adding CHT as an induction or as CHRT after surgery may improve treatment results [57,58]. Three of our patients underwent surgery followed by RT, and CHRT was given to one patient. The main reason for the failure of this malignancy is the local recurrence or distant spread of the disease [59]. Although all our patients were locoregionally cured, one of them died due to distant metastases.

5.7. Sinonasal Mucoepidermoid Carcinoma

Mucoepidermoid carcinoma is a common salivary gland malignancy that rarely arises in the sinonasal region. This malignancy was found in only 3% of the patients in our group. Maxilla is the most typical primary site for this tumor [60], and all our cases were localized in maxilla. Generally, treatment includes surgery followed by RT. Trantafilou et al. reported results of treatment for 164 patients with 1, 2, and 5 years of OS of 83%, 77.0%, and 57%, respectively [60]. Such therapy was effective for our patients, and none of them experienced treatment failure.

5.8. Acinic Cell Carcinoma

Acinic cell carcinoma is a rare cancer of this region. A review of the National Cancer Database reported 28 such patients treated between 2004 and 2016. Most of these tumors arose in the nasal cavity [61], and this was also the primary site of the tumor in our patient. Biron et al. pointed out that all 18 of his cases were low-grade [62]. Surgery alone was the main treatment option in a cohort described by Khirsagar et al. [61]. Overall survival at 1, 5, and 10 years was 100%, 84.3%, and 52.3–72.2%, respectively [61,62]. A meta-analysis of survival from cases in the literature performed by Biron et al. estimated 10 year recurrence-free survival at 92.9% [62]. Our patient presented with 14 years of OS, despite local recurrences for the last 10 years that had been treated subsequently. A good result from a few salvage attempts was probably due to the low grade of this tumor. Our result confirms that it is a rare entity with relatively good long-term outcomes, and salvage may be effective [61,62].

Patients suffering from MSTT require a multidisciplinary team approach not only at diagnosis but also during follow-up. Multidisciplinary care of patients with their survivorship issues is needed including rehabilitation or comprehensive nutritional assessment. Of special importance is support in the management of the consequences of surgery or RT, including the prevention of delayed radiation-induced complications (second malignancies, hypothyroidism, and tissue necrosis). Moreover, surveillance is also significant because it helps facilitate an early diagnosis of recurrence. Our data indicates that salvage is effective, but often a multimodal and multidisciplinary team should decide what salvage option is optimal for a particular patient in an individual clinical situation, taking into account stereotactic radiosurgery and intensity-modulated particle therapy (i.e., protons and ^{12}C-carbon ions) [16,63]. Due to the rarity and heterogeneity of MSTT cancer registries, international clinical studies dedicated to patients with MSTT could be proposed as a solution for this rare disease [64].

This study has several limitations common to retrospective studies, which are even more pronounced here due to the diverse pathology and low number of cases. On the other hand, even a few cases of a rare pathology well described in a clinical scenario could be beneficial. We believe that our data will support general knowledge about this disease and may add value to the discussion about the management of patients with MSTT in the future.

6. Conclusions

Patients with non-SCC MSTT present a diverse prognosis that is related to several clinical and tumor-related factors. In most cases, a multimodal primary treatment is suggested to decrease the risk of local recurrence, which is the main reason for failure. Recommendations are, however, sparse due to the rarity of such malignancies and the almost complete absence of clinical trials. In this study, we indicate that salvage is possible in most patients with non-SCC MSTT with locoregional failure and may significantly prolong their overall survival.

Author Contributions: Data collection, results elaboration, writing—manuscript preparation, literature review, U.K.; design, data completion, results elaboration, statistical calculation, writing—manuscript editing of the final version, T.W.R.; data collection, M.K.; elaboration of histopathological data, E.C.; elaboration of radiodiagnostic data, B.B.-B.; elaboration of surgical data, C.S.; consultation of design and revision of the final version of the manuscript, K.S. All authors have read and agreed to the published version of the manuscript.

Funding: This research received no external funding.

Institutional Review Board Statement: The study was conducted according to the guidelines of the Declaration of Helsinki and approved by the Ethics Committee of the Maria Skłodowska-Curie National Research In-stitute of Oncology, Gliwice Branch (decision code: KB/430-73/21; date of approval: 10 May 2021).

Informed Consent Statement: Patient consent was waived due to retrospective data and they could not be identified.

Data Availability Statement: The data are available upon request from the corresponding author.

Conflicts of Interest: The authors declare no conflict of interest.

References

1. Dulguerov, P.; Jacobsen, M.S.; Allal, A.S.; Lehmann, W.; Calcaterra, T. Nasal and paranasal sinus carcinoma: Are we making progress? A series of 220 patients and a systematic review. *Cancer* **2001**, *92*, 3012–3029. [CrossRef]
2. Kaplan, D.J.; Kim, J.H.; Wang, E.; Snyderman, C. Prognostic Indicators for Salvage Surgery of Recurrent Sinonasal Malignancy. *Otolaryngol. Neck Surg.* **2015**, *154*, 104–112. [CrossRef]
3. Abdelmeguid, A.S.; Teeramatwanich, W.; Roberts, D.B.; Amit, M.; Ferraroto, R.; Glisson, B.S.; Kupferman, M.E.; Su, S.Y.; Phan, J.; Garden, A.S.; et al. Neoadjuvant chemotherapy for locoregionally advanced squamous cell carcinoma of the paranasal sinuses. *Cancer* **2021**, *127*, 1788–1795. [CrossRef]
4. Thompson, L.D.R.; Franchi, A. New tumor entities in the 4th edition of the World Health Organization classification of head and neck tumors: Nasal cavity, paranasal sinuses and skull base. *Virchows Arch.* **2017**, *472*, 315–330. [CrossRef] [PubMed]
5. Turri-Zanoni, M.; Gravante, G.; Castelnuovo, P. Molecular Biomarkers in Sinonasal Cancers: New Frontiers in Diagnosis and Treatment. *Curr. Oncol. Rep.* **2022**, *24*, 55–67. [CrossRef]
6. Gore, M.R. Survival in sinonasal and middle ear malignancies: A population-based study using the SEER 1973–2015 database. *BMC Ear Nose Throat Disord.* **2018**, *18*, 13. [CrossRef]
7. Thorup, C.; Sebbesen, L.; Danø, H.; Leetmaa, M.; Andersen, M.; von Buchwald, C.; Kristensen, C.A.; Bentzen, J.; Godballe, C.; Johansen, J.; et al. Carcinoma of the nasal cavity and paranasal sinuses in Denmark 1995–2004. *Acta Oncol.* **2009**, *49*, 389–394. [CrossRef] [PubMed]
8. Jégoux, F.; Métreau, A.; Louvel, G.; Bedfert, C. Paranasal sinus cancer. *Eur. Ann. Otorhinolaryngol. Head Neck Dis.* **2013**, *130*, 327–335. [CrossRef] [PubMed]
9. Youlden, D.R.; Cramb, S.M.; Peters, S.; Porceddu, S.V.; Møller, H.; Fritschi, L.; Baade, P.D. International comparisons of the incidence and mortality of sinonasal cancer. *Cancer Epidemiol.* **2013**, *37*, 770–779. [CrossRef] [PubMed]
10. Thawani, R.; Kim, M.S.; Arastu, A.; Feng, Z.; West, M.T.; Taflin, N.F.; Thein, K.Z.; Li, R.; Geltzeiler, M.; Lee, N.; et al. The contemporary management of cancers of the sinonasal tract in adults. *CA A Cancer J. Clin.* **2022**, *73*, 72–112. [CrossRef]
11. Patel, N.N.; Maina, I.W.; Kuan, E.C.; Triantafillou, V.; Trope, M.A.; Carey, R.M.; Workman, A.D.; Tong, C.C.; Kohanski, M.A.; Palmer, J.N.; et al. Adenocarcinoma of the Sinonasal Tract: A Review of the National Cancer Database. *J. Neurol. Surg. Part B Skull Base* **2019**, *81*, 701–708. [CrossRef]

12. van der Laan, T.P.; Bij, H.P.; van Hemel, B.M.; Plaat, B.E.C.; Wedman, J.; van der Laan, B.F.A.M.; Halmos, G.B. The importance of multimodality therapy in the treatment of sinonasal neuroendocrine carcinoma. *Eur. Arch. Oto-Rhino-Laryngol.* **2013**, *270*, 2565–2568. [CrossRef] [PubMed]
13. Amsbaugh, M.J.; Yusuf, M.; Silverman, C.; Bumpous, J.; Perez, C.A.; Potts, K.; Tennant, P.; Redman, R.; Dunlap, N. Organ preservation with neoadjuvant chemoradiation in patients with orbit invasive sinonasal cancer otherwise requiring exenteration. *Radiat. Oncol. J.* **2016**, *34*, 209–215. [CrossRef] [PubMed]
14. Koivunen, P.; Mäkitie, A.A.; Bäck, L.; Pukkila, M.; Laranne, J.; Kinnunen, I.; Aitasalo, K.; Grénman, R. A national series of 244 sinonasal cancers in Finland in 1990–2004. *Eur. Arch. Oto-Rhino-Laryngol.* **2011**, *269*, 615–621. [CrossRef] [PubMed]
15. Hu, W.; Hu, J.; Huang, Q.; Gao, J.; Yang, J.; Qiu, X.; Kong, L.; Lu, J.J. Particle beam radiation therapy for sinonasal malignancies: Single institutional experience at the Shanghai Proton and Heavy Ion Center. *Cancer Med.* **2020**, *9*, 7914–7924. [CrossRef] [PubMed]
16. Ferrari, M.; Taboni, S.; Carobbio, A.; Emanuelli, E.; Maroldi, R.; Bossi, P.; Nicolai, P. Sinonasal Squamous Cell Carcinoma, a Narrative Reappraisal of the Current Evidence. *Cancers* **2021**, *13*, 2835. [CrossRef]
17. Sakata, K.; Maeda, A.; Rikimaru, H.; Ono, T.; Koga, N.; Takeshige, N.; Tokutomi, T.; Umeno, H.; Kiyokawa, K.; Morioka, M. Advantage of Extended Craniofacial Resection for Advanced Malignant Tumors of the Nasal Cavity and Paranasal Sinuses: Long-Term Outcome and Surgical Management. *World Neurosurg.* **2016**, *89*, 240–254. [CrossRef]
18. Doescher, J.; Veit, J.A.; Hoffmann, T.K. Die 8. Ausgabe der TNM-Klassifikation. *HNO* **2017**, *65*, 956–961. [CrossRef]
19. Robin, T.P.; Jones, B.; Ba, O.M.G.; Phan, A.; Abbott, D.; McDermott, J.D.; Goddard, J.A.; Raben, D.; Lanning, R.M.; Karam, S.D. A comprehensive comparative analysis of treatment modalities for sinonasal malignancies. *Cancer* **2017**, *123*, 3040–3049. [CrossRef]
20. Dirix, P.; Nuyts, S.; Geussens, Y.; Jorissen, M.; Poorten, V.V.; Fossion, E.; Hermans, R.; Bogaert, W.V.D. Malignancies of the Nasal Cavity and Paranasal Sinuses: Long-Term Outcome with Conventional or Three-Dimensional Conformal Radiotherapy. *Int. J. Radiat. Oncol.* **2007**, *69*, 1042–1050. [CrossRef]
21. Hafström, A.; Sjövall, J.; Persson, S.S.; Nilsson, J.S.; Svensson, C.; Brun, E.; Greiff, L. Outcome for sinonasal malignancies: A population-based survey. *Eur. Arch. Oto-Rhino-Laryngol.* **2021**, *279*, 2611–2622. [CrossRef]
22. Nightingale, J.; Lum, B.; Ladwa, R.; Simpson, F.; Panizza, B. Adenoid cystic carcinoma: A review of clinical features, treatment targets and advances in improving the immune response to monoclonal antibody therapy. *Biochim. et Biophys. Acta Rev. Cancer* **2021**, *1875*, 188523. [CrossRef] [PubMed]
23. Castelnuovo, P.; Turri-Zanoni, M.; Battaglia, P.; Antognoni, P.; Bossi, P.; Locatelli, D. Sinonasal Malignancies of Anterior Skull Base: Histology-driven Treatment Strategies. *Otolaryngol. Clin. N. Am.* **2016**, *49*, 183–200. [CrossRef] [PubMed]
24. Arnold, A.; Ziglinas, P.; Ochs, K.; Alter, N.; Geretschläger, A.; Lädrach, K.; Zbären, P.; Caversaccio, M. Therapy options and long-term results of sinonasal malignancies. *Oral Oncol.* **2012**, *48*, 1031–1037. [CrossRef]
25. Mattavelli, D.; Tomasoni, M.; Ferrari, M.; Compagnoni, A.; Schreiber, A.; Taboni, S.; Rampinelli, V.; Marazzi, E.; Raffetti, E.; de Zinis, L.O.R.; et al. Salvage surgery in recurrent sinonasal cancers: Proposal for a prognostic model based on clinicopathologic and treatment-related parameters. *Head Neck* **2022**, *44*, 1857–1870. [CrossRef]
26. Filtenborg, M.V.; Lilja-Fischer, J.K.; Sharma, M.B.; Primdahl, H.; Kjems, J.; Plaschke, C.C.; Wessel, I.; Kristensen, C.A.; Andersen, M.; Andersen, E.; et al. Sinonasal cancer in Denmark 2008–2015: A population-based phase-4 cohort study from DAHANCA. *Acta Oncol.* **2021**, *60*, 333–342. [CrossRef]
27. Wong, D.J.; Smee, R.I. Sinonasal carcinomas–A single-centre experience at Prince of Wales Hospital, Sydney, Australia, from 1994 to 2016. *J. Med. Imaging Radiat. Oncol.* **2020**, *64*, 450–459. [CrossRef]
28. Mirghani, H.; Mortuaire, G.; Armas, G.L.; Hartl, D.; Aupérin, A.; El Bedoui, S.; Chevalier, D.; Lefebvre, J.L. Sinonasal cancer: Analysis of oncological failures in 156 consecutive cases. *Head Neck* **2013**, *36*, 667–674. [CrossRef]
29. Zocchi, J.; Pietrobon, G.; Campomagnani, I.; Riggi, E.; Veronesi, G.; Borchini, R.; Pellini, R.; Volpi, L.; Bignami, M.; Castelnuovo, P. The role of a post therapeutic surveillance program for sinonasal malignancies: Analysis of 417 patients. *Head Neck* **2019**, *42*, 963–973. [CrossRef]
30. Hanna, E.; DeMonte, F.; Ibrahim, S.; Roberts, D.; Levine, N.; Kupferman, M. Endoscopic Resection of Sinonasal Cancers with and without Craniotomy. *Arch. Otolaryngol. Neck Surg.* **2009**, *135*, 1219–1224. [CrossRef]
31. Blanch, J.L.; Ruiz, A.M.; Alos, L.; Traserra-Coderch, J.; Bernal-Sprekelsen, M. Treatment of 125 Sinonasal Tumors: Prognostic Factors, Outcome, and Follow-up. *Otolaryngol. Neck Surg.* **2004**, *131*, 973–976. [CrossRef]
32. Myers, L.L.; Nussenbaum, B.; Bradford, C.R.; Teknos, T.N.; Esclamado, R.M.; Wolf, G.T. Paranasal Sinus Malignancies: An 18-Year Single Institution Experience. *Laryngoscope* **2002**, *112*, 1964–1969. [CrossRef]
33. Flynn, C.; Khaouam, N.; Gardner, S.; Higgins, K.; Enepekides, D.; Balogh, J.; MacKenzie, R.; Singh, S.; Davidson, J.; Poon, I. The Value of Periodic Follow-up in the Detection of Recurrences after Radical Treatment in Locally Advanced Head and Neck Cancer. *Clin. Oncol.* **2010**, *22*, 868–873. [CrossRef] [PubMed]
34. Kacorzyk, U.; Rutkowski, T.W. The Role of Salvage in the Management of Patients with Sinonasal Squamous Cell Carcinoma. *Biomedicines* **2022**, *10*, 1266. [CrossRef]
35. Michel, G.; Joubert, M.; Delemazure, A.; Espitalier, F.; Durand, N.; Malard, O. Adenoid cystic carcinoma of the paranasal sinuses: Retrospective series and review of the literature. *Eur. Ann. Otorhinolaryngol. Head Neck Dis.* **2013**, *130*, 257–262. [CrossRef] [PubMed]

36. Hoppe, B.S.; Stegman, L.D.; Zelefsky, M.J.; Rosenzweig, K.E.; Wolden, S.L.; Patel, S.G.; Shah, J.P.; Kraus, D.H.; Lee, N.Y. Treatment of nasal cavity and paranasal sinus cancer with modern radiotherapy techniques in the postoperative setting—The MSKCC experience. *Int. J. Radiat. Oncol.* **2007**, *67*, 691–702. [CrossRef] [PubMed]
37. Abdelmeguid, A.S.; Bell, D.; Hanna, E.Y. Sinonasal Undifferentiated Carcinoma. *Curr. Oncol. Rep.* **2019**, *21*, 26. [CrossRef] [PubMed]
38. Jiang, G.; Ang, K.; Peters, L.; Wendt, C.; Oswald, M.; Goepfert, H. Maxillary sinus carcinomas: Natural history and results of postoperative radiotherapy. *Radiother. Oncol.* **1991**, *21*, 193–200. [CrossRef] [PubMed]
39. Jeremic, B.; Shibamoto, Y.; Milicic, B.; Nikolic, N.; Dagovic, A.; Aleksandrovic, J.; Vaskovic, Z.; Tadic, L. Elective ipsilateral neck irradiation of patients with locally advanced maxillary sinus carcinoma. *Cancer* **2000**, *88*, 2246–2251. [CrossRef]
40. Kim, G.E.; Chung, E.J.; Lim, J.J.; Keum, K.C.; Lee, S.W.; Cho, J.H.; Lee, C.G.; Choi, E.C. Clinical significance of neck node metastasis in squamous cell carcinoma of the maxillary antrum. *Am. J. Otolaryngol.* **1999**, *20*, 383–390. [CrossRef]
41. Cantù, G.; Bimbi, G.; Miceli, R.; Mariani, L.; Colombo, S.; Riccio, S.; Squadrelli, M.; Battisti, A.; Pompilio, M.; Rossi, M. Lymph Node Metastases in Malignant Tumors of the Paranasal Sinuses. *Arch. Otolaryngol. Neck Surg.* **2008**, *134*, 170–177. [CrossRef] [PubMed]
42. Atallah, S.; Casiraghi, O.; Fakhry, N.; Wassef, M.; Uro-Coste, E.; Espitalier, F.; Sudaka, A.; Kaminsky, M.C.; Dakpe, S.; Digue, L.; et al. A prospective multicentre REFCOR study of 470 cases of head and neck Adenoid cystic carcinoma: Epidemiology and prognostic factors. *Eur. J. Cancer* **2020**, *130*, 241–249. [CrossRef] [PubMed]
43. Chen, A.M.; Bucci, M.K.; Weinberg, V.; Garcia, J.; Quivey, J.M.; Schechter, N.R.; Phillips, T.L.; Fu, K.K.; Eisele, D.W. Adenoid cystic carcinoma of the head and neck treated by surgery with or without postoperative radiation therapy: Prognostic features of recurrence. *Int. J. Radiat. Oncol.* **2006**, *66*, 152–159. [CrossRef]
44. van Weert, S.; Bloemena, E.; van der Waal, I.; de Bree, R.; Rietveld, D.H.; Kuik, J.D.; Leemans, C.R. Adenoid cystic carcinoma of the head and neck: A single-center analysis of 105 consecutive cases over a 30-year period. *Oral Oncol.* **2013**, *49*, 824–829. [CrossRef] [PubMed]
45. Ciccolallo, L.; Licitra, L.; Cantú, G.; Gatta, G. Survival from salivary glands adenoid cystic carcinoma in European populations. *Oral Oncol.* **2009**, *45*, 669–674. [CrossRef]
46. Lehmann, A.E.; Remenschneider, A.; Dedmon, M.; Meier, J.; Gray, S.T.; Lin, D.T.; Chambers, K.J. Incidence and Survival Patterns of Sinonasal Undifferentiated Carcinoma in the United States. *J. Neurol. Surg. Part B Skull Base* **2014**, *76*, 94–100. [CrossRef]
47. Kuo, P.; Manes, R.P.; Schwam, Z.G.; Judson, B.L. Survival Outcomes for Combined Modality Therapy for Sinonasal Undifferentiated Carcinoma. *Otolaryngol. Head Neck Surg.* **2017**, *156*, 132–136. [CrossRef]
48. Amit, M.; Abdelmeguid, A.S.; Watcherporn, T.; Takahashi, H.; Tam, S.; Bell, D.; Ferrarotto, R.; Glisson, B.; Kupferman, M.E.; Roberts, D.B.; et al. Induction Chemotherapy Response as a Guide for Treatment Optimization in Sinonasal Undifferentiated Carcinoma. *J. Clin. Oncol.* **2019**, *37*, 504–512. [CrossRef]
49. Thomas, T.V.; Abraham, A.; Bhanat, E.; Al Hmada, Y.; Albert, A.; Vijayakumar, S.; Stinger, S.P.; Packianathan, S. Malignant peripheral nerve sheath tumor of nasal cavity and paranasal sinus with 13 years of follow-up—A case report and review of literature. *Clin. Case Rep.* **2019**, *7*, 2194–2201. [CrossRef]
50. Andrä, C.; Rauch, J.; Li, M.; Ganswindt, U.; Belka, C.; Saleh-Ebrahimi, L.; Ballhausen, H.; Nachbichler, S.B.; Roeder, F. Excellent local control and survival after postoperative or definitive radiation therapy for sarcomas of the head and neck. *Radiat. Oncol.* **2015**, *10*, 140. [CrossRef]
51. Koontz, B.F.; Miles, E.F.; Rubio, M.A.D.; Madden, J.F.; Fisher, S.R.; Scher, R.L.; Brizel, D. Preoperative radiotherapy and bevacizumab for angiosarcoma of the head and neck: Two case studies. *Head Neck* **2008**, *30*, 262–266. [CrossRef]
52. Gullane, P.; Kraus, D.; Weber, R. Soft tissue sarcoma. *Head Neck* **2002**, *24*, 296–300. [CrossRef] [PubMed]
53. Dulguerov, P.; Allal, A.S.; Calcaterra, T.C. Esthesioneuroblastoma: A meta-analysis and review. *Lancet Oncol.* **2001**, *2*, 683–690. [CrossRef] [PubMed]
54. Bhayani, M.K.; Yilmaz, T.; Sweeney, A.; Calzada, G.; Roberts, D.B.; Levine, N.B.; DeMonte, F.; Hanna, E.Y.; Kupferman, M.E. Sinonasal adenocarcinoma: A 16-year experience at a single institution. *Head Neck* **2014**, *36*, 1490–1496. [CrossRef]
55. Meccariello, G.; Deganello, A.; Choussy, O.; Gallo, O.; Vitali, D.; De Raucourt, D.; Georgalas, C. Endoscopic nasal versus open approach for the management of sinonasal adenocarcinoma: A pooled-analysis of 1826 patients. *Head Neck* **2015**, *38*, E2267–E2274. [CrossRef] [PubMed]
56. Faisal, M.; Haider, I.; Adeel, M.; Waqas, O.; Hussain, R.; Jamshed, A. Small cell neuroendocrine carcinoma of nose and paranasal sinuses: The Shaukat Khanum Memorial Cancer Hospital experience and review of literature. *J. Pak. Med. Assoc.* **2018**, *68*, 133–136.
57. Bhattacharyya, N.; Thornton, A.F.; Joseph, M.P.; Goodman, M.L.; Amrein, P.C. Successful Treatment of Esthesioneuroblastoma and Neuroendocrine Carcinoma with Combined Chemotherapy and Proton Radiation: Results in 9 Cases. *Arch. Otolaryngol. Neck Surg.* **1997**, *123*, 34–40. [CrossRef]
58. Fitzek, M.M.; Thornton, A.F.; Varvares, M.; Ancukiewicz, M.; Mcintyre, J.; Adams, J.; Rosenthal, S.; Joseph, M.; Amrein, P. Neuroendocrine tumors of the sinonasal tract. *Cancer* **2002**, *94*, 2623–2634. [CrossRef]
59. Babin, E.; Rouleau, V.; Vedrine, O.P.; Toussaint, B.; De Raucourt, D.; Malard, O.; Cosmidis, A.; Makaeieff, M.; Dehesdin, D. Small cell neuroendocrine carcinoma of the nasal cavity and paranasal sinuses. *J. Laryngol. Otol.* **2006**, *120*, 289–297. [CrossRef]

60. Triantafillou, V.; Maina, I.W.; Kuan, E.C.; Kohanski, M.A.; Tong, C.C.; Patel, N.N.; Carey, R.M.; Workman, A.D.; Palmer, J.N.; Adappa, N.D.; et al. Sinonasal mucoepidermoid carcinoma: A review of the National Cancer Database. *Int. Forum Allergy Rhinol.* **2019**, *9*, 1046–1053. [CrossRef]
61. Kshirsagar, R.S.; Eide, J.G.; Brant, J.A.; Palmer, J.N.; Adappa, N.D. Sinonasal Acinic Cell Carcinoma: A Review of the National Cancer Database. *Am. J. Rhinol. Allergy* **2022**, *36*, 741–746. [CrossRef]
62. Biron, V.L.; Lentsch, E.J.; Gerry, D.R.; Bewley, A.F. Case-control analysis of survival outcomes in sinonasal acinic cell carcinoma. *Int. Forum Allergy Rhinol.* **2014**, *4*, 507–511. [CrossRef] [PubMed]
63. Orlandi, E.; Iacovelli, N.A.; Ingargiola, R.; Resteghini, C.; Bossi, P.; Licitra, L.; Ferrari, M.; Nicolai, P. Treatment Options for Recurrent Anterior Skull Base Tumors. *Anterior Skull Base Tumors* **2020**, *84*, 231–245. [CrossRef]
64. Gronchi, A.; Haas, R.L.; Bonvalot, S. Cancer registries and randomised clinical trials in rare tumours: At the two extremes of daily clinical practice. *Eur. J. Cancer* **2016**, *64*, 113–115. [CrossRef] [PubMed]

Disclaimer/Publisher's Note: The statements, opinions and data contained in all publications are solely those of the individual author(s) and contributor(s) and not of MDPI and/or the editor(s). MDPI and/or the editor(s) disclaim responsibility for any injury to people or property resulting from any ideas, methods, instructions or products referred to in the content.

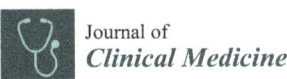

Article

Functioning Endocrine Outcome after Endoscopic Endonasal Transsellar Approach for Pituitary Neuroendocrine Tumors

Gabriele Molteni *, Nicole Caiazza, Gianfranco Fulco, Andrea Sacchetto, Antonio Gulino and Daniele Marchioni

Division of Otorhinolaryngology, Department of Surgery, Dentistry, Gynecology, and Pediatrics, University of Verona, University Hospital of Verona, Piazzale L.A. Scuro, 10, 37134 Verona, Italy
* Correspondence: gabbomolteni@gmail.com; Tel.: +39-0458128333

Abstract: Background: The endoscopic endonasal approach (EEA) is a well-established technique for the treatment of pituitary neuroendocrine tumor Preservation of normal gland tissue is crucial to retain effective neuroendocrine pituitary function. The aim of this paper is to analyze pituitary endocrine secretion after EEA for pituitary neuroendocrine tumor to identify potential predictors of functioning gland recovery. Methods: Patients who underwent an exclusive EEA for pituitary neuroendocrine tumors between October 2014 and November 2019 were reviewed. Patients were divided into groups according to postoperative pituitary function (Group 1, unchanged; group 2, recovering; group 3, worsening). Results: Among the 45 patients enrolled, 15 presented a silent tumor and showed no hormonal impairment, and 30 patients presented pituitary dysfunction. A total of 19 patients (42.2%) were included in group 1, 12 (26.7%) patients showed pituitary function recovery after surgery (group 2), and 14 patients (31.1%) exhibited the onset of new pituitary deficiency postoperatively (group 3). Younger patients and those with functioning tumor were more likely to have complete pituitary hormonal recovery ($p = 0.0297$ and $p = 0.007$, respectively). No predictors of functional gland worsening were identified. Conclusion: EEA for pituitary neuroendocrine tumor is a reliable and safe technique regarding postoperative hormonal function. Preserving pituitary function after tumor resection should be a primary goal in a minimally invasive approach.

Keywords: pituitary neoplasms; pituitary disease; endoscopy; hypopituitarism; treatment outcome

1. Introduction

In recent years, the endoscopic endonasal approach (EEA) has become a well-established and safe technique for the treatment of pituitary neuroendocrine tumor (PitNET) [1–6]. The primary goal of this kind of surgery is the decompression of neurovascular structures surrounding the sellar space, such as the cerebral trunk or optic chiasm; therefore, many studies have been published evaluating factors affecting the extent of resection and clinical recovery from symptoms such as headache and disturbance of visual and olfactory function [7–9]. Concurrent with tumor removal, preservation of normal gland tissue is crucial to provide an effective neuroendocrine pituitary function after surgery, thus avoiding the need for supplementary hormonal therapy. Investigation of pituitary secretion is therefore mandatory to correctly assess the effects of surgery and yet few reports have been published on this topic [10–13].

The aim of this preliminary report is to analyze pituitary endocrine secretion after EEA for pitNET performed at our institution in order to identify potential predictors of functional gland recovery or worsening.

2. Materials and Methods

A retrospective chart review was conducted on patients who underwent an EEA for treatment of pitNET between October 2014 and November 2019 at our Referral Skull Base Center. Inclusion criteria were: (1) exclusive EEA approach to the tumor, (2) tumor

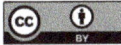

diameter > 1 cm in any plane, (3) postoperative histologically confirmed diagnosis of pitNET. Pituitary microadenomas were excluded because their small size prevents a mass effect on the surrounding normal gland tissue; therefore, in these cases, preoperative and postoperative hormonal impairment related to mass effect and surgical maneuvers, respectively, are generally not observed.

Patients underwent a preoperative and postoperative (3 months after surgery) dedicated magnetic resonance imaging (MRI) pituitary protocol. Radiological characteristics were evaluated first by one of the authors and then validated by a second observer with emphasis on T1 contrast enhanced and T2 sequences in axial, coronal, and sagittal images. Tumor size was assessed by measuring its major axis in any plane. Cavernous sinus invasion was graded according to the modified Knosp score [14,15] and this grading was confirmed in all cases by surgical evidence, intraoperatively.

The extent of resection was classified, based on the 3-month postoperative MRI, as follows: (1) Gross total resection (GTR), when there was absence of residual tumoral tissue, (2) Near-total resection (NTR), in cases showing a small tumoral residual, recognized in at least two consecutive MRI slices and in two different planes, close to neurovascular structures (optic chiasm, healthy pituitary gland, internal carotid artery), despite the fact that a complete resection had been planned, (3) Subtotal resection (STR), when only a debulking was preoperatively planned for a giant invasive pituitary tumor. In these patients, the main goal was decompression of neurovascular structures to restore or prevent worsening of neurological symptoms.

Laboratory tests were used to define hormonal pituitary assessment; pituitary function was evaluated preoperatively and 6 months postoperatively in all patients. No dynamic measurements were performed. Thyroid gland-related hypothyroidism was not contemplated as a defect in this study.

Endocrine evaluation included five adeno–pituitary axes: adrenocorticotropic hormone (ACTH, reference values between 1.80 and 13.20 pmol/L) and cortisol (reference values between 133 and 537 nmol/L); thyroid-stimulating hormone (TSH, reference values between 0.30 and 4.20 mUI/L) and free T4 (reference values between 11.0 and 22.0 pmol/L); growth hormone (GH, reference value lower than 7.00 microg/L) and insulin-like growth factor 1 (IGF-1, reference values between 8.00 and 26.00 nmol/L); prolactin (PRL, reference values between 102 and 496 mIU/L); follicle-stimulating hormone (FSH, reference value according to the ovarian cycle), and luteinizing hormone (LH, reference value according to ovarian cycle), and, depending on patient sex, estradiol and/or free and total testosterone. To assess ACTH deficiency and the presence of ACTH secerning tumor, ACTH and cortisol blood levels were analyzed [16]. To determine GH deficiency, the measurements of IGF-1 were considered. Low serum IGF-I levels in patients with ≥3 additional pituitary hormone deficiencies after pituitary surgery diagnosed GH deficiency in the absence of GH stimulation testing [17,18].

To evaluate posterior pituitary gland function, urine osmolarity was checked. The diagnosis of postoperative insipidus diabetes was based on polyuria with low urine osmolarity [19].

Data were collected in a Microsoft Excel (Microsoft Corp., Redmond, WA, USA) spreadsheet and updated periodically.

Patients were divided into three groups based on their postoperative pituitary function compared to the preoperative function, as follows. Unchanging group (group 1): patients showing unchanged pituitary function after surgery. Recovering group (group 2): patients with a postoperative improvement in pituitary function. Worsening group (group 3): patients with postoperative worsening of pituitary function.

We decided to evaluate the factors which could be potential predictors of gland recovery or deficiency after surgery. We analyzed the impact of sex, age, maximum tumor diameter, Knosp grade, presence of tumoral residual, presence of functioning tumor, previous surgery, and intraoperative cerebrospinal fluid (CSF) leakage.

Statistical analysis was performed by Fisher's exact test and Student's t-test to assess differences between groups. Statistical significance was assessed at the level $\alpha = 0.05$. The normality of data distribution was assessed with the Kolmogorov-Smirnov test. The assessment of the normality of data distribution was performed as a prerequisite for Fisher's exact test and Student's t-test.

3. Results

Among a total of 47 patients who underwent an EEA for pitNET at our Referral Skull Base Center in the period examined, based on inclusion criteria, 45 were admitted to this study.

3.1. Patient Demographics

Out of 45 patients enrolled, 26 were male (57.7%), and 19 were female (42.3%). Age at time of surgery ranged from 21 to 79 years (mean age 56.9, SD 14.5).

3.2. Radiological Characteristics: Tumor Size and Knosp Grade

Preoperative MRI demonstrated a mean maximum tumor diameter of 28.13 mm (range, 12–79 mm, SD 14.24).

Knosp grade was 0 in 9 patients (20%), 1 in 12 patients (26.7%), 2 in 12 patients (26.7%), 3 in 1 patient (2.2%) and 4 in 11 patients (24.4%). Cavernous sinus invasion (Knosp grade 3 and 4) was observed radiographically in 12 patients (26.7%).

3.3. Extent of Resection

A standard fully endoscopic transsphenoidal transsellar approach was conducted in most cases (73.3%, 33 patients). The remaining 12 patients (26.7%) underwent an expanded transsellar-trans-planum approach. GTR was achieved in 33 (73.3%) patients, NTR in 10 (22.2%) patients and STR in 2 (4.4%) patients. Suprasellar cistern invasion was seen in 16 patients (35.5%). Therefore, the presence of residual tumoral tissue was observed overall in 12 (26.7%) patients.

3.4. History of Previous Pituitary Surgery

A total of eight patients (17.8%) had presented with recurrent tumors after previous transsphenoidal surgery at another hospital center.

3.5. Preoperative Pituitary Function

Among the 45 patients, 15 presented with a silent tumor and showed no hormonal impairment, while 30 patients presented with preoperative pituitary dysfunction: 16 patients presented a functioning tumor and 14 patients presented a silent tumor with a deficit disorder in at least 1 hormonal release.

Among the functioning tumor patients (16), 7/16 presented growth hormone (GH) secreting tumors, 7/16 medically resistant prolactinomas (PRL), 1/16 thyroid-stimulating hormone (TSH) and 1/16 adrenocorticotrophic hormone (ACTH) secreting tumor. Four out of 16 patients also had hypofunctional pituitary changes, with deficit disorders in at least 1 hormone.

Among the silent tumor patients (29), 15/29 presented no hormonal impairment and 14/29 a deficit disorder, 8/14 presented hypogonadism, 8/14 hypothyroidism, 6/14 hypoadrenalism, and 3/14 GH-deficit. PRL was oversecreted in 3/14 patients (due to pituitary stalk compression) and under-secreted in 3/14 patients. No patient presented diabetes insipidus.

3.6. Postoperative Pituitary Function

Overall, postoperative pituitary function in our series was unchanged or improved in 21 patients (46.7%), whereas in 24 patients (53.3%) a new hormonal deficiency was observed in at least one hormonal axis. The mean functional deficiency was 2.7 hormones, with the loss of at least three hormones in 8 (17.8%) patients. Considering the type of hormonal imbalance after surgery, we reported 17 patients (37.7%) with hypoadrenalism, 11 patients (24.4%) with hypogonadism, 19 patients (42.2%) with hypothyroidism, three patients (6.6%) with GH deficit, and three patients (6.6%) with PRL deficit. Finally, two patients (4.4%) developed persistent diabetes insipidus, treated continuously with desmopressin.

Among the 16 patients with functioning tumor, eight cases showed a normalization of pituitary function after surgery. Eight patients presented a deficiency in at least one hormonal axis: in three patients the hormonal deficiency was also present before surgery, while five patients developed a new deficit in one or more hormonal release after the transsphenoidal transsellar approach. Out of the last wight patients with pituitary deficiency, four patients showed the persistence of hormonal hypersecretion observed preoperatively (one GH and three PRL secreting tumor).

Among the 29 patients affected by a silent tumor, nine patients showed a new deficit in at least in one hormonal axis postoperatively. Nine patients with normal preoperative pituitary function did not show any deficit after surgery, seven patients with a preoperatively deficit in at least one hormonal release maintained the same deficiency after surgery, while four patients, with at least one preoperative hormonal deficiency, exhibited a completely pituitary gland recovery after EEA. Further details regarding all patients' hormonal results are reported in the Supplementary Materials.

Patients were sub-classified into three groups according to hormonal secretion detected preoperatively and 6 months after surgery.

A total of 19 patients (42.2%) were included in the unchanging group (group 1): in nine cases (20%), a normal preoperative pituitary function persisting after surgery was observed, whereas in 10 patients (22.2%), the hormonal deficiency detected before surgery remained unchanged postoperatively. The recovering group (group 2) consisted of 12 (26.7%) patients showing pituitary function normalization postoperatively. A total of 14 patients (31.1%) were included in the worsening group (group 3), exhibiting the onset of a new pituitary deficiency postoperatively.

3.7. Recovering Group Characteristics (Group 2)

The characteristics of the 12 patients who presented complete pituitary recovery after surgery in terms of demographics, secreting tumor, tumor size, and extent of resection are shown in Table 1.

Table 1. Features' description for patients who showed a pituitary gland recovery after endoscopic transsphenoidal surgery (group 2).

#	Age	Sex	Maximum Diameters (mm)	KNOSP Grade	Resection	Functioning pitNET	Prior Surgery	Intraoperative CSF Leak	Type of Impairment after Surgery
1	53	M	15	1	GTR	Yes (GH)	No	No	-
2	43	M	19	0	GTR	No	No	No	-
3	43	F	20	0	NTR	No	No	No	-
4	47	M	25	2	GTR	No	No	No	-
5	33	M	51	4	NTR	Yes (TSH)	No	No	-
6	50	F	18	0	GTR	Yes (ACTH)	No	No	-
7	58	F	42	4	GTR	Yes (PRL)	No	No	-
8	30	F	18	1	GTR	No	No	No	-
9	69	M	12	1	GTR	Yes (GH)	No	No	-
10	72	F	13	1	GTR	Yes (GH)	No	No	-
11	64	F	12	0	GTR	Yes (GH)	No	No	-
12	25	F	21	1	GTR	Yes (PRL)	No	Yes	-

3.8. Worsening Group Characteristics (Group 3)

Out of 14 patients, five (35.7%) presented a functioning tumor. The mean age was 59 years (S.D. ± 14.3). The mean maximum diameter of treated pitNET was 29.1 mm (S.D. ± 15.6 mm). Knosp grade was 0 in two patients (14.3%), 1 in two patients (14.3%), 2 in six patients (42.9%), 3 in one patient (7.1%) and 4 in three patients (21.4%). Eleven patients underwent GTR, in two patients we performed a near total resection and in one patient a debulking of the lesion. The mean hormone deficiency was 2.7 and the hormones involved were TSH in 12/14, ACTH in 11/14, and gonadotropin in 7/14. Impairment in GH/IGF-1 release was detected in three patients; prolactin deficiency was found in three patients. No diabetes insipidus was identified in this group. Among this group, two patients had undergone previous surgery. Intraoperative CSF leak was observed in four patients. The features of patients in group 3 are summarized in Table 2.

Table 2. Features' description for patients who exhibited the onset of new pituitary deficiency after endoscopic transsphenoidal surgery (group 3). Legend: ↓: under the reference value; ↑: over the reference value.

#	Age	Sex	Maximum Diameters (mm)	KNOSP Grade	Resection	Functioning pitNET	Prior Surgery	Intraoperative CSF Leak	Type of Impairment after Surgery
1	21	M	21	0	GTR	Yes (PRL)	No	No	TSH, LH/FSH ↓ PRL ↑
2	60	M	58	2	NTR	No	No	Yes	ACTH, TSH, LH/FSH ↓
3	52	M	12	0	GTR	Yes (GH)	No	No	TSH, PRL ↓ GH/IGF-1 ↑
4	49	M	32	2	GTR	No	No	No	ACTH, TSH, LH/FSH, PRL ↓
5	65	M	62	3	NTR	No	Yes	Yes	ACTH, TSH, LH/FSH and GH/IGF-1 ↓
6	67	F	17	2	GTR	No	Yes	No	TSH ↓
7	64	F	22	2	GTR	Yes (PRL)	No	No	ACTH, TSH ↓
8	53	M	15	1	GTR	Yes (GH)	No	No	ACTH, TSH, LH/FSH, PRL ↓
9	55	M	24	2	GTR	No	No	No	ACTH, TSH, LH/FSH, GH/IGF-1 ↓
10	77	M	25	4	GTR	No	No	No	ACTH ↓
11	51	M	15	2	GTR	Yes (GH)	No	No	ACTH, TSH ↓
12	66	M	31	1	GTR	No	No	No	ACTH ↓
13	67	F	28	4	GTR	No	No	Yes	ACTH, TSH ↓
14	79	M	45	4	STR	No	No	Yes	ACTH, TSH, LH/FSH, GH/IGF-1 ↓

3.9. Predictors of Pituitary Function Recovery or Worsening

Sex, maximum diameter, Knosp grade, tumoral residual and intraoperative CSF leak were not predictors of gland recovery. Younger patients ($p = 0.0297$) and those with functioning tumor ($p = 0.007$) were more likely to have complete pituitary hormonal recovery, as shown in Table 3.

Table 3. Predictors of gland recovery following transsphenoidal surgery. p values < 0.05 are shown in bold.

Predictor	Group 1	Group 2	p Value
N. patients	19	12	
Age in years, mean (±SD)	60.5 (±12.7)	48.9 (±15.1)	**0.0297**
Male sex, number (%)	11 (57.9%)	4 (33.3%)	0.2734
Maximum diameter, mm mean (±SD)	31.2 (±13.9)	22 (±12.1)	0.0753
KNOSP grade			
0–2	13	10	0.4325
3–4	6	2	
Tumoral residual	7	2	0.4184
Functioning pitNET	3	8	**0.007**
Prior surgery	6	0	0.0585
Intraoperative CSF leak	4	1	0.6236

The results were not statistically significant for all the factors tested ($p > 0.2$ in all cases) with regard to pituitary gland worsening (Table 4).

Table 4. Predictors of new pituitary gland deficiency following transsphenoidal surgery.

Predictor	Group 1	Group 3	p Value
N. patients	19	14	
Age in years, mean (±SD)	60.5 (±12.7)	59 (±14.3)	0.7577
Male sex, n (%)	11 (57.9%)	11 (78.6%)	0.2783
Maximum diameter, mm mean (±SD)	31.2 (±13.9)	29.1 (±15.6)	0.6819
KNOSP grade			
0–2	13	10	1
3–4	6	4	
Tumoral residual	7	3	0.4551
Functioning pitNET	3	5	0.2379
Prior surgery	6	2	0.4157
Intraoperative CSF leak	4	4	0.6951

3.10. Patients Affected by Silent and Functioning Tumor: Sub-Classification into the Three Groups According to Hormonal Secretion

Among the 29 patients affected by silent tumors, 16 (55.2%) presented an unchanged pituitary function after surgery (group 1), nine (31%) showed a postoperative new hormonal deficiency (group 3) and only four (13.8%) exhibited a completely pituitary gland recovery (group 2).

The 16 patients affected by functioning tumors demonstrated a complete normalization of the pituitary function postoperatively (group 2) in eight cases (50%); three (18.7%) patients were included in the unchanged group (group 1) and five (31.3%) patients developed a deficiency in at least one hormonal release (group 3) after EEA.

The features of each group according to sex, age at time of surgery, maximum diameter, Knosp grade and tumoral residual are displayed in Table 5. Because of the limited sample size, the comparison between groups did not provide statistically significant data.

Table 5. Features' description for silent tumors and functioning tumors' patients subclassified into three groups according to postoperative pituitary gland function.

	Silent Tumors (29 Patients)		
Variables	Group 1	Group 2	Group 3
N. patients	16	4	9
Age in years, mean (± SD)	64.5 (±9.1)	40.75 (±7.41)	65 (±9.55)
Male sex, number (%)	9 (56.25%)	2 (50%)	7 (77.8%)
Maximum diameter, mm mean (± SD)	31.81 (±15.17)	20.5 (±3.10)	35.8 (±15.69)
KNOSP grade			
0–2	12	4	5
3–4	4	0	4
Tumoral residual	6	1	3
	Functioning Tumors (16 Patients)		
Variables	Group 1	Group 2	Group 3
N. patients	3	8	5
Age in years, mean (±SD)	39 (±3.60)	53 (±16.71)	48.2 (±16.08)
Male sex, number (%)	2 (66.7%)	2 (25%)	4 (80%)
Maximum diameter, mm mean (±SD)	28 (±1.73)	23 (±15.02)	17 (±4.30)
KNOSP grade			
0–2	1	6	5
3–4	2	2	0
Tumoral residual	1	1	0

4. Discussion

Since its first report in 1992, a fully endoscopic endonasal approach to sellar lesions has become increasingly common and is actually considered the first choice for surgical treatment of pitNET [20]. In fact, the EEA shows similar rates of GTR and perioperative mortality [21–25] as for classic craniofacial approaches and ensures a better quality of life [1,13,26,27]. The main goal of these approaches is to remove pathological tissue to reduce the mass effect on critical neurovascular structures in close relationship to sellar space, especially the optic chiasm, interpeduncular and prepontine cisterns and brainstem. On this basis, in the last decade, many reports have been published on the outcomes of this surgery, with special regard to the extent of resection and its relationship to recovery from symptoms, especially headache, and disturbance of visual and olfactory function [7,8]. In addition, another key point during surgical maneuvers is the visualization and preservation of the unaffected gland tissue encased or displaced by the pathological tissue. This step is crucial in providing an effective neuroendocrine pituitary function after surgery, thus avoiding the need for supplementary hormonal therapy. The analysis of hormonal secretion is therefore a necessary step to correctly assess the effects of this kind of surgery on pituitary function, and several reports have been published on this topic [10–13].

Among the 45 patients in this study, 14 (31.1%) displayed a postoperative loss in at least one hormone (worsening group, group 3), 12 patients (26.7%) with preoperative hormonal impairment showed complete recovery of hormonal secretion (recovering group, group 2), whereas in 19 patients (42.2%), no change in gland functioning was detected (unchanging group, group 1). A multicenter prospective study conducted by Little et al. (2019) [13] reported that 21.1% of patients (20/95) experienced recovery in at least one axis, whereas 9.7% of patients (14/145) had developed at least one new deficiency. Elshazly et al. [28] evaluated 55 patients with giant pituitary tumor (>4 cm in maximum diameter) who underwent surgery with an EEA. A new hormonal deficit occurred in eight patients, whereas recovery of one or more hormonal axis deficits occurred in six patients. In the study conducted by Do et al. [29] on recurrent pituitary tumor, 14.8% of patients (9/61) developed single or multiple new anterior pituitary deficits after first surgical treatment.

With regard to the onset of new postoperative hormonal deficiency, the rate of hormonal loss observed in our experience was higher than in the aforementioned reports. Despite a challenging comparison, due to the absence of standardized benchmarks, we analyzed the patients in the worsening group to clarify these data. In 42.8% of cases (6/14 patients), a supradiaphragmatic or para-sellar space invasion was observed. Although the relationship with suprasellar involvement and Knosp grade was not statistically significant, this result supports the idea that increasing tumor mass may lead to ischemic injury or direct destruction of healthy pituitary parenchyma, thus resulting in hormonal loss. This claim clearly needs to be verified by studies with a larger sample size, but nonetheless it is in agreement with the findings of other authors [27].

Regarding the type of hormonal deficiencies observed in the worsening group, in our study population the most common deficit reported was thyrotropin hormone (TSH), followed by adrenocortical hormone (ACTH) and gonadotropin (FSH/LH). This result is in contrast to other reports [30], where ACTH was the most frequently detected deficit after surgery, but at present there is insufficient data to clarify these differences.

An intriguing argument concerns the onset of postoperative diabetes insipidus, a rare complication of the EEA that is most frequently found in its transient form. Nayak et al. [31] revealed permanent diabetes insipidus onset in 4% of patients who underwent EEA. In their series of 271 patients, the presence of visual abnormalities, suprasellar extension, and maximal tumor diameter was significantly associated with an increased incidence of postoperative diabetes insipidus, both transient and permanent. In our series, no patient presented insipidus diabetes preoperatively. Because of the laboratory tests for hormonal pituitary assessment at 6 months postoperatively, transient diabetes insipidus was not evaluated in this study. Two patients (4.4%) developed persistent insipidus diabetes after surgery, treated continuously with desmopressin. Given the small sample size, it is not possible to perform a statistical analysis. Nonetheless, it is interesting to note that diabetes insipidus occurred in two patients with giant tumor with suprasellar involvement, and in which a CFS leak emerged during surgery. In our opinion, this finding suggests that extensive surgical manipulation, as in the event of a CSF leak, can lead to trauma to the gland or infundibulum tissue.

With regard to the recovering group, our findings are in accordance with those reported in several studies, in which recovery of preoperative hormonal deficits occurred in 10–30% of cases, varying from type to involvement of the lesions [12,28,30,32]. As a further observation, considering both the recovering and unchanging groups, in 68.9% of cases, no worsening of pituitary function was observed.

To better clarify the data analysis, we decided to focus our attention on selected potential predictors of postoperative function recovery or worsening. Considering tumor size, Fatemi et al. [10] demonstrated that, the larger the tumor, the greater the risk of pituitary gland failure; they indicated a size of 20 mm as the upper limit; beyond 20 mm, the pituitary failure rate is increased. In our cohort, among the 31 patients with tumor size > 20 mm, 10 experienced postoperative new hormonal loss (32.2%), whereas out of 14 patients with tumor size <20 mm, four (28.6%) showed a new deficiency. Even though this result was not statistically significant, we believe this finding is probably related to the greater surgical handling occurring in larger tumors. In addition, as previously reported by Nomikos et al. [27], it is interesting to observe that tumor size affected gonadotropin release more than other hormonal axes. In fact, we detected 11 cases with postoperative gonadal loss and these patients presented a mean maximum tumor diameter of 38.2 mm.

While surgery to an increasing size of tumor has a negative impact on the function of healthy gland tissue postoperatively, removal of that tumor mass may lead to a greater improvement in hormonal release, due to the mass decompression effect. In this regard, the main regularized hormone after surgery in our series was prolactin, followed by stabilization of gonadotropin and adrenocortical hormone deficiency. Previous studies on this topic [27,33] observed that preoperative hyperprolactinemia typically results from compression of the pituitary stalk, and decompression maneuvers mainly affect prolactin release compared with other hormones; thus, prolactin blood level could be considered a useful predictor of postoperative recovery of pituitary function [27,33]. Infundibular compression is the main mechanism, affecting the delivery of hypothalamic hormones and determining hypopituitarism, thus explaining the better recovery rate in these patients.

Regarding the role of functioning tumor in conditioning postoperative gland function, a few studies have evaluated the impact of the EEA on enhanced hormonal secretion. In a series of 142 prolactinomas, Akin et al. [34] showed that 74.6% of patients went into remission after the EEA. Concerning GH-secreting pitNET, endocrinological cure was achieved in 46–61% of patients after the EEA [35–38]. The presence of a functioning tumor was a strong predictor of postoperative gland recovery ($p = 0.007$). According to the authors, this result was not related to tumor size, but to the earlier diagnosis in functioning compared to silent tumors.

Furthermore, in agreement with the report by Webb and colleagues [30], the rate of complete hypopituitarism recovery in patients with GH releasing tumor was greater than in the other patients (4/7); these patients were typically younger, and both the hormonal therapy before surgery and their high IGF-1 levels helped to preserve pituitary gland activity.

As reported by other authors [10,27], in our cohort, age was a significant predictor of pituitary restoration ($p = 0.0297$): younger patients presented a better pituitary function after endoscopic surgery compared to the others, despite preoperative pituitary gland status or tumor size.

The last noteworthy consideration concerns the role of the intraoperative CSF leak. Fatemi et al. [10] observed that this is related to a worse hormonal postoperative function and reflects the more extensive surgical manipulation of the infundibulum and gland. Although, in our series, the statistical analysis did not reveal a significant result, among nine patients who experienced intraoperative CSF leak, only one presented postoperative pituitary gland recovery. Furthermore, this finding could be predictive of permanent diabetes insipidus [39]. In fact, both patients who developed persistent diabetes insipidus showed a dural defect with an intraoperative CSF leak.

This study may help to establish standardized benchmarks in the evaluation of functional pituitary outcome after endoscopic approaches to pitNET.

The absence of hormones' dynamic measurements and the low sample size are the main limitations of this study, and these preliminary results need to be validated in studies with a larger sample size.

5. Conclusions

This preliminary report confirms that EEA for pitNET is a reliable technique with regard to postoperative hormonal function. This is supported by the finding that only a minority of patients needed replacement hormonal therapy after surgery. The young age and the presence of functioning tumor proved to be predictors of functional gland recovery after surgery. No predictors of functional gland worsening were identified in our cohort. Nonetheless, the increasing size of the tumor and the presence of intraoperative CSF leak may play a role in the development of new postoperative hormonal loss. This finding could be related to more extensive surgical manipulation, as already reported in other experiences. Preserving pituitary function after pitNET resection is crucial for patients' hormonal balance and this should be a primary goal in a minimally invasive approach.

Supplementary Materials: The following supporting information can be downloaded at: https://www.mdpi.com/article/10.3390/jcm12082986/s1.

Author Contributions: G.M.: Conceptualization, Supervision; N.C.: Methodology, Data curation, Writing—Original draft preparation, Visualization; G.F.: Data curation, Writing—Original draft preparation; A.S.: Reviewing; A.G.: Conceptualization, Reviewing; D.M.: Supervision, Investigation. All authors have read and agreed to the published version of the manuscript.

Funding: The authors did not receive any grant for this study from funding agencies in the public, commercial or not-for profit sectors.

Institutional Review Board Statement: All procedures performed in studies involving human participants were in accordance with the ethical standards of the institutional and national research committee and with the 1964 Helsinki Declaration.

Informed Consent Statement: Informed consent was obtained from all individual participants included in the study.

Data Availability Statement: Full data are available from the corresponding author upon request.

Conflicts of Interest: The authors declare that the study was conducted in the absence of any commercial or financial relationships that could be construed as a potential conflict of interest.

References

1. Gao, Y.; Zhong, C.; Wang, Y.; Xu, S.; Guo, Y.; Dai, C.; Zheng, Y.; Wang, Y.; Luo, Q.; Jiang, J. Endoscopic versus microscopic transsphenoidal pituitary adenoma surgery: A meta-analysis. *World J. Surg. Oncol.* **2014**, *12*, 94. [CrossRef] [PubMed]
2. Goudakos, J.K.; Markou, K.D.; Georgalas, C. Endoscopic versus microscopic trans-sphenoidal pituitary surgery: A systematic review and meta-analysis. *Clin. Otolaryngol.* **2011**, *36*, 212–220. [CrossRef] [PubMed]
3. Frank, G.; Pasquini, E.; Farneti, G.; Mazzatenta, D.; Sciarretta, V.; Grasso, V.; Faustini Fustini, M. The endoscopic versus the traditional approach in pituitary surgery. *Neuroendocrinology* **2006**, *83*, 240–248. [CrossRef] [PubMed]
4. DeKlotz, T.R.; Chia, S.H.; Lu, W.; Makambi, K.H.; Aulisi, E.; Deeb, Z. Meta-analysis of endoscopic versus sublabial pituitary surgery. *Laryngoscope* **2012**, *122*, 511–518. [CrossRef] [PubMed]
5. Liu, H.; Zhou, Y.; Chen, Y.; Wang, Q.; Zhang, H.; Xu, Y. Treatment outcomes of neuroendoscopic and microscopic trans-sphoidal pituitary adenomectomies and the effects on hormone levels. *Minerva Surg.* **2023**. [CrossRef]
6. Molteni, G.; Sacchetto, A.; Saccardo, T.; Gulino, A.; Marchioni, D. Quality of Life Evaluation After Trans-Nasal Endoscopic Surgery for Skull Base Tumors. *Am. J. Rhinol. Allergy* **2021**, *35*, 507–515. [CrossRef]
7. Dallapiazza, R.F.; Grober, Y.; Starke, R.M.; Laws, E.R.; Jane, J.A. Long-term results of endonasal endoscopic transsphenoidal resection of nonfunctioning pituitary macroadenomas. *Neurosurgery* **2015**, *76*, 42–52; discussion 52–53. [CrossRef]
8. Netuka, D.; Masopust, V.; Fundová, P.; Astl, J.; Školoudík, D.; Májovský, M.; Beneš, V. Olfactory Results of Endoscopic Endonasal Surgery for Pituitary Adenoma: A Prospective Study of 143 Patients. *World Neurosurg.* **2019**, *129*, e907–e914. [CrossRef]
9. Layard Horsfall, H.; Lawrence, A.; Venkatesh, A.; Loh, R.T.S.; Jayapalan, R.; Koulouri, O.; Sharma, R.; Santarius, T.; Gurnell, M.; Dorward, N.; et al. Reported outcomes in transsphenoidal surgery for pituitary adenomas: A systematic review. *Pituitary* **2023**. [CrossRef]
10. Fatemi, N.; Dusick, J.R.; Mattozo, C.; McArthur, D.L.; Cohan, P.; Boscardin, J.; Wang, C.; Swerdloff, R.S.; Kelly, D.F. Pituitary hormonal loss and recovery after transsphenoidal adenoma removal. *Neurosurgery* **2008**, *63*, 709–718; discussion 718–719. [CrossRef]
11. Iglesias, P.; Arcano, K.; Triviño, V.; García-Sancho, P.; Díez, J.J.; Cordido, F.; Villabona, C. Non-functioning pituitary adenoma underwent surgery: A multicenter retrospective study over the last four decades (1977–2015). *Eur. J. Intern. Med.* **2017**, *41*, 62–67. [CrossRef] [PubMed]
12. Laws, E.R.; Iuliano, S.L.; Cote, D.J.; Woodmansee, W.; Hsu, L.; Cho, C.H. A Benchmark for Preservation of Normal Pituitary Function After Endoscopic Transsphenoidal Surgery for Pituitary Macroadenomas. *World Neurosurg.* **2016**, *91*, 371–375. [CrossRef] [PubMed]
13. Little, A.S.; Gardner, P.A.; Fernandez-Miranda, J.C.; Chicoine, M.R.; Barkhoudarian, G.; Prevedello, D.M.; Yuen, K.C.J.; Kelly, D.F.; TRANSSPHER Study Group. Pituitary gland recovery following fully endoscopic transsphenoidal surgery for nonfunctioning pituitary adenoma: Results of a prospective multicenter study. *J. Neurosurg.* **2019**, *133*, 1732–1738. [CrossRef] [PubMed]
14. Knosp, E.; Steiner, E.; Kitz, K.; Matula, C. Pituitary adenomas with invasion of the cavernous sinus space: A magnetic resonance imaging classification compared with surgical findings. *Neurosurgery* **1993**, *33*, 610–617; discussion 617–618. [CrossRef]
15. Micko, A.S.G.; Wöhrer, A.; Wolfsberger, S.; Knosp, E. Invasion of the cavernous sinus space in pituitary adenomas: Endoscopic verification and its correlation with an MRI-based classification. *J. Neurosurg.* **2015**, *122*, 803–811. [CrossRef]
16. van Aken, M.O.; Lamberts, S.W.J. Diagnosis and treatment of hypopituitarism: An update. *Pituitary* **2005**, *8*, 183–191. [CrossRef]
17. Tritos, N.A.; Biller, B.M.K. Current concepts of the diagnosis of adult growth hormone deficiency. *Rev. Endocr. Metab. Disord.* **2021**, *22*, 109–116. [CrossRef]

18. Hartman, M.L.; Crowe, B.J.; Biller, B.M.K.; Ho, K.K.Y.; Clemmons, D.R.; Chipman, J.J.; HyposCCS Advisory Board; U.S. HypoCCS Study Group. Which patients do not require a GH stimulation test for the diagnosis of adult GH deficiency? *J. Clin. Endocrinol. Metab.* **2002**, *87*, 477–485. [CrossRef]
19. Lamas, C.; del Pozo, C.; Villabona, C. Neuroendocrinology Group of the SEEN Clinical guidelines for management of diabetes insipidus and syndrome of inappropriate antidiuretic hormone secretion after pituitary surgery. *Endocrinol. Nutr. Organo Soc. Espanola Endocrinol. Nutr.* **2014**, *61*, e15–e24. [CrossRef]
20. Jho, H.-D.; Carrau, R.L. Endoscopic endonasal transsphenoidal surgery: Experience with 50 patients. *J. Neurosurg.* **1997**, *87*, 44–51. [CrossRef]
21. Graffeo, C.S.; Dietrich, A.R.; Grobelny, B.; Zhang, M.; Goldberg, J.D.; Golfinos, J.G.; Lebowitz, R.; Kleinberg, D.; Placantonakis, D.G. A panoramic view of the skull base: Systematic review of open and endoscopic endonasal approaches to four tumors. *Pituitary* **2014**, *17*, 349–356. [CrossRef] [PubMed]
22. Komotar, R.J.; Starke, R.M.; Raper, D.M.S.; Anand, V.K.; Schwartz, T.H. Endoscopic skull base surgery: A comprehensive comparison with open transcranial approaches. *Br. J. Neurosurg.* **2012**, *26*, 637–648. [CrossRef] [PubMed]
23. Batra, P.S.; Luong, A.; Kanowitz, S.J.; Sade, B.; Lee, J.; Lanza, D.C.; Citardi, M.J. Outcomes of minimally invasive endoscopic resection of anterior skull base neoplasms. *Laryngoscope* **2010**, *120*, 9–16. [CrossRef] [PubMed]
24. Asemota, A.O.; Ishii, M.; Brem, H.; Gallia, G.L. Comparison of Complications, Trends, and Costs in Endoscopic vs Microscopic Pituitary Surgery: Analysis from a US Health Claims Database. *Neurosurgery* **2017**, *81*, 458–472. [CrossRef] [PubMed]
25. Azad, T.D.; Lee, Y.-J.; Vail, D.; Veeravagu, A.; Hwang, P.H.; Ratliff, J.K.; Li, G. Endoscopic vs. Microscopic Resection of Sellar Lesions-A Matched Analysis of Clinical and Socioeconomic Outcomes. *Front. Surg.* **2017**, *4*, 33. [CrossRef]
26. Hansasuta, A.; Pokanan, S.; Punyawai, P.; Mahattanakul, W. Evolution of Technique in Endoscopic Transsphenoidal Surgery for Pituitary Adenoma: A Single Institution Experience from 220 Procedures. *Cureus* **2018**, *10*, e2010. [CrossRef]
27. Nomikos, P.; Ladar, C.; Fahlbusch, R.; Buchfelder, M. Impact of primary surgery on pituitary function in patients with non-functioning pituitary adenomas—A study on 721 patients. *Acta Neurochir.* **2004**, *146*, 27–35. [CrossRef]
28. Elshazly, K.; Kshettry, V.R.; Farrell, C.J.; Nyquist, G.; Rosen, M.; Evans, J.J. Clinical Outcomes After Endoscopic Endonasal Resection of Giant Pituitary Adenomas. *World Neurosurg.* **2018**, *114*, e447–e456. [CrossRef]
29. Do, H.; Kshettry, V.R.; Siu, A.; Belinsky, I.; Farrell, C.J.; Nyquist, G.; Rosen, M.; Evans, J.J. Extent of Resection, Visual, and Endocrinologic Outcomes for Endoscopic Endonasal Surgery for Recurrent Pituitary Adenomas. *World Neurosurg.* **2017**, *102*, 35–41. [CrossRef]
30. Webb, S.M.; Rigla, M.; Wägner, A.; Oliver, B.; Bartumeus, F. Recovery of hypopituitarism after neurosurgical treatment of pituitary adenomas. *J. Clin. Endocrinol. Metab.* **1999**, *84*, 3696–3700. [CrossRef]
31. Nayak, P.; Montaser, A.S.; Hu, J.; Prevedello, D.M.; Kirschner, L.S.; Ghalib, L. Predictors of Postoperative Diabetes Insipidus Following Endoscopic Resection of Pituitary Adenomas. *J. Endocr. Soc.* **2018**, *2*, 1010–1019. [CrossRef] [PubMed]
32. Yildirim, A.E.; Sahinoglu, M.; Ekici, I.; Cagil, E.; Karaoglu, D.; Celik, H.; Nacar, O.A.; Belen, A.D. Nonfunctioning Pituitary Adenomas Are Really Clinically Nonfunctioning? Clinical and Endocrinological Symptoms and Outcomes with Endoscopic Endonasal Treatment. *World Neurosurg.* **2016**, *85*, 185–192. [CrossRef] [PubMed]
33. Arafah, B.M.; Nekl, K.E.; Gold, R.S.; Selman, W.R. Dynamics of prolactin secretion in patients with hypopituitarism and pituitary macroadenomas. *J. Clin. Endocrinol. Metab.* **1995**, *80*, 3507–3512. [CrossRef]
34. Akin, S.; Isikay, I.; Soylemezoglu, F.; Yucel, T.; Gurlek, A.; Berker, M. Reasons and results of endoscopic surgery for prolactinomas: 142 surgical cases. *Acta Neurochir.* **2016**, *158*, 933–942. [CrossRef] [PubMed]
35. Shin, S.S.; Tormenti, M.J.; Paluzzi, A.; Rothfus, W.E.; Chang, Y.-F.; Zainah, H.; Fernandez-Miranda, J.C.; Snyderman, C.H.; Challinor, S.M.; Gardner, P.A. Endoscopic endonasal approach for growth hormone secreting pituitary adenomas: Outcomes in 53 patients using 2010 consensus criteria for remission. *Pituitary* **2013**, *16*, 435–444. [CrossRef] [PubMed]
36. Jane, J.A.; Starke, R.M.; Elzoghby, M.A.; Reames, D.L.; Payne, S.C.; Thorner, M.O.; Marshall, J.C.; Laws, E.R.; Vance, M.L. Endoscopic transsphenoidal surgery for acromegaly: Remission using modern criteria, complications, and predictors of outcome. *J. Clin. Endocrinol. Metab.* **2011**, *96*, 2732–2740. [CrossRef]
37. Hofstetter, C.P.; Mannaa, R.H.; Mubita, L.; Anand, V.K.; Kennedy, J.W.; Dehdashti, A.R.; Schwartz, T.H. Endoscopic endonasal transsphenoidal surgery for growth hormone-secreting pituitary adenomas. *Neurosurg. Focus* **2010**, *29*, E6. [CrossRef]
38. Campbell, P.G.; Kenning, E.; Andrews, D.W.; Yadla, S.; Rosen, M.; Evans, J.J. Outcomes after a purely endoscopic transsphenoidal resection of growth hormone-secreting pituitary adenomas. *Neurosurg. Focus* **2010**, *29*, E5. [CrossRef]
39. Nemergut, E.C.; Zuo, Z.; Jane, J.A.; Laws, E.R. Predictors of diabetes insipidus after transsphenoidal surgery: A review of 881 patients. *J. Neurosurg.* **2005**, *103*, 448–454. [CrossRef]

Disclaimer/Publisher's Note: The statements, opinions and data contained in all publications are solely those of the individual author(s) and contributor(s) and not of MDPI and/or the editor(s). MDPI and/or the editor(s) disclaim responsibility for any injury to people or property resulting from any ideas, methods, instructions or products referred to in the content.

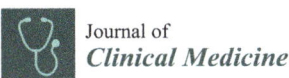

Systematic Review

Transoral Robotic Surgery in the Management of Submandibular Gland Sialoliths: A Systematic Review

Marta Rogalska [1,*], Lukasz Antkowiak [2], Anna Kasperczuk [3], Wojciech Scierski [4] and Maciej Misiolek [4]

1. Faculty of Medicine, Medical University of Warsaw, 02-091 Warsaw, Poland
2. Department of Pediatric Neurosurgery, Medical University of Silesia in Katowice, 40-752 Katowice, Poland; lukaszantkowiak7@gmail.com
3. Faculty of Mechanical Engineering, Institute of Biomedical Engineering, Bialystok University of Technology, 15-351 Bialystok, Poland; a.kasperczuk@pb.edu.pl
4. Department of Otorhinolaryngology and Oncological Laryngology, Faculty of Medical Sciences in Zabrze, Medical University of Silesia in Katowice, 41-800 Zabrze, Poland; wojciech.scierski@sum.edu.pl (W.S.); maciej.misiolek@sum.edu.pl (M.M.)
* Correspondence: rogalska_marta@wp.pl

Abstract: This study aimed to systematically review the literature to determine the efficacy and safety of transoral robotic surgery (TORS) in the management of submandibular gland (SMG) sialolithiasis. PubMed, Embase, and Cochrane were searched for English-language articles evaluating TORS in the management of SMG stones published up to 12 September 2022. Nine studies with a total of 99 patients were included. Eight patients underwent TORS followed by sialendoscopy (TS); 11 patients underwent sialendoscopy followed by TORS and sialendoscopy (STS); 4 patients underwent sialendoscopy followed by TORS only (ST); and 4 patients underwent TORS without sialendoscopy (T). The mean operative time amounted to 90.97 min. The mean procedure success rate reached 94.97%, with the highest for ST (100%) and T (100%), followed by the TS (95.04%) and STS (90.91%) variants. The mean follow-up time was 6.81 months. Transient lingual nerve injury occurred in 28 patients (28.3%) and was resolved in all of them within the mean of 1.25 months. No permanent lingual nerve injury was reported. TORS is a safe and effective management modality for hilar and intraparenchymal SMG sialoliths, with high procedural success in terms of successful sialolith removal, SMG preservation, and reduced risk of permanent postoperative lingual nerve damage.

Keywords: sialolithotomy; sialendoscopy; robot-assisted; sialolithiasis; submandibular stones; lingual nerve

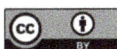

1. Introduction

Sialolithiasis represents the most common cause of obstructive salivary gland disorders [1]. While postmortem studies indicate a 0.115% prevalence of sialoliths in the general population, their clinical (symptomatic) prevalence amounts to 0.45% [1–3]. Most salivary stones (as high as 80–90% of cases) affect the submandibular gland (SMG), with a preferential location in the distal third of the Wharton's duct, at the hilum or in the hilo-parenchymal area of the SMG [1].

The removal of large proximal or hilo-parenchymal SMG sialoliths has traditionally been managed by means of transcervical sialoadenectomy, which carries a significant risk to the marginal mandibular nerve and might lead to an aesthetically unappealing scar [1,4]. With the advancement of sialendoscopy, a combined approach (CA) technique incorporating sialendoscopy and transoral sialolithotomy has enabled SMG preservation with a procedure success rate ranging from 90% to 100% [5–11]. Notably, transoral duct surgery with interventional sialendoscopy, as well as intraductal shock wave lithotripsy (ISWL) can be performed in local anesthesia, the latter of which has reported success rates above 90% [12–14].

Despite being superior to the previous non-gland-sparing modalities, the CA sialolithotomy poses several challenges, which are magnified the closer the SMG stone is to the hilum. The higher risk of lingual nerve damage due to its intimate relationship with Wharton's duct near its exit point at the SMG hilum contributes to the 2% rate of permanent tongue paresthesia reported after the CA procedure [15]. Furthermore, poor visualization and limited space for instrumentation, amplified in the presence of unfavorable anatomy and physical features such as obesity, reduced mouth opening, and prominent teeth, represent additional considerable drawbacks of the CA technique [16].

Recently, the application of robotic technology in the treatment of various head and neck disorders (obstructive sleep apnea, and pathologies involving the thyroid, parathyroid, oropharynx, hypopharynx, and supraglottis [17]) has favored the spread of this procedure for the removal of proximal hilar submandibular duct sialoliths. Since the initial experiences with robot-assisted SMG sialolithotomy, as well as its outcomes and advantages compared to the CA technique, have been reported, the purpose of the present study was to systematically review the literature to determine the efficacy and safety of transoral robotic surgery (TORS) in the management of SMG sialolithiasis.

2. Materials and Methods

2.1. Study Guidance

The review was conducted according to the PRISMA (Preferred Reporting Items for Systematic Reviews and Meta-Analyses) guidelines [18]. The study protocol was registered with the International Platform of Registered Systematic Review and Meta-analysis Protocols (INPLASY) under the number INPLASY202330068 [19].

2.2. Search Strategy and Criteria

The PubMed, Embase, and Cochrane databases were searched by two authors (M.R. and L.A.) independently for English-language full-text papers published from inception until 16 September 2022. Comprehensive electronic search strategies included terms for submandibular gland sialoliths ("submandibular" OR "salivary" OR "gland" OR "sialolithiasis" OR "sialolith" OR "megalith" OR "stone") AND terms for operative technique ("sialolithotomy" OR "sialoendoscopy" OR "sialendoscopy" OR "transoral") AND terms for robotic assistance ("robot" OR "robotic" OR "robot-assisted" OR "robotic assisted").

After duplicate removal, all studies were screened by two authors (M.R. and L.A.) independently, based on the title and the abstract. Inclusion criteria comprised clinical studies, case series, and case reports evaluating TORS in the management of submandibular gland stones. Contrarily, publications with an unrelated topic as well as conference papers, review articles, commentaries, and letters to the editor, were excluded. Additionally, the reference lists in all preselected articles were screened for further relevant papers.

2.3. Eligibility Criteria

The study was found eligible if it described the application of robot-assisted sialolithotomy (RAS) in the removal of the submandibular gland sialoliths.

2.4. Data Extraction and Analysis

From the included studies, the following data were extracted: first author and publication year, study design, number of patients, sialolith location(s), sialolith size(s), used robotic surgical system, variation of TORS-assisted sialolithotomy (i.e., (1) TORS immediately followed by sialendoscopy (TS); (2) sialendoscopy immediately followed by TORS and subsequent sialendoscopy (STS); (3) sialendoscopy immediately followed by TORS only (ST); TORS without sialendoscopy (T)), procedure success rate, procedure duration, intraoperative complications, postoperative complications, and time until symptom resolution. If RAS consisted of more than one step (i.e., TS, STS, ST), all of them were performed within the same surgical procedure. Procedure success was defined as a successful sialolith removal with submandibular gland preservation and absence of symptom recurrence at the latest available follow-up. In order to calculate the weighted averages of all available quantitative parameters, weights were selected proportionally to the sample size.

3. Results

3.1. Study Selection

The literature search yielded 638 articles, including 293 from PubMed, 333 from Embase, and 12 from Cochrane. After the removal of 527 duplicate records, 111 studies were screened. Three non-English studies and 70 articles with an irrelevant topic were excluded, as well as 23 conference papers and 6 review articles. The remaining nine articles [4,15,16,20–25] were found eligible and included in the further analysis. Figure 1 shows the entire literature selection process.

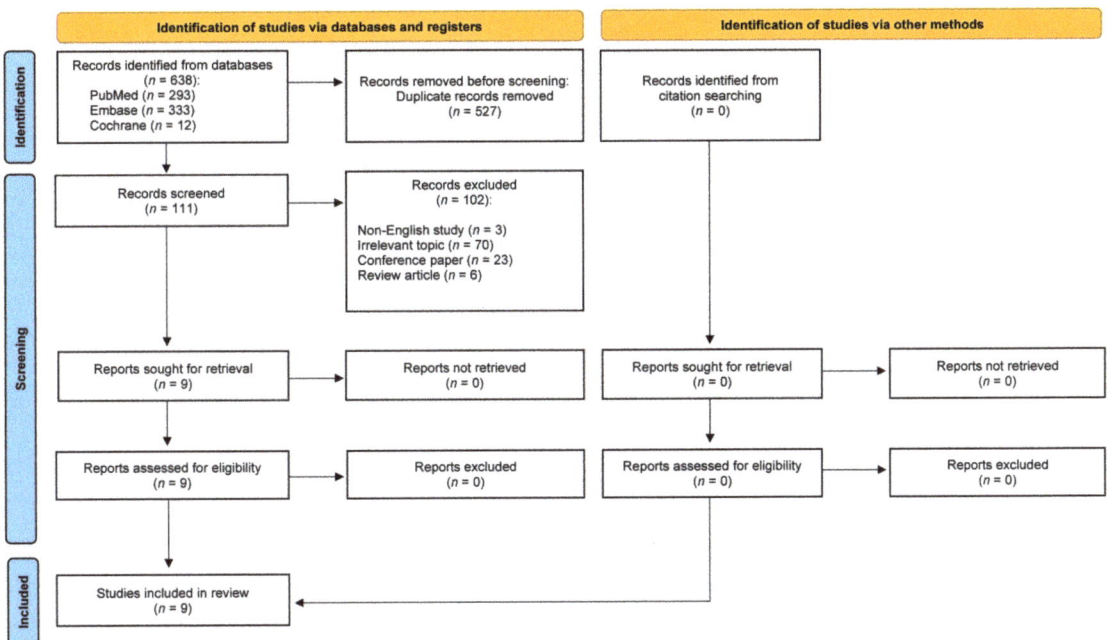

Figure 1. PRISMA flowchart of the medical database search strategy.

3.2. Study Characteristics

The included studies involved a total of 99 patients. Eight patients from four studies [4,15,20,22] underwent TORS followed by sialendoscopy (TS). In eleven patients from two studies [4,23], sialendoscopy followed by TORS and sialendoscopy (STS) was performed. Four patients from two studies [4,16] underwent sialendoscopy followed by TORS only (ST), whereas in the remaining four patients from three studies [21,24,25], TORS without sialendoscopy (T) was performed. Complete study characteristics are presented in Table 1.

Table 1. Characteristics of studies included in the systematic review.

First Author (year)	No. of Patients	Sialolith Size, Mean (Range) (mm)	Sialolith Location	Robotic Surgical System	Procedure Success Rate (%)	Procedure Duration, Mean (Range) (min)	Follow-Up Time, Mean (Range)	Transient Lingual Nerve Injury (%)	Duration of Transient Lingual Nerve Injury, Mean (Range)	Permanent Lingual Nerve Injury (%)
ST											
Wen (2021) [4]	3	8.7	hilar or intraglandular	da Vinci Si or da Vinci SP (Intuitive Surgical Inc., Sunnyvale, CA, USA)	100%	213 (157–283)	2.8 months	-	-	0%
Walvekar (2011) [16]	1	19	hilo-parenchymal	da Vinci Si (Intuitive Surgical Inc., Sunnyvale, CA, USA)	100%	120	-	0%	-	0%
STS											
Wen (2021) [4]	10	8.6	hilar or intraglandular	da Vinci Si or da Vinci SP (Intuitive Surgical Inc., Sunnyvale, CA, USA)	90.0%	190 (88–301)	12.9 months	-	-	0%
Vergez (2021) [23]	1	10	hilar	da Vinci Si (Intuitive Surgical Inc., Sunnyvale, CA, USA)	100%	50	-	0%	-	0%
TS											
Razavi (2016) [15]	22	12.3 (5–20)	hilar	da Vinci Si (Intuitive Surgical Inc., Sunnyvale, CA, USA)	100%	67 (38–143)	14 (5–25) months	18%	2.5 (2–3) weeks	0%
Tampio (2021) [20]	33	8.9 (5–20)	hilar	da Vinci Si (Intuitive Surgical Inc., Sunnyvale, CA, USA)	94%	62 (13–111) *	19 (14–21) days	15.1%	54 (30–84) days	0%
Wen (2021) [4]	24	14.5	hilar or intraglandular	da Vinci Si or da Vinci SP (Intuitive Surgical Inc., Sunnyvale, CA, USA)	91.7%	103 (57–184)	7.2 months	-	-	0%
Frost (2020) [22]	1	19	hilar	da Vinci SP (Intuitive Surgical Inc., Sunnyvale, CA, USA)	100%	-	3 months	100%	-	-
T											
Capaccio (2019) [21]	1	15	hilo-parenchymal	da Vinci Si (Intuitive Surgical Inc., Sunnyvale, CA, USA)	100%	55	3 months	0%	-	0%

Table 1. *Cont.*

First Author (year)	No. of Patients	Sialolith Size, Mean (Range) (mm)	Sialolith Location	Robotic Surgical System	Procedure Success Rate (%)	Procedure Duration, Mean (Range) (min)	Follow-Up Time, Mean (Range)	Transient Lingual Nerve Injury (%)	Duration of Transient Lingual Nerve Injury, Mean (Range)	Permanent Lingual Nerve Injury (%)
Capaccio (2019) [21]	1	8	hilo-parenchymal	da Vinci Si (Intuitive Surgical Inc., Sunnyvale, CA, USA)	100%	45	3 months	0%	-	0%
Capaccio (2021) [24]	1	15	hilo-parenchymal	Flex Robotic System (Medrobotics Inc., Raynham, MA, USA)	100%	130 (bilateral)	3 months	100%	1 month	0%
Capaccio (2022) [25]	1	25	hilo-parenchymal	Flex Robotic System (Medrobotics Inc., Raynham, MA, USA)	100%	30	3 months	0%	-	0%

Legend: TORS, transoral robotic surgery; TS, TORS followed by sialendoscopy; ST, sialendoscopy followed by TORS and sialendoscopy followed by TORS; T, TORS without sialendoscopy. * calculated based on 32 patients since one patient underwent TS on the left and an additional sialendoscopy with wire basket retrieval of a contralateral submandibular gland stone. This patient's procedure time was excluded from the analysis.

3.3. Sialolith Size

Sialolith size was evaluated in all nine studies [4,15,16,20–25]. The mean sialolith size amounted to 11.46 mm (range 4–28 mm).

3.4. Aim of Sialendoscopy

Sialendoscopy prior to the sialolith removal was performed to facilitate sialolith localization in 15 patients [4,16,23]. In Wen et al.'s study [4], a sialendoscopy-first approach (ST or STS) was selected in case of non-palpable or multiple sialoliths. In a patient described by Vergez et al., sialendoscopy allowed the identification of a hilar sialolith impacted beyond proximal ductal stenosis [23]. In 91 patients [4,15,20,22,23], after the successful sialolith removal, the ductal system was explored with a sialendoscope to ensure the submandibular duct patency by identifying any additional sialoliths, remaining stone fragments, or areas of ductal stenosis.

3.5. Procedure Duration Time

Procedure duration time was reported in all nine studies [4,15,16,20–25]. The mean operative time amounted to 90.97 min (range 13–143 min) and was the shortest for the T (43.33 min), followed by the TS (76.03 min), STS (177.27 min), and ST (189.75 min) techniques.

3.6. Procedure Success Rate

Procedural success was described in all nine studies [4,15,16,20–25]. The mean procedure success rate reached 94.97%, with the highest for the ST (100%) and T (100%), followed by the TS (95.04%) and STS (90.91%) variants.

3.7. Follow-Up Time

The duration of the follow-up was reported in seven studies [4,15,20–22,24,25]. The mean follow-up time was 6.81 months (range 0.35–65.53 months).

3.8. Complications

Transient lingual nerve injury occurred in 28 patients (28.3%) from five studies [4,15,20,22,24] and resolved in all of them within the mean of 1.25 months (range 0.5–2.8 months). No permanent lingual nerve injury was described in the included studies.

4. Discussion

The initial implementation of robotic assistance in head and neck surgery has concerned predominantly oncologic indications since it reduced hospitalization length and enabled access to tumors in challenging anatomic locations [26]. However, numerous authors have recently emphasized the benefits of incorporating TORS in the management of non-oncologic pathologies located in areas with poor operative exposure, including large proximal, hilar, or hilo-parenchymal SMG sialoliths [4,15,20].

The advantages of robot-assisted surgery might result from the magnified three-dimensional view of the surgical field, which allows the surgeon to have an accurate anatomical delineation and enhanced perception of the depth of the oral floor, lingual nerve, Wharton's duct, and hilo-parenchymal SMG region [15,20,21]. Furthermore, the heightened operative visualization facilitates the use of smaller incisions, allows the better identification of vital structures (such as the lingual nerve), and enables decreased manipulation of Wharton's duct. The functional preservation of the main submandibular duct simplifies sialendoscopic access through its natural ostium in case of residual microliths [21]. Additionally, due to the medicolegal ramifications of the lingual nerve injury, the video documentation of an intact nerve, available by means of the RAS procedure, is crucial, even if, at certain stages of the procedure, its mobilization is unavoidable [4]. Moreover, since all surgical steps are visible to the whole operating room staff, the crowding around the operating space is reduced, and the use of the robotic unit can serve as an excellent teaching tool for residents and medical students [4,16].

Increased dexterity and precision due to the 360° range of motion provided by the robotic instrumentation result in improved tissue manipulation, less unnecessary trauma to the local structures, and a safer dissection of the lingual nerve and Wharton's duct at the SMG hilum. Razavi et al. suggested that the abovementioned advantages might partially prevent postoperative ductal scarring and stenosis, which may ultimately enable the avoidance of symptom recurrence and the necessity of reoperation [15]. Furthermore, contrarily to the CA technique, RAS allows for the greater involvement of a surgical assistant without compromising the operative field visually or spatially [15]. Thus, the assistant surgeon can simultaneously perform the suction, tissue traction, and push-up of the SMG from the neck in order to better expose the parenchyma in the oral floor [21].

Another significant but frequently overlooked advantage of robotic surgery is the benefit of improved surgical ergonomics [27]. A comfortable seated position and decreased prolonged neck strain might reduce the frequency of work-related musculoskeletal disorders among ENT specialists and ultimately lead to the increased career length of a head and neck surgeon.

The numerous abovementioned technical advantages of RAS compared to the CA technique might contribute to the higher success rate of the robot-assisted approach (94.97% vs. 75–87% [15,28], respectively). Notably, of the five patients in our review where RAS was unsuccessful, three individuals experienced symptom recurrence [4]. Two of them required sialendoscopy for recurrent sialoliths removal; in one of them, SMG excision was ultimately necessitated, during which frank purulence, SMG fibrosis, and a 5 mm intraparenchymal stone were discovered [4]. Of the remaining two patients, in one individual, the sialolith could not be localized on sialendoscopy due to the extensive scarring of the surgical field [20]. This prompted SMG excision, which revealed three sialoliths within the SMG parenchyma and the proximal Wharton's duct [20]. In the other patient, who suffered from frequent sialadenitis secondary to sialolithiasis, significant inflammation and fibrosis of the SMG and surrounding tissues made the localization of the sialolith unfeasible, and SMG removal was eventually required [20]. Given these failures, the robot-assisted technique might be less successful in the case of deep parenchymal localization of the sialoliths and considerable SMG fibrosis resulting from chronic inflammation.

Additionally, due to the significant discrepancies in sample sizes between the applied TORS variations (T, TS, ST, STS), care must be taken when interpreting the differences in their success rates. Although the success rates of the ST and T techniques (amounting to 100%) were higher than the success rates of the TS variations (95.04%), the ST and T groups were considerably smaller than the TS sample (4 patients vs. 80 patients, respectively). With larger sample sizes in the ST and T groups, their actual success rate could noticeably decrease, thus reducing the difference between the effectiveness of each technique. Furthermore, the success rates of various TORS modifications should not be juxtaposed since each management method was applied for specific indications (single vs. multiple, palpable vs. non-palpable, hilar vs. hilo-parenchymal sialoliths). Generally, palpable sialoliths and those ≥5 mm on imaging were treated by the TORS-first approach, whereas, in the case of multiple or unpalpable SMG stones, the sialendoscopy-first approach was selected, similarly to the algorithm proposed by Quiz et al. [4,5]. Based on the results of our review, we state that all techniques proved to be highly effective, taking into account the indications for their implementation. Nonetheless, randomized control trials with patients anonymously assigned to each group (ST, STS, TS, or T) regardless of the sialolithiasis characteristics are necessary to compare the success rates of TORS variations.

Despite the often-cited belief that the employment of the robot in SMG sialolithotomy increases the operative time, our analysis revealed the mean procedure time amounted to 90.97 min, which is similar to or slightly shorter than the average of 90 to 113 min for the conventional CA technique [27,29]. Nonetheless, due to the scarcity of the literature describing CA procedure times and the fact that the available reports date back to the time when CAS was a more novel procedure, the actual CA operative time could have decreased with greater surgical experience.

Additionally, our results suggest a lower incidence of permanent lingual nerve damage with RAS compared to the CA technique (0% vs. 2%, respectively). Importantly, the literature regarding the presence of lingual nerve injury after sialolith removal via the CA technique includes both patients with hilar and ductal SMG sialoliths, the latter of which are not as intimately related to the lingual nerve as those in the hilar location. Nevertheless, even considering the higher inherent risk to the lingual nerve in our review due to the hilar or intraparenchymal localization of all sialoliths, permanent lingual nerve damage was omitted in all cases.

Despite many advantages of robotic assistance in SMG sialolithotomy, the lack of tactile feedback and the necessity of greater reliance on visual cues constitute one of its significant limitations [15,20,23]. However, this disadvantage might be partially mitigated through intraoperative stone palpation by the assistant surgeon and due to the fixed position of most hilar SMG sialoliths [15]. Tissue mobility might be interpreted as a haptic sense, but only by an experienced robotic surgeon; therefore, the incorporation of the preoperative ultrasonography and Cone Beam CT might be mandatory to successfully pursue the excision of purely unpalpable parenchymal SMG sialoliths [5,30,31].

Furthermore, according to our analysis, the mean sialolith size was greater than that reported in the literature regarding the sialolith excision via the non-robotic transoral technique [5,7,8,10,11,32–34]. With the increase in the sialolith size, the necessity of tactile feedback diminishes, which facilitates the robotic removal of SMG stones. Contrarily, smaller sialoliths impose the importance of stone palpation, which cannot be provided by RAS.

Notably, the possible traumatic mechanical effect of robotic instruments during RAS might contribute to the high rate of postsurgical transient lingual nerve injury (28.3%) in our review. Although our results are higher than those reported in the literature regarding the CA technique [7,9,33,35,36], patients from the included studies were considered to suffer from transient lingual nerve injury, even if the lingual paresthesia remained very subtle. Additionally, all patients in our review were treated with the Da Vinci Si and SP robot (Intuitive Surgical Inc., Sunnyvale, CA, USA), or Flex Robotic system (Medrobotics Inc., Raynham, MA, USA). Notably, Da Vinci Si (Intuitive Surgical Inc., Sunnyvale, CA, USA) has recently been replaced by the more advanced Da Vinci Xi robotic system (Intuitive Surgical Inc., Sunnyvale, CA, USA). The difference in the instrument sizes between the robotic systems might influence their handling and associated tissue damage during the procedure [37]. We hypothesize that the transient lingual nerve injury rate could be decreased by the wider application of RAS, which would improve the learning curve of head and neck surgeons.

Furthermore, RAS remains a reasonable approach mainly for large, deeply located sialoliths, and when unfavorable conditions such as pharyngeal reflex are present. In challenging anatomic conditions (e.g., markedly reduced mouth opening), RAS, as with other transoral approaches, might not be technically feasible. Another significant disadvantage of RAS is the necessity of performing the surgery under general anesthesia.

Finally, a considerable drawback of robotic assistance is the limited availability of the device in rural areas. Additionally, significant costs associated with the RAS procedure limit its wide applicability across multiple institutions. Conversely to tertiary medical centers, where this technology is utilized in multiple surgical specialties, smaller hospitals with a lower case volume might find this technology financially disadvantageous [20,23].

Limitations

Our systematic review comprises mainly case series and non-randomized, retrospective, single-center studies with limited sample sizes; thus, we advocate caution in interpreting the results. Moreover, the exclusion of non-English-language papers could have restricted the already scarce literature describing RAS in the management of patients with SMG sialolithotomy. Additionally, although the mean follow-up time in our review amounting to 6.81 months is long enough to capture postoperative complications such as lingual nerve damage, it might be insufficient to describe the actual rate of SMG sialolithiasis recurrence.

5. Conclusions

RAS is a safe and effective management modality for hilar and intraparenchymal SMG sialoliths, with a high procedural success in terms of successful sialolith removal and SMG preservation, and a vastly reduced risk of permanent postoperative lingual nerve damage. Future prospective studies with expanded RAS cohorts and longer follow-up times are highly warranted to precisely define the extent of RAS utility and reliability in the management of patients with SMG sialoliths.

Author Contributions: Conceptualization, M.R.; methodology, M.R., L.A. and A.K.; formal analysis, M.R. and L.A.; data curation, M.R. and L.A.; writing—original draft preparation, M.R. and L.A.; writing—review and editing, W.S. and M.M.; visualization, M.R. and L.A.; supervision, W.S. and M.M. All authors have read and agreed to the published version of the manuscript.

Funding: This research received no external funding.

Institutional Review Board Statement: Not applicable.

Informed Consent Statement: Not applicable.

Data Availability Statement: The data generated during this study are available within the article. Datasets analyzed during the current study preparation are available from the corresponding author on reasonable request.

Conflicts of Interest: The authors declare no conflict of interest.

References

1. Capaccio, P.; Torretta, S.; Ottavian, F.; Sambataro, G.; Pignataro, L. Modern management of obstructive salivary diseases. *Acta Otorhinolaryngologica Italica* **2007**, *27*, 161–172. [PubMed]
2. McGurk, M.; Escudier, M.P.; Brown, J.E. Modern management of salivary calculi. *Br. J. Surg.* **2005**, *92*, 107–112. [CrossRef] [PubMed]
3. Sánchez Barrueco, Á.; Santillán Coello, J.M.; González Galán, F.; Alcalá Rueda, I.; Aly, S.O.; Sobrino Guijarro, B.; Mahillo Fernández, I.; Cenjor Español, C.; Villacampa Aubá, J.M. Correction to: Epidemiologic, radiologic, and sialendoscopic aspects in chronic obstructive sialadenitis. *Eur. Arch. Oto-Rhino-Laryngol.* **2023**, *280*, 2061–2062. [CrossRef] [PubMed]
4. Wen, C.Z.; Douglas, J.E.; Elrakhawy, M.; Paul, E.A.; Rassekh, C.H. Nuances and Management of Hilar Submandibular Sialoliths with Combined Transoral Robotic Surgery-Assisted Sialolithotomy and Sialendoscopy. *Otolaryngol.—Head Neck Surg.* **2021**, *165*, 76–82. [CrossRef]
5. Quiz, J.; Gillespie, M.B. Transoral Sialolithotomy Without Endoscopes: An Alternative Approach to Salivary Stones. *Otolaryngol. Clin. N. Am.* **2021**, *54*, 553–565. [CrossRef]
6. Sproll, C.; Naujoks, C.; Holtmann, H.; Kübler, N.R.; Singh, D.D.; Rana, M.; Lommen, J. Removal of stones from the superficial lobe of the submandibular gland (SMG) via an intraoral endoscopy-assisted sialolithotomy. *Clin. Oral Investig.* **2019**, *23*, 4145–4156. [CrossRef]
7. Jadu, F.M.; Jan, A.M. A meta-analysis of the efficacy and safety of managing parotid and submandibular sialoliths using sialendoscopy assisted surgery. *Saudi Med. J.* **2014**, *35*, 1188–1194.
8. Ziegler, C.M.; Steveling, H.; Seubert, M.; Mühling, J. Endoscopy: A minimally invasive procedure for diagnosis and treatment of diseases of the salivary glands. *Br. J. Oral Maxillofac. Surg.* **2004**, *42*, 1. [CrossRef]
9. Nahlieli, O.; Shacham, R.; Zagury, A.; Bar, T.; Yoffe, B. The Ductal Stretching Technique: An Endoscopic-Assisted Technique for Removal of Submandibular Stones. *Laryngoscope* **2007**, *117*, 1031–1035. [CrossRef]
10. Liu, D.; Zhang, Z.; Zhang, Y.; Zhang, L.; Yu, G. Diagnosis and management of sialolithiasis with a semirigid endoscope. *Oral Surg. Oral Med. Oral Pathol. Oral Radiol. Endodontol.* **2009**, *108*, 9–14. [CrossRef]
11. Su, Y.; Liao, G.; Zheng, G.; Liu, H.; Liang, Y.; Ou, D. Sialoendoscopically Assisted Open Sialolithectomy for Removal of Large Submandibular Hilar Calculi. *J. Oral Maxillofac. Surg.* **2010**, *68*, 68–73. [CrossRef] [PubMed]
12. Koch, M.; Mantsopoulos, K.; Müller, S.; Sievert, M.; Iro, H. Treatment of Sialolithiasis: What Has Changed? An Update of the Treatment Algorithms and a Review of the Literature. *J. Clin. Med.* **2021**, *11*, 231. [CrossRef] [PubMed]
13. Koch, M.; Schapher, M.; Mantsopoulos, K.; von Scotti, F.; Goncalves, M.; Iro, H. Multimodal treatment in difficult sialolithiasis: Role of extracorporeal shock-wave lithotripsy and intraductal pneumatic lithotripsy: ESWL and IPL in Difficult Sialolithiasis. *Laryngoscope* **2018**, *128*, E332–E338. [CrossRef]

14. Koch, M.; Schapher, M.; Mantsopoulos, K.; Goncalves, M.; Iro, H. Intraductal Pneumatic Lithotripsy after Extended Transoral Duct Surgery in Submandibular Sialolithiasis. *Otolaryngol. Neck Surg.* **2019**, *160*, 63–69. [CrossRef]
15. Razavi, C.; Pascheles, C.; Samara, G.; Marzouk, M. Robot-assisted sialolithotomy with sialendoscopy for the management of large submandibular gland stones. *Laryngoscope* **2016**, *126*, 345–351. [CrossRef] [PubMed]
16. Walvekar, R.R.; Tyler, P.D.; Tammareddi, N.; Peters, G. Robotic-assisted transoral removal of a submandibular megalith. *Laryngoscope* **2011**, *121*, 534–537. [CrossRef] [PubMed]
17. Garas, G.; Arora, A. Robotic Head and Neck Surgery: History, Technical Evolution and the Future. *ORL J. Oto-Rhino-Laryngol. Its Relat. Spec.* **2018**, *80*, 117–124. [CrossRef]
18. Page, M.J.; McKenzie, J.E.; Bossuyt, P.M.; Boutron, I.; Hoffmann, T.C.; Mulrow, C.D.; Shamseer, L.; Tetzlaff, J.M.; Akl, E.A.; Brennan, S.E.; et al. The PRISMA 2020 statement: An updated guideline for reporting systematic reviews. *BMJ* **2021**, *372*, n71. [CrossRef]
19. Rogalska, M.; Antkowiak, L.; Kasperczuk, A.; Scierski, W.; Misiolek, M. *Transoral Robotic Surgery in the Management of Submandibular Gland Sialoliths: A Systematic Review*; INPLASY—International Platform of Registered Systematic Review and Meta-Analysis Protocols: Middletown, DE, USA, 2023. [CrossRef]
20. Tampio, A.J.F.; Marzouk, M.F. Robot-assisted sialolithotomy with sialoendoscopy: A review of safety, efficacy and cost. *J. Robot. Surg.* **2021**, *15*, 229–234. [CrossRef]
21. Capaccio, P.; Montevecchi, F.; Meccariello, G.; D'Agostino, G.; Cammaroto, G.; Pelucchi, S.; Vicini, C. Transoral robotic surgery for hilo-parenchymal submandibular stones: Step-by-step description and reasoned approach. *Int. J. Oral Maxillofac. Surg.* **2019**, *48*, 1520–1524. [CrossRef]
22. Frost, A.S.; Byrnes, Y.M.; Wen, C.Z.; Rassekh, C.H. Single-port transoral robotic combined approach with sialendoscopy for sialolithiasis: Case report and review of the literature. *Head Neck* **2020**, *42*, E12–E15. [CrossRef] [PubMed]
23. Vergez, S.; Cheval, M.; Chabrillac, E. Transoral robotic removal of submandibular sialolith combined with sialendoscopic assistance. *Eur. Ann. Otorhinolaryngol. Head Neck Dis.* **2021**, *138* (Suppl. S2), 65–66. [CrossRef] [PubMed]
24. Capaccio, P.; Cammarota, R.; Riva, G.; Albera, A.; Albera, R.; Pecorari, G. Transoral robotic surgery for bilateral parenchymal submandibular stones: The Flex Robotic System. *B-ENT* **2021**, *17*, 45–48. [CrossRef]
25. Capaccio, P.; Riva, G.; Cammarota, R.; Gaffuri, M.; Pecorari, G. Minimally invasive transoral robotic surgery for hiloparenchymal submandibular stone: Technical note on Flex Robotic System. *Clin. Case Rep.* **2022**, *10*, e04529. [CrossRef]
26. Chung, T.K.; Rosenthal, E.L.; Magnuson, J.S.; Carroll, W.R. Transoral robotic surgery for oropharyngeal and tongue cancer in the United States. *Laryngoscope* **2015**, *125*, 140–145. [CrossRef]
27. Walvekar, R.R.; Bomeli, S.R.; Carrau, R.L.; Schaitkin, B. Combined approach technique for the management of large salivary stones. *Laryngoscope* **2009**, *119*, 1125–1129. [CrossRef]
28. Schwartz, N.; Hazkani, I.; Goshen, S. Combined approach sialendoscopy for management of submandibular gland sialolithiasis. *Am. J. Otolaryngol.* **2015**, *36*, 632–635. [CrossRef]
29. Wallace, E.; Tauzin, M.; Hagan, J.; Schaitkin, B.; Walvekar, R.R. Management of giant sialoliths: Review of the literature and preliminary experience with interventional sialendoscopy. *Laryngoscope* **2010**, *120*, 1974–1978. [CrossRef]
30. Vicini, C.; Cammaroto, G.; Meccariello, G.; Iannella, G.; Goldenberg, D.; Pignataro, L.; Torretta, S.; Maniaci, A.; Cocuzza, S.; Capaccio, P. Trans-oral robotic surgery for Hilo-parenchymal submandibular stones. *Oper. Tech. Otolaryngol.-Head Neck Surg.* **2021**, *32*, 174–178. [CrossRef]
31. Costan, V.V.; Ciocan-Pendefunda, C.C.; Sulea, D.; Popescu, E.; Boisteanu, O. Use of Cone-Beam Computed Tomography in Performing Submandibular Sialolithotomy. *J. Oral Maxillofac. Surg.* **2019**, *77*, 1656.e1–1656.e8. [CrossRef]
32. Saga-Gutierrez, C.; Chiesa-Estomba, C.M.; Larruscain, E.; González-García, J.Á.; Sistiaga, J.A.; Altuna, X. Transoral Sialolitectomy as an Alternative to Submaxilectomy in the Treatment of Submaxillary Sialolithiasis. *Ear Nose Throat J.* **2019**, *98*, 287–290. [CrossRef] [PubMed]
33. Liu, D.-G.; Jiang, L.; Xie, X.-Y.; Zhang, Z.-Y.; Zhang, L.; Yu, G.-Y. Sialoendoscopy-assisted sialolithectomy for submandibular hilar calculi. *J. Oral Maxillofac. Surg. Off. J. Am. Assoc. Oral Maxillofac. Surg.* **2013**, *71*, 295–301. [CrossRef] [PubMed]
34. Zhao, Y.-N.; Zhang, Y.-Q.; Zhang, L.-Q.; Xie, X.-Y.; Liu, D.-G.; Yu, G.-Y. Treatment strategy of hilar and intraglandular stones in wharton's duct: A 12-year experience. *Laryngoscope* **2020**, *130*, 2360–2365. [CrossRef] [PubMed]
35. Nahlieli, O. Complications of traditional and modern therapeutic salivary approaches. *Acta Otorhinolaryngol. Ital.* **2017**, *37*, 142–147. [CrossRef] [PubMed]
36. Nahlieli, O. Complications of Sialendoscopy: Personal Experience, Literature Analysis, and Suggestions. *J. Oral Maxillofac. Surg.* **2015**, *73*, 75–80. [CrossRef]
37. Fiacchini, G.; Vianini, M.; Dallan, I.; Bruschini, L. Is the Da Vinci Xi system a real improvement for oncologic transoral robotic surgery? A systematic review of the literature. *J. Robot. Surg.* **2021**, *15*, 1–12. [CrossRef]

Disclaimer/Publisher's Note: The statements, opinions and data contained in all publications are solely those of the individual author(s) and contributor(s) and not of MDPI and/or the editor(s). MDPI and/or the editor(s) disclaim responsibility for any injury to people or property resulting from any ideas, methods, instructions or products referred to in the content.

Communication

Multi-Level 3D Surgery for Obstructive Sleep Apnea: Could It Be the Future?

Angelo Eplite [1,*], Claudio Vicini [2], Giuseppe Meccariello [2], Giannicola Iannella [3], Antonino Maniaci [4], Angelo Cannavicci [2], Francesco Moretti [5], Fabio Facchini [5], Tommaso Mazzocco [5] and Giovanni Cammaroto [2]

1. Department of Biomedical and Clinical Sciences "Luigi Sacco", University of Milan, Via GB Grassi 74, 20154 Milan, Italy
2. Department of Head-Neck Surgery, Otolaryngology, Head-Neck and Oral Surgery Unit, Morgagni Pierantoni Hospital, Via Carlo Forlanini 34, 47121 Forlì, Italy; claudio@claudiovicini.com (C.V.); drmeccariello@gmail.com (G.M.); a.cannavicci.md@gmail.com (A.C.); giovanni.cammaroto@hotmail.com (G.C.)
3. Department of 'Organi di Senso', University "Sapienza", Viale dell'Università 33, 00185 Rome, Italy; giannicola.iannella@uniroma.it
4. Department of Medical and Surgical Sciences and Advanced Technologies "GF Ingrassia", ENT Section, University of Catania, Piazza Università 2, 95100 Catania, Italy; tonymaniaci@hotmail.it
5. Department ENT & Audiology, University of Ferrara, Via Savonarola 9, 44121 Ferrara, Italy; francesco.moretti@unife.it (F.M.); fabio.facchini@unife.it (F.F.); tommaso.mazzocco@unife.it (T.M.)
* Correspondence: angelo.epli@gmail.com; Tel.: +39-34-88-54-8906

Abstract: (1) Background: Obstructive sleep apnea (OSA) is the most common sleep-related breathing disorder and is characterized by recurrent episodes of complete or partial obstruction of the upper airway, leading to reduced or absent breathing during sleep. A nocturnal upper airway collapse is often multi-levelled. The aim of this communication is to describe a 3D multi-level surgery setting in OSA pathology, introducing new surgical approaches, such as 4K-3D endoscopic visualization for the tongue base approach with the aid of a coblator and exoscopic visualization in the palatal approach. (2) Methods: Seven patients affected by OSA underwent 3D Barbed Reposition Pharyngoplasty (BRP) surgery associated with transoral coblation tongue base reduction and nose surgery. (3) Results: No patients experienced intra-operative, post-operative or delayed complications. For OSA multi-level 3D surgery, it took less than 2 h: the median 3D system setting time was 12.5 ± 2.3 min; the overall procedure time was 59.3 ± 26 min. (4) Conclusions: The use of the 4K-3D endoscope and coblator for tongue base resectioning and of the 3D exoscope for lateral pharyngoplasty represents an excellent system in multi-level OSA related surgery that could reduce the time and the costs compared to those of robotic surgery.

Keywords: 3D surgery; coblator; 3D tongue base resection; 3D barbed reposition pharyngoplasty

1. Introduction

Obstructive sleep apnea (OSA) syndrome is a respiratory sleep disorder characterized by partial or complete recurrent episodes of upper airway collapses that occur during the night [1]. A nocturnal upper airway collapse is often multi-levelled. Several surgical procedures have been developed in recent years to correct retrolingual and retropalatal collapses [2]. In the last 15 years, TORS has been widely used for the resectioning of excess baselingual lymphatic tissue, which causes secondary epiglottis, as well as in epiglottoplasty in cases of primary epiglottis [3]. The use of robotic surgery and innovative surgery on the soft palate called "Barbed Reposition Pharyngoplasty" (BRP) represent the fundamental points of multi-level surgery on OSA patients [4].

Recently, our group introduced new surgical approaches using, i.e., 4K-3D endoscopic visualization for the tongue base approach and exoscopic visualization for the palatal approach. Hereafter, we describe the technique of a multi-level surgery setting and report on its feasibility and safety.

2. Material and Methods

This study was approved by the Ethics Committee of the Morgagni-Pierantoni Hospital (rif. 34/2022) on 10 March 2022. Prior to the study, all individual participants included signed an informed consent form.

Each patient (of the seven recruited) was placed in the supine position on the operating table. In multi-level surgery for obstructive sleep apnea, including septal correction, tongue base and palatal surgeries, general anesthesia was given via orotracheal intubation.

A 4K-3D videoendoscope with a 10 mm diameter and a 30° field of view for the tongue base approach was assembled on a mechanical holder, and then attached to the bed using an autostatic arm (Figure 1). The 3D exoscopic system for the BRP (after palatine tonsillectomy) was fixed to the Versacrane™ holding system, which was positioned on one side of the surgeon; the exoscope and the Versacrane™ holding arm were connected to a clamping jaw.

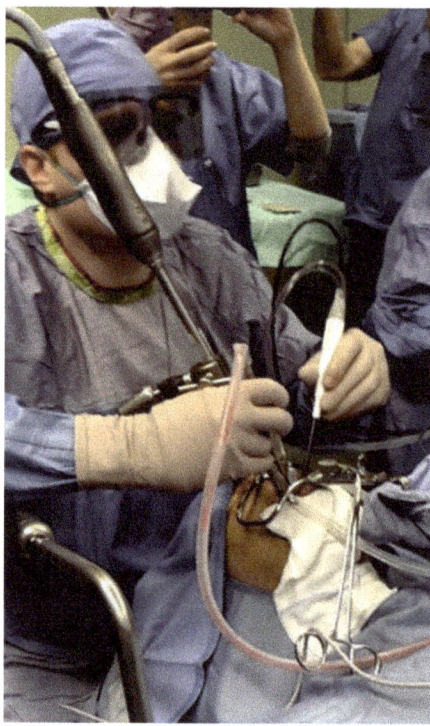

Figure 1. The 4K-3D videoendoscope with 10 mm diameter and 30° field of view used for the base tongue approach was assembled on a mechanical holder, and then attached to the bed using an autostatic arm. The first surgeon stood near the patient's head, facing a 3D monitor placed beside the operating table toward its end in order to visualize the anatomical structures in a defined way.

All patients were in a "sniffing position" (neck flexed and head extended): the exposure of the tongue base was achieved with a single silk suture in the oral tongue, which was tractioned outside the mouth. There are several types of mouth gags and retractors, depending on the type of procedure. We used the Davis Meyer mouth gag, which was suspended by an ordinary Mayo stand. These mouth gags come with two types of tongue blades. Russel Davis blades with a groove for the endotracheal tube allow the tube to be fixed along the midline, and they are typically used for tonsillectomies and palatal surgery. Flat blades, instead, have a lower profile and allow there to be more space in the oral cavity, but require an endotracheal tube to be fixed to the side of the oral cavity. Flat blades also have two suction pumps for smoke evacuation.

Once the patient was ready and draped, the videoendoscope was positioned in the center of the patient's mouth, while the exoscope was clothed with a sterile cover and positioned directly above the surgical field in a distance of 30–50 cm in order to have enough space for instrument handling (Figure 2). The main 3D monitor (55″) was placed beside the operating table toward its end and directly in front of the first surgeon, while a secondary 3D monitor was set in front of the second surgeon. The first surgeon stood at the patient's head, facing the monitor. The second surgeon sat behind, using the controller (joystick) and maintained the focus of the camera on the surgical field, adjusting the optical magnification. All surgeons and nurses wore 3D passive polarized glasses, so that the entire surgical team could benefit from the presence of 3D vision during the execution of the procedure.

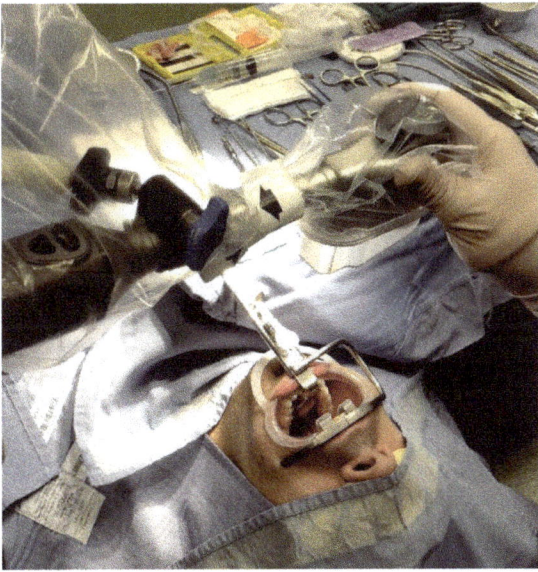

Figure 2. Storz Crowe–Davis mouth gag with a wide and hollow blade was placed and suspended using a lifting Mayo stand. A plastic cheek retractor was also used to make wider the oral opening and protect oral commissure. The exoscope was positioned directly above the surgical field at a distance of 3050 cm.

We used the coblator as an operative instrument; we chose to perform surgery with EVac 70 Xtra HP® as the coblation wand for either ablation or resection, which was used also for tongue base surgery and tontillectomy, which was executed before the lateral pharyngoplasty. It was used at a power of 7 ablation/5 coagulation.

Patients underwent the ablation of 1 cm of tongue base lymphatic tissue on each side of the midline split (2 cm width and 1 cm depth of tissue ablation). The margins of resection include the anterosuperior sulcus terminalis, lateral amygdalo-glossus sulcus and posteroinferior glosso-epiglottic sulcus. Then, the ablation of each palatine tonsil was meticulously realized (Figure 3), sparing the palatopharyngeus muscles and the utmost mucosa covering both pillars in order to perform Barbed Reposition Pharingoplasty. The whole operating room team could see the surgical steps on 3D monitors (Figure 4).

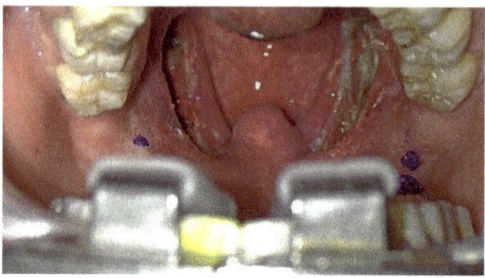

Figure 3. Palatal operative field visualized with the exoscope: the first step of BRP surgery is tonsillectomy, saving as much of the muscular component of the lateral walls of the pharynx as possible.

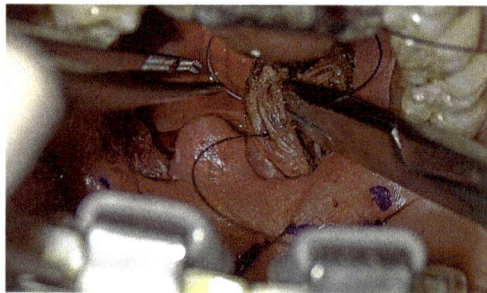

Figure 4. One of the most important step of BRP surgery: the needle must be introduced, from the lateral to the medial regions, posterior to the palato-pharyngeal muscle bundle, which is most commonly at the junction between the superior third and the inferior two thirds of it. The technique requires a second passage at the back, lateral to the raphe and the application of proper tension to the suture in order to reposition the palatopharyngeal muscle more laterally and more anteriorly.

3. Results

Currently, seven patients affected by OSA underwent 3D surgery with BRP associated with transoral coblation tongue base reduction and nose surgery. The median age was 53 years (range 40–66), and the median preoperative apnoea–hypopnea index (AHI) and body mass index (BMI) were 30.7 (2536) and 28.9 (23.7–31.5), respectively. The median preoperative Epworth Sleepiness Scale (ESS) score was 10 (6–14). The median 3D system setting time was 12.5 ± 2.3 min. The overall procedure time was 59.3 ± 26 min.

No patients experienced intra-operative, post-operative or delayed complications.

Only one patient experienced a transient dysphagia that spontaneously resolved within one month.

4. Discussion

Preliminary evaluations allow us to make some important considerations.

No significant differences were found in the setup times and preparation of the room, both in case of the use of the robot and the coblator (despite the initial difficulties related to the use of a new surgical instrument compared to those of the robot, which has been used for years). The robotic operating room setup times briefly include: docking (the patient side cart was moved to the edge of the patient bed and aligned at a 30° angle from the long axis of the patient surgical bed); exposure of the operative field with Crowe–Davis retractor in order to place the robotic arms in the patient's mouth: the camera's endoscope arm was positioned in the center of the patient's mouth, while the right and left instrument arms were the operative tools used for tissue dissection.

Even the exposure qualities in order to optimally operate are not significantly different despite the two different methods. The 3D visualization of the robot makes it possible to acknowledge small details, such as vascular and nerve structures, which would be difficult to see with the naked eye, allowing a precise and sometimes almost completely bloodless resection to be performed. The quality of visualization using the 4K-3D endoscope, on the other hand, allows the optimal assessment of the depth of field, enabling the surgeon to be attentive and accurate in the resection, despite the initial discomfort/difficulty encountered in coordinating the visualization of the monitor in front of them and gestures linked to the use of the coblator via the transoral route. The similar quality of exposure and visualization means that the resection times are comparable between the two sides, averaging around 10 min for the removal of a lingual tonsil.

The differences between the two approaches are mainly related to the introduction of a new surgical instrument, such as the coblator and the 3D 4K endoscope/exoscope, in the operating field. Therefore, it was harder to prepare the operating field and performing the resection of the baselingual lymphatic tissue, especially for the first patients. It should also be considered, as already mentioned, the initial difficulties related to the innovative use of the coblator on the base tongue and the correct coordination between visual feedback, while the operator's head is extended in order to correctly view the surgical field on the monitor in front of them with 3D polarized glasses, as well as tactile feedback, which is given via the direct contact between the surgeon and the oropharyngeal district. With the robot, as we know, there is no direct contact between the first operator and the patient.

Other major differences were found considering the extent of resection, which according to a first subjective judgement of the surgeon, was greater for the robot. As a matter of fact, robotic baselingual resection has become by now a standard procedure: the identification of the midline of the superior (terminal sulcus), lateral (amygdala-glossal sulcus) and inferior margins (glossoepiglottic sulcus). With both procedures, a similar number of small intraoperative bleeding events occurred, which were slightly more common when they were performed using the coblator (about 3 on average versus 12 bleedings, or sometimes, complete exsanguination), and which could be easily managed by the second operator handling bipolar forceps, while using the robot, or letting the bleedings clot, while using the coblator.

This allows us to underline further differences between the two systems, as well as the need in robotic surgery for two operators to work together during the surgical procedure. As mentioned above, the second operator has a very important role in order to eliminate any issues that may arise by using robotic arms and to aspirate fumes that may obstruct the view of the first surgeon or to control small intraoperative bleedings with bipolar forceps.

The last difference is the possibility with the robot to obtain samples that can be histologically evaluated, contrary to the coblator, whose main task is linked to the production of bioproducts that determine cellular destruction and allows the tissue resection to be macroscopically performed. This leads us to understand how much more useful the coblator can be in functional surgery compared to neoplastic pathology in which the production of an operative piece is fundamental for the performance of a histological examination.

A very important aspect that should not be overlooked is the difference in the costs between the two technologies. The price of the Da Vinci Robot is around EUR 2,000,000, with annual maintenance costs of around EUR 200,000; each intervention, depending on the type, has a cost that varies from EUR 4500 to 6500. The endoscope + exoscope 4K-3D system has a much lower price, around EUR 200,000, with an additional EUR 20,000 for the purchase of the coblator and an intervention's cost of less than EUR 1000. Furthermore, the possibility of using 4K-3D technology not only for rhonchi surgery, but also for salivary gland [5], thyroid and ear surgeries in ENT pathology [6,7], as well as laparoscopic approaches in general surgery and gynecology [8], makes it possible to quickly bring down the initial purchase costs.

Finally, the possibility of using Vitom in palatal surgery, although it may seem to be "excessive" and expensive, fulfils an important didactic function: it allows the whole surgical team to visualize a very deep and dark anatomical region, such as the soft palate. Everyone can, therefore, follow the fundamental steps of isolating the palate-pharyngeal muscle and anchoring it to the pterygomandibular raphe on a 3D monitor using polarized glasses in order to stabilize the lateral walls of the pharynx.

5. Conclusions

In conclusion, the use of the 4K-3D endoscope and coblator for tongue base resectioning and of the 3D exoscope for lateral pharyngoplasty represents an excellent alternative system in multi-level OSA-related surgery that could reduce the costs of robotic surgery. Furthermore, it also can be used to teach and involve everyone in the surgical team and let them become more aware of the various steps of the surgical act.

Author Contributions: Conceptualization, C.V.; methodology, C.V.; software, A.E.; validation, C.V. and G.M.; formal analysis, A.E. and G.I.; investigation, G.C.; resources, A.C., A.M. and T.M.; data curation, F.M. and F.F.; writing—original draft preparation, A.E.; writing—review and editing, G.C.; visualization, G.M.; supervision, C.V.; project administration, C.V. and G.M.; funding acquisition, G.C. All authors have read and agreed to the published version of the manuscript.

Funding: This research received no external funding.

Institutional Review Board Statement: The study was conducted in accordance with the Declaration of Helsinki, and approved by the Institutional Review Board (or Ethics Committee of the Morgagni-Pierantoni Hospital) (rif. 34/2022 on 10 March 2022).

Informed Consent Statement: Informed consent was obtained from all individual participants included in the study. My manuscript has no associated data.

Data Availability Statement: Not applicable.

Conflicts of Interest: All authors certify that they have no affiliations with or involvement in any organization or entity with any financial interest (such as honoraria; educational grants; participation in speakers' bureaus; membership, employment, consultancies, stock ownership, or other equity interest; and expert testimony or patent-licensing arrangements), or non-financial interest (such as personal or professional relationships, affiliations, knowledge or beliefs) in the subject matter or materials discussed in this manuscript.

References

1. Iannella, G.; Magliulo, G.; Greco, A.; de Vincentiis, M.; Ralli, M.; Maniaci, A.; Pace, A.; Vicini, C. Obstructive Sleep Apnea Syndrome: From Symptoms to Treatment. *Int. J. Environ. Res. Public Health* **2022**, *19*, 2459. [CrossRef] [PubMed]
2. Crawford, J.A.; Montevecchi, F.; Vicini, C.; Magnuson, J.S. Transoral robotic sleep surgery: The obstructive sleep apnea-hypopnea syndrome. *Otolaryngol. Clin. N. Am.* **2014**, *47*, 397–406. [CrossRef]
3. Vicini, C.; Montevecchi, F.; Gobbi, R.; De Vito, A.; Meccariello, G. Transoral robotic surgery for obstructive sleep apnea syndrome: Principles and technique. *World J. Otorhinolaryngol. Head Neck Surg.* **2017**, *3*, 97–100. [CrossRef] [PubMed]
4. Vicini, C.; Meccariello, G.; Cammaroto, G.; Rashwan, M.; Montevecchi, F. Barbed reposition pharyngoplasty in multilevel robotic surgery for obstructive sleep apnoea. *Acta Otorhinolaryngol. Ital.* **2017**, *37*, 214–217. [CrossRef] [PubMed]
5. Mincione, A.; Lepera, D.; Rizzi, L. VITOM 3D System in Parotid Gland Surgery: Our Experience. *J. Craniofac. Surg.* **2021**, *32*, e138–e141. [CrossRef] [PubMed]
6. Kullar, P.; Tanna, R.; Ally, M.; Vijendren, A.; Mochloulis, G. VITOM 4K 3D Exoscope: A Preliminary Experience in Thyroid Surgery. *Cureus* **2021**, *13*, e12694. [CrossRef] [PubMed]
7. Tan, S.H.; Kulasegarah, J.; Prepageran, N. A three-dimensional exoscope system for bilateral simultaneous cochlear implant surgery: How I do it. *J. Laryngol. Otol.* **2022**, *136*, 360–362. [CrossRef] [PubMed]
8. Taylor, B.; Myers, E.M. Initial Gynecologic Experience Using the VITOM® HD Exoscope for Vaginal Surgery. *J. Minim. Invasive Gynecol.* **2015**, *22*, S103. [CrossRef] [PubMed]

Disclaimer/Publisher's Note: The statements, opinions and data contained in all publications are solely those of the individual author(s) and contributor(s) and not of MDPI and/or the editor(s). MDPI and/or the editor(s) disclaim responsibility for any injury to people or property resulting from any ideas, methods, instructions or products referred to in the content.

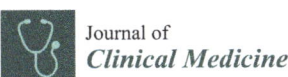

Systematic Review

Radiomics-Based Analysis in the Prediction of Occult Lymph Node Metastases in Patients with Oral Cancer: A Systematic Review

Serena Jiang [1,*], Luca Giovanni Locatello [2], Giandomenico Maggiore [1] and Oreste Gallo [1]

1. Department of Otorhinolaryngology, Careggi University Hospital, Largo Brambilla 3, 50134 Florence, Italy
2. Department of Otorhinolaryngology, University Hospital "Santa Maria Della Misericordia", Azienda Sanitaria Universitaria Friuli Centrale (ASUFC), 33100 Udine, Italy; locatello.lucagiovanni@gmail.com
* Correspondence: serena.jiang@unifi.it; Tel.: +39-0557947989

Abstract: Background: Tumor extension and metastatic cervical lymph nodes' (LNs) number and dimensions are major prognostic factors in patients with oral squamous cell carcinoma (OSCC). Radiomics-based models are being integrated into clinical practice in the prediction of LN status prior to surgery in order to optimize the treatment, yet their value is still debated. Methods: A systematic review of the literature was conducted according to the PRISMA guideline. Baseline study characteristics, and methodological items were extracted and summarized. Results: A total of 10 retrospective studies were included into the present study, each of them exploiting a single imaging modality. Data from a cohort of 1489 patients were analyzed: the highest AUC value was 99.5%, ACC ranges from 68% to 97.5%, and sensibility and specificity were over 0.65 and 0.70, respectively. Conclusion: Radiomics may be a noninvasive tool to predict occult LN metastases (LNM) in OSCC patients prior to treatment; further prospective studies are warranted to create a reproducible and reliable method for the detection of LNM in OSCC.

Keywords: radiomics; head and neck; cancer; oral squamous cell carcinoma; oral carcinoma artificial intelligence

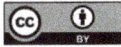

1. Introduction

Oral squamous cell carcinoma (OSCC) is the eighth most common malignancy worldwide [1]. It has a poor prognosis, with an overall 5-year survival rate of around 45–55% depending on the series considered [2]. This figure is much lower (around 20–30% at five years) especially in advanced stages according to the eighth edition of the AJCC/UICC [3]. The major prognostic factors are depth of invasion (DOI) > 5 mm, extranodal extension, positive or close surgical margins, pT3 or pT4 tumor (i.e., larger than 4 cm or infiltrating bony structures such as the mandible), pN2 or pN3 nodal disease, perineural invasion, vascular invasion, and lymphatic invasion. In particular, the presence of lymph node metastases (LNM) alone is known to reduce survival by approximately 50% [4].

The standard of care for OSCC is complete surgical resection with sufficient surgical margins (at least 5 mm are deemed necessary), followed by adjuvant radio-/chemotherapy in properly selected cases where the aforementioned adverse prognostic features are present. The following therapeutic strategies are currently available in managing a clinically negative (cN0) neck in early stage OSCCs [5]:

1. Elective neck dissection (ND): which is associated with esthetic and functional morbidity and it represents a procedure that may affect negatively the quality of life of the patient; the decision on whether to perform or not ND in all cases of cN0 neck is still under debate [6];

2. Watch and wait policy: this is currently disregarded as a valid option because it was substantially demonstrated that elective neck dissection resulted in longer overall and disease-free survival than did therapeutic neck dissection after nodal relapse [7];
3. Sentinel node biopsy (SNB): in 2015, the Sentinel European Node Trial (SENT) reported an overall sensitivity and negative predictive value of 86% and 95%, respectively [8], and this strategy may be considered the current gold standard for early stage OSCC [9].

The introduction of artificial intelligence (AI) and its application to clinical decision-making in order to individualize patient care has become a major topic of discussion. Radiomics is a machine-learning (ML) approach for image analyses using advanced mathematical analysis [10].

In recent years, due to the development of ML algorithms coupled with more accessible digital data, more and more researchers have begun to focus on predicting molecular biomarkers, therapeutic responses, and survival prognostic factors in patients with head and neck (HN) carcinomas by extracting radiomics information features (e.g., shape description, intensity, or texture characteristics) from different imaging patterns (e.g., CT, MRI, PET, ultrasound images) [11]; in Mossinelli's [12] retrospective study on 79 patients with oral tongue squamous cell carcinoma (OTSCC) MRI-based radiomics represents a promising noninvasive method of precision medicine, improving prognosis prediction before surgery.

Different non-invasive strategies exist for the prediction of LN status: clinical examination by digital palpation, neck imaging by ultrasound/CT/MRI potentially coupled with fine-needle aspiration of the suspected nodes, DNA microarray gene-expression profiling [13], nuclear medicine techniques such as positron emission tomography, the degree of differentiation of the primary tumor or the depth of invasion [14], but the gold standard is postoperative histopathological examination of the LNs. As a matter of fact, only a detailed (by simple microscopy and by techniques of immunohistochemistry) examination of the excised specimens can allow a surgical pathologist to identify micrometastases, which would have otherwise been overlooked. Despite the fact that ND is associated with many potential surgical complications, it remains true that up to 30% of early stage disease has occult cervical micrometastatic disease [15].

If we rely only upon preoperative standard imaging techniques, we know that lymph nodes larger than 10 mm are considered abnormal, yet around 20% of such nodes are pathologically free of disease, while up to 23% of nodes that show histological extracapsular spread measure less than 10 mm. Other features such as the presence of intranodal necrosis or irregular margins may indicate cancerous involvement but with variable accuracy [16,17].

In order to improve the diagnostic yield of these techniques, radiomics analyses have been successfully applied to predict the LN status of colorectal [18], cervical [19], and bladder cancer [20]. The role of radiomics in the assessment of occult lymph nodes in OSCCs patients have never been addressed to the best of our knowledge, and the aim of the present systematic review is to summarize the currently available clinical evidence on this topic while highlighting the unmet needs in this context.

2. Materials and Methods

2.1. Searching Strategy and Selection Criteria

Following the Preferred Reporting Items for Systematic Reviews and Meta-Analyses (PRISMA) guideline [21] we conducted a literature search of articles published from the beginning up to February 2023, using PubMed, Embase, Cochrane Library, and Scopus in order to identify the relevant studies. The following keywords were used: "radiomics AND oral cancer OR tumor".

We included all original studies that implemented radiomics-based algorithms for analyzing preoperative imaging in patients with proven histology of OSCC. Articles were excluded based on the following criteria: studies with less than 10 patients or case reports, meeting abstracts, review/meta-analysis, and data not clearly stating the diagnostic performance.

The present systematic review is unregistered.

2.2. Data Collection

The title and abstract of the selected papers were carefully read according to the inclusion and exclusion criteria and duplicates were removed. We extracted data from each study, which were reviewed for consistency among the authors, and any discrepancies were resolved by consensus. The full text of the included studies was then read in order to extract the following data:

Reference: first author, year of publication, and country;
Study design (retrospective, prospective);
Preoperative imaging technique;
Where the predictive imaging features were extracted from (primary tumor, cervical lymph nodes);
Software used for the radiomics-based analysis;
Recruitment time span;
Sample size: divided into primary/train cohort and validation/test cohort;
Tumoral subsite of the oral cavity and staging (TNM 8th edition);
Number of positive and negative LNs or number of patients with positive and negative nodes;
Diagnostic quantitative data: sensitivity, specificity, accuracy (ACC), area under the receiving operator curve (AUC).

2.3. Definition of the Outcomes, Synthesis of the Literature, and Meta-Analysis

In manuscripts where multiple ML models were implemented, we have chosen the one with the highest AUC value. Due to the heterogeneity of the preoperative imaging techniques, the segmentation and features extraction, it was not possible to meta-analyze the papers; it was thus decided to critically discuss all the articles qualitatively.

2.4. Quality Assessment and Statistical Methods

The quality and the risk of bias of the articles included in this review were evaluated by the Quality In Prognosis Studies (QUIPS) tool with any discrepancies resolved by consensus by the authors [22]. Visualization of the risk-of-bias assessments was performed by creating a traffic lights plot using the robvis tool (version 0.3.0.900) [23].

3. Results

A flowchart of the study selection process is reported in Figure 1. We identified a total of 419 articles, we excluded 35 duplicates and 301 records because they were not relevant; out of the 63 papers screened, a total of 10 manuscripts were selected for in-depth analysis as shown in Table 1.

The majority of the articles (70%) were published in 2022, one in 2020, one in 2021 and one in 2019, while none of the included articles was published before 2019.

All the studies were retrospective in nature and most of them were based on single-center evaluation with a variable number of patients (total n = 1489; range = 40–313). The preoperative imaging study was made using MRI in five studies, CT in four, and PET in a remaining one.

A total of 60% of the articles focused on primary carcinoma of the tongue, amongst other oral cavity subsites (gingiva, floor of mouth), with a predictable spotlight on early stages (stage I–II).

In more than half of the cases, a validation cohort was screened using the same criteria as that for the primary cohort. Where the segmentation subsite was the tumor, the partition into the validation and the primary cohort was made among the patients; on the contrary, when the subsite was the LN, the division was made among the examined LNs.

In 60% of the included articles, the predictive features for occult LNM were derived from radiological features of the primary tumor, while in 30% they were derived from the features of the LNs; overall, the most accurate diagnostic models were derived using tumor-based features.

The diagnostic performances of the included studies are summarized in Table 2. Wang et al. [26] reported the highest AUC value (0.995), meanwhile, the least value was observed by Kudoh [30] (0.79); ACC ranges from 0.68 to 0.975; sensibility and specificity, when reported, are over 0.65 and 0.70, respectively, in two out of seven they were above 0.90.

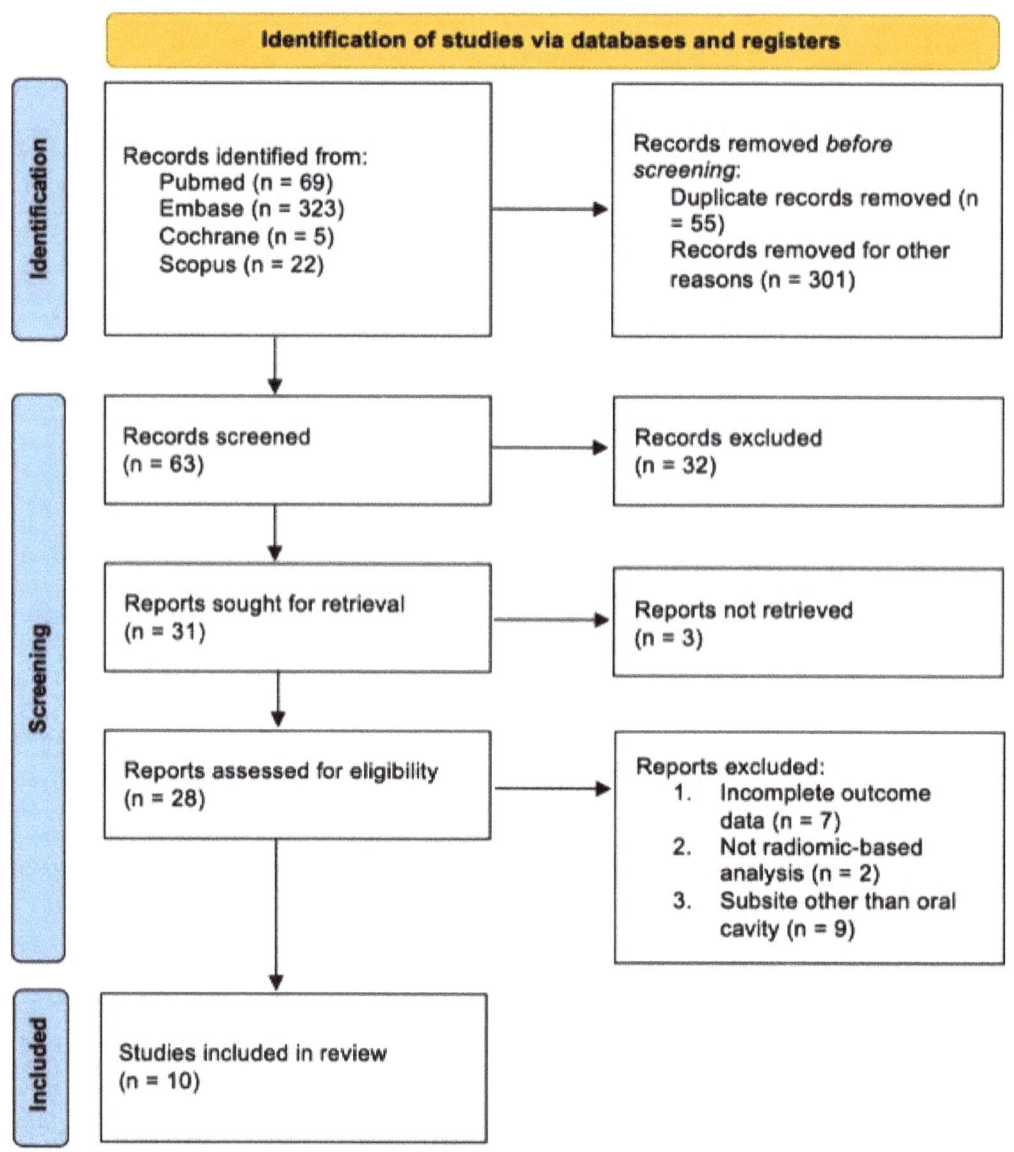

Figure 1. PRISMA flow diagram.

Table 1. Characteristics of the included studies. MRI, magnetic resonance imaging; CT, computed tomography; PET, positron emission tomography; LN, lymph node; NA, not available; pts, patients.

Study	Country	Study Type (Retrospective R, Prospective P)	Imaging Technique (MRI 1, CT 2, PET 3)	Feature Extraction	Software	Year of Recruitment	Sample Size (n)	Primary/Train Cohort (%)	Validation/Test Cohort (%)	Subsite (%)	Staging	Positive LNs (n)	Negative LNs (n)
Wang Y et al., 2022 [24]	China	R	1	LN	LIFEx (EVOMICS)	2013–2021	160	75	25	100 oral cavity (70.1 tongue)	61 I–II 39 III–IV	NA	NA
Tomita et al., 2021 [25]	Japan	R	2	LN	Python	2013–2017	44	70	30	100 oral (tongue, gingiva, floor of mouth)	I–IV	51	150
Wang F et al., 2022 [26]	China	R	1	Tumor	Python (version 3.5.2)	2012–2019	236	67	33	100 tongue	I–IV	99	137
Kubo et al., 2022 [27]	Japan	R	2	LN	Python (Pyradiomics software)	2008–2019	161	NA	NA	100 tongue	I–III	63	NA
Zhong et al., 2022 [28]	China	R	2	Tumor	Matlab 2018b (MathWork)	2013–2018	313	60	40	100 tongue	I–IV	143	170
Committeri et al., 2022 [29]	Italy	R	2	Tumor	PyRadiomics	2016–2020	81	80	20	100 tongue	I–II	NA	NA
Kudoh et al., 2022 [30]	Japan	R	3	Tumor	Matlab	2015–2019	40	80	20	100 tongue	15 I, 30 II, 18 III, 37 IV	19 pts	21 pts
Traverso et al., 2020 [31]	Multicentric	R	1	NA	PyRadiomics v2.1.2	2003–2017	243	70	30	100 oral	NA	NA	NA
Traverso et al., 2019 [32]	Multicentric	R	1	Tumor	PyRadiomics	NA	134	80	20	100 oral	NA	NA	NA
Ren et al., 2022 [33]	China	R	1	Tumor	Pyradiomics	2015–2021	55	NA	NA	100 tongue	I–II	21 pts	34 pts

Table 2. Diagnostic performance of the included studies. ACC, accuracy; AUC, Area Under the Curve; NA, not available.

Study	Sensitivity	Specificity	ACC (95%CI)	AUC (95%CI)
Wang Y et al., 2022 [24]	0.85	0.71	0.79	0.82
Tomita et al., 2021 [25]	0.74	0.88	0.85	0.85
Wang F et al., 2022 [26]	0.95	0.98	0.97	0.99
Kubo et al., 2022 [27]	NA	NA	0.85	0.92
Zhong et al., 2022 [28]	0.82	0.87	0.84	0.91
Committeri et al., 2022 [29]	0.94	0.98	0.96	0.93
Kudoh et al., 2022 [30]	0.65	0.70	0.68 ± 0.13	0.79
Traverso et al., 2020 [31]	NA	NA	0.70 (0.67–0.71)	NA
Traverso et al., 2019 [32]	NA	NA	NA	0.83
Ren et al., 2022 [33]	0.79	0.86	0.82	0.87 (0.77–0.96)

Only three studies included a comparative analysis of the ML model with the radiologists' evaluation: Committeri et al. [29] demonstrated a better performance of radiomics over the clinician's performance, in Ren's study [33] they were similar, and Wang Y [24] reported slightly worse values for ML model. Expectedly, the combination of clinical and ML models outperformed the single modality.

A traffic lights plot was created to visualize the risk-of-bias assessment (Figure 2), with a moderate-to-low risk of bias among all the included studies.

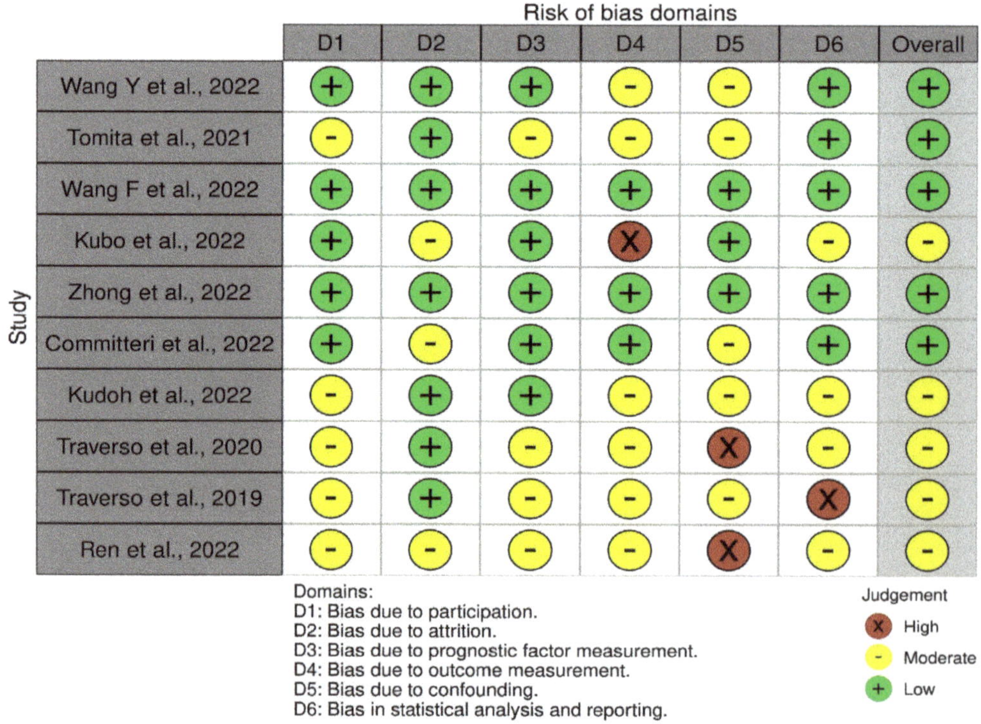

Figure 2. Traffic lights plot [24–33].

4. Discussion

In the present systematic review, we examined the use of radiomics-based analysis for the detection of occult neck metastasis in OSCC. Given the prognostic value of any nodal metastasis, early detection of OSCC and a comprehensive therapeutic strategy for both the primary tumor and the associated lymph nodes are of utmost importance.

Radiomics is a growing area of research that extracts and models medical image features using ML methods. Its goal is to implement AI algorithms in order to create a more accurate, cost-effective, and patient-tailored diagnostic and/or therapeutic tool. In the literature there are multiple studies that use radiomics for HN tumors: various authors critically reviewed the developments in diagnostic and therapeutic approaches in nasopharyngeal [34], laryngeal [35], thyroid [36], and salivary gland tumors [37]. Giannitto et al. [38] focused the attention on the diagnostic accuracy and methodological quality items in radiomics-based ML for the diagnosis of LNM in patients with HN cancer; however, the review did not discriminate outcomes based on tumor subsite, with almost half of the patients being affected by thyroid tumor. Additionally, Romeo et al. [39] used a similar approach in the prediction of tumor grade and nodal status on oropharyngeal and oral carcinomas.

ML models can be applied potentially to all imaging techniques, although it is preferentially used for more standardizable and reproducible ones, such as CT and MR. In the included papers, only Kudoh et al. [30] processed PET images and, interestingly, they reported the lowest diagnostic performance. Moreover, like the vast majority of studies of radiomics in HN, the studies herein analyzed are based on a single imaging modality.

Apart from the chosen imaging protocol, methodological heterogeneity is present also in the delineation of the region of interest (ROI), in the software used for image elaboration and radiomics feature extraction and processing.

Useful data on nodal status can be obtained even from the primary tumor mass because it is probably related to tumor biological heterogeneity and aggressiveness. As a matter of fact, the majority of the studies in our review extracted features from tumors (6), while only three were from LNs.

By focusing on these latter, in Wang's article [24] the inclusion criteria were as follows: histopathologically proven OSCC who underwent ND and preoperative MRI contrast-enhanced scans of the head and neck. The LN with the "largest volume or with unclear edges and internal necrosis", that is radiologically suspicious lymph nodes, were selected as the ROI. Only eight features were used to build the radiomics model. Tomita's study [25] also included patients with histologically proven OSCC with benign or metastatic cervical LNs and available preoperative contrast-enhanced CT data. ROIs were drawn across all slices of the cross-sectional areas of the targeted LNs, that is those levels that were known to harbor micrometastases at final histopathology. For the evaluation of the CT scans, three radiologists independently assessed the LN status using specific criteria to determine if they were considered metastatic. The AUC values of the best ML-based model were superior to those of each individual human reader ($p < 0.05$); additionally, there were significant differences in specificity and diagnostic accuracy rates between them, demonstrating the potential of radiomics analysis in improving the accuracy of LN status assessment compared to human readers. Lastly, Kubo et al. [27] focused on cN0 patients diagnosed with tongue cancer who received treatment aimed at the primary tumor site without additional therapies (elective ND, chemotherapy). For patients that developed occult cervical LNM, but with no recurrence of the primary tumor, salvage surgery was performed, and histological analysis confirmed the presence of metastatic squamous cell carcinoma in these LNs. To analyze the CT scans, two radiation oncologists manually contoured each neck node level slice by slice in the axial plane rather than the primary tumor. It is crucial to point out that Wang Y [24] and Tomita [25] conducted an analysis on patients with suspicious LN that could be detected preoperatively on the radiological scans and then underwent ND. By comparing the results of AI-based analysis with clinical assessments, they can evaluate the potential of ML-based models as a tool in diagnosing and predicting malignancy in patients with positive LNs. Unsurprisingly, the choice of the ROI where to perform the extraction of the features was performed retrospectively. ML has the main objective to identify occult nodal disease: even if the exact ROI may be ambiguous where no radiologically suspicious region exists by definition, the anatomical levels most at risk (e.g., ipsilateral I-II-III levels for a cancer of the lateral tongue margin) remain those to assess with the focus on LNs rather than the primary tumor site, the researchers aim to improve the accuracy of cervical nodal staging; furthermore, the primary tumor itself could sometimes be challenging to contour accurately due to artifacts or its small size [27], while contouring neck nodes could be a more standardized process with fewer variations among different individuals.

Divergence in the qualitative items comes along with quantitative differences (e.g., number of images and/or features extracted). It is misleading to evaluate the performance of ML when diverse choices, selection methods, and classifiers are applied because the resulting models become sensitive to perturbation, contamination, and leakage of data.

Concerning the performance evaluation, and by excluding Kudoh's results [30], AUC is over 82% in the reviewed studies. Only three out of ten conducted generalizability assessment with an independent ($n = 1$) or an external validation cohort.

There are many articles that introduce conventional imaging methods to predict cervical LN status early in OSCC. Van den Brekel et al. [40] compared the performance of ultrasound, CT, and MRI in 88 cN0 necks: sensitivity, specificity, and accuracy were for ultrasound 58%, 75%, and 68%, for CT 49%, 78%, and 66%, for MRI 55%, 88%, and 75%, respectively; FDG-PET studies reported sensitivity and specificity are quite variable: although this imaging modality is very useful in differentiating between benign and metastatic cervical LNs, inflammation and small nodal size can affect the nodal status assessment [41].

The current review found five studies that reported the traditional diagnostic performance of the radiologists; it is interesting to note that the average AUC, ACC, sensibility, and specificity curves of the clinicopathological factors were not always lower than those of the radiomics features. Wang Y et al. [24] found that the AUC of the model of MRI radiomic features was 0.88, which was better than that of the ADC and LN size; also Tomita [25] claimed that the radiomics approach yielded better diagnostic performance for differentiating between benign and metastatic cervical LNs than conventional CT; in Wang's article [26] multivariate logistic regression analysis identified MRI-reported LN status (OR 2.432, 95% CI, 1.093–5.411) as an independent predictor of LNM. Kudoh [30] demonstrated that the 18F-FDG PET-based model had better potential for diagnosing cervical LNM and predicting late LNM in patients with OSCC than the clinicopathological factors model. Eventually, none of them performed a decision curve analysis to offer clinical guidelines for the preoperative management of the patient.

The specificity of ultrasound-guided FNAC is approximately 100%, advantages of the technique are its relatively low cost, lack of radiation exposure, and low-threshold availability; the main drawbacks are the sampling error of the aspirate due to the small size or inaccessibility of the LN and the operator-dependent nature of the procedure. If radiomic features of the primary tumor can outperform diagnostic assessment of the neck with imaging or ultrasound-guided FNAC is a demanding query to which we cannot give an answer yet [42]. However, cross-sectional imaging has the advantage to perform a full assessment of the lymph nodes, while FNAC is capable to sample only a part of it where the tumoral cells might not be identified.

The ambition of AI-based models is to help clinical evaluations in detecting occult LNM in OSCCs and unfortunately, a meta-analysis could not be conducted for the aforementioned methodological issues: this is the first limitation of our work.

Other limitations that must be acknowledged are the failure to validate model performance on a large, independent, external data set that prevents the applicability of findings to populations at large scale; the absence of well-structured, public/open, and worldwide "big data", and of the methods used for training. AI-based algorithms notably require an enormous quantity of input information, therefore even in the face of over a thousand patients, we are far from reaching a definite answer in this field [43]. In this regard, the standardization of the automated methods, and the availability of high-quality open-source data seem imperative. Moreover, no prospective studies have been conducted and there is still the problem of "overfitting" which happens when AI gives undue importance to spurious correlations within past data.

All the reviewed articles are retrospective and they support and echo these findings.

This systematic review is poor in terms of clinical utility evaluation. We conducted a meticulous and independent search, according to PRISMA guidelines, of multiple online-available databases in order to provide an overview of the best performance of radiomics in LN status characterization in OSCCs; we wanted to highlight the strengths of this analysis but also the weak points, in order to create a shared approach in terms of both feature computation and methodology that will hopefully move this field of research to the routine clinical practice.

This is a rapidly evolving research area. Nowadays, we can talk about "multi-omics" data analysis (radiomics, genomics, proteomics, and metabolomics) that can be integrated with clinicopathological factors to help in accurate disease prediction, patient stratification, and delivery of precision medicine [44].

Radiomics prediction model has the potential to become a non-invasive diagnostic tool for HN cancer and LN status before treatment. By digitizing and analyzing the medical image data, the model's predictions become more objective and standardized, thus reducing potential subjectivity in the diagnosis process and human error. Secondly, models can be validated and modified as more data becomes available, further enhancing its accuracy and reliability; moreover, AI may support inexperienced doctors in the assessment of lesions. This possibility also introduces medico-legal issues since the medical human judgment can fail as well as the AI: who would be liable if a mistake is made during AI-enhanced decision-making—such as ML-aided radiological diagnosis [45,46].

Cost-effective AI models can allow hospitals to incorporate the latter into daily clinical use; in order to make it happen, in addition to the development of a shared database of different medical centers from all over the world, prospective studies with a uniform and standardized imaging and processing protocol applied on a large and homogeneous cohort with an independent and/or external validation cohort should be conducted.

5. Conclusions

This systematic review provides an overview of the performance of radiomics-based models concerning the LN status in OSCCs. From our preliminary findings, the addition of AI-based models in the assessment of preoperative imaging may satisfactorily improve the detection of pathological lymph nodes in OSCC's patients. Future reproduction of our results in other cohorts and by a uniform analytical protocol is anticipated. Finally, a proper clinical validation of these models in terms of oncological endpoints such as survival and disease-free recurrence is needed before incorporating these models in the decision-making process for these patients.

Author Contributions: S.J.: data curation, formal analysis, investigation, methodology, validation, visualization, and writing—original draft. L.G.L. and G.M.: conceptualization, project administration, validation, visualization, supervision, review, and editing. O.G.: Conceptualization, project administration, resources, supervision, review, and editing. All authors have read and agreed to the published version of the manuscript.

Funding: This research received no external funding.

Institutional Review Board Statement: Not applicable. The study protocol was performed in accordance with the Declaration of Helsinki.

Informed Consent Statement: Informed consent was obtained from all subjects involved in the study.

Data Availability Statement: The data that support the findings of this study are openly available in Pubmed, Embase, Scholar.

Conflicts of Interest: The authors declare no conflict of interest.

References

1. Elaiwy, O.; El Ansari, W.; AlKhalil, M.; Ammar, A. Epidemiology and pathology of oral squamous cell carcinoma in a multi-ethnic population: Retrospective study of 154 cases over 7 years in Qatar. *Ann. Med. Surg.* **2020**, *60*, 195–200. [CrossRef] [PubMed]
2. Abati, S.; Bramati, C.; Bondi, S.; Lissoni, A.; Trimarchi, M. Oral Cancer and Precancer: A Narrative Review on the Relevance of Early Diagnosis. *Int. J. Environ. Res. Public Health* **2020**, *17*, 9160. [CrossRef] [PubMed]
3. Amin, M.B.; Edge, S.; Greene, F.; Byrd, D.R.; Brookland, R.K.; Washington, M.K.; Gershenwald, J.E.; Compton, C.C.; Hess, K.R.; Sullivan, D.C.; et al. *AJCC Cancer Staging Manual*, 8th ed.; Springer: Chicago, IL, USA, 2009.
4. Matos, L.L.; Guimarães, Y.L.M.; Leite, A.K.; Cernea, C.R. Management of Stage III Oral Cavity Squamous Cell Carcinoma in Light of the New Staging System: A Critical Review. *Curr. Oncol. Rep.* **2023**, *25*, 107–113. [CrossRef]
5. Vassiliou, L.V.; Acero, J.; Gulati, A.; Hölzle, F.; Hutchison, I.L.; Prabhu, S.; Testelin, S.; Wolff, K.-D.; Kalavrezos, N. Management of the clinically N0 neck in early-stage oral squamous cell carcinoma (OSCC). An EACMFS position paper. *J. Cranio-Maxillofac. Surg.* **2020**, *48*, 711–718. [CrossRef]
6. De Bree, R.; Takes, R.P.; Shah, J.P.; Hamoir, M.; Kowalski, L.P.; Robbins, K.T.; Rodrigo, J.P.; Sanabria, A.; Medina, J.E.; Rinaldo, A.; et al. Elective neck dissection in oral squamous cell carcinoma: Past, present and future. *Oral Oncol.* **2019**, *90*, 87–93. [CrossRef]
7. Ren, Z.-H.; Xu, J.-L.; Li, B.; Fan, T.-F.; Ji, T.; Zhang, C.-P. Elective versus therapeutic neck dissection in node-negative oral cancer: Evidence from five randomized controlled trials. *Oral Oncol.* **2015**, *51*, 976–981. [CrossRef] [PubMed]
8. Gupta, T.; Maheshwari, G.; Kannan, S.; Nair, S.; Agarwal, J.P. Should Sentinel Lymph Node Biopsy Be Considered the New Standard of Care for Early-Stage Clinically Node-Negative Oral Squamous Cell Carcinoma? *J. Clin. Oncol.* **2022**, *40*, 1706–1709. [CrossRef]
9. Schilling, C.; Stoeckli, S.J.; Haerle, S.K.; Broglie, M.A.; Huber, G.F.; Sorensen, J.A.; Bakholdt, V.; Krogdahl, A.; von Buchwald, C.; Bilde, A.; et al. Sentinel European Node Trial (SENT): 3-year results of sentinel node biopsy in oral cancer. *Eur. J. Cancer* **2015**, *51*, 2777–2784. [CrossRef] [PubMed]
10. Van Dijk, L.V.; Fuller, C.D. Artificial Intelligence and Radiomics in Head and Neck Cancer Care: Opportunities, Mechanics, and Challenges. *Am. Soc. Clin. Oncol. Educ. Book* **2021**, *41*, e225–e235. [CrossRef]
11. Peng, Z.; Wang, Y.; Wang, Y.; Jiang, S.; Fan, R.; Zhang, H.; Jiang, W. Application of radiomics and machine learning in head and neck cancers. *Int. J. Biol. Sci.* **2021**, *17*, 475–486. [CrossRef] [PubMed]
12. Mossinelli, C.; Tagliabue, M.; Ruju, F.; Cammarata, G.; Volpe, S.; Raimondi, S.; Zaffaroni, M.; Isaksson, J.L.; Garibaldi, C.; Cremonesi, M.; et al. The role of radiomics in tongue cancer: A new tool for prognosis prediction. *Head Neck* **2023**, *45*, 849–861. [CrossRef] [PubMed]
13. Roepman, P.; Wessels, L.F.A.; Kettelarij, N.; Kemmeren, P.; Miles, A.J.; Lijnzaad, P.; Tilanus, M.G.J.; Koole, R.; Hordijk, G.-J.; van der Vliet, P.C.; et al. An expression profile for diagnosis of lymph node metastases from primary head and neck squamous cell carcinomas. *Nat. Genet.* **2005**, *37*, 182–186. [CrossRef]
14. Faisal, M.; Abu Bakar, M.; Sarwar, A.; Adeel, M.; Batool, F.; Malik, K.I.; Jamshed, A.; Hussain, R. Depth of invasion (DOI) as a predictor of cervical nodal metastasis and local recurrence in early stage squamous cell carcinoma of oral tongue (ESSCOT). *PLoS ONE* **2018**, *13*, e0202632. [CrossRef]
15. Jang, S.S.; Davis, M.E.; Vera, D.R.; Lai, S.Y.; Guo, T.W. Role of sentinel lymph node biopsy for oral squamous cell carcinoma: Current evidence and future challenges. *Head Neck* **2023**, *45*, 251–265. [CrossRef] [PubMed]
16. Chong, V. Cervical lymphadenopathy: What radiologists need to know. *Cancer Imaging* **2004**, *4*, 116–120. [CrossRef] [PubMed]
17. van den Brekel, M.W.; Stel, H.V.; Castelijns, J.A.; Nauta, J.J.; van der Waal, I.; Valk, J.; Meyer, C.J.; Snow, G.B. Cervical lymph node metastasis: Assessment of radiologic criteria. *Radiology* **1990**, *177*, 379–384. [CrossRef] [PubMed]
18. Zhao, J.; Wang, H.; Zhang, Y.; Wang, R.; Liu, Q.; Li, J.; Li, X.; Huang, H.; Zhang, J.; Zeng, Z.; et al. Deep learning radiomics model related with genomics phenotypes for lymph node metastasis prediction in colorectal cancer. *Radiother. Oncol.* **2022**, *167*, 195–202. [CrossRef]
19. Li, H.; Zhu, M.; Jian, L.; Bi, F.; Zhang, X.; Fang, C.; Wang, Y.; Wang, J.; Wu, N.; Yu, X. Radiomic Score as a Potential Imaging Biomarker for Predicting Survival in Patients with Cervical Cancer. *Front. Oncol.* **2021**, *11*, 706043. [CrossRef]
20. Wu, S.; Zheng, J.; Li, Y.; Yu, H.; Shi, S.; Xie, W.; Liu, H.; Su, Y.; Huang, J.; Lin, T. A Radiomics Nomogram for the Preoperative Prediction of Lymph Node Metastasis in Bladder Cancer. *Clin. Cancer Res.* **2017**, *23*, 6904–6911. [CrossRef]
21. Liberati, M.; Tetzlaff, J.; Altman, D.G.; PRISMA Group. Preferred reporting items for systematic reviews and meta-analyses: The PRISMA statement. *PLoS Med.* **2009**, *6*, e1000097. [CrossRef] [PubMed]
22. Hayden, J.A.; Van Der Windt, D.A.; Cartwright, J.L.; Côté, P.; Bombardier, C. Assessing Bias in Studies of Prognostic Factors. *Ann. Intern. Med.* **2013**, *158*, 280–286. [CrossRef]

23. McGuinness, L.A.; Higgins, J.P.T. Risk-of-bias VISualization (robvis): An R package and Shiny web app for visualizing risk-of-bias assessments. *Res. Synth. Methods* **2021**, *12*, 55–61. [CrossRef] [PubMed]
24. Wang, Y.; Yu, T.; Yang, Z.; Zhou, Y.; Kang, Z.; Wang, Y.; Huang, Z. Radiomics based on magnetic resonance imaging for preoperative prediction of lymph node metastasis in head and neck cancer: Machine learning study. *Head Neck* **2022**, *44*, 2786–2795. [CrossRef] [PubMed]
25. Tomita, H.; Yamashiro, T.; Heianna, J.; Nakasone, T.; Kimura, Y.; Mimura, H.; Murayama, S. Nodal-based radiomics analysis for identifying cervical lymph node metastasis at levels I and II in patients with oral squamous cell carcinoma using contrast-enhanced computed tomography. *Eur. Radiol.* **2021**, *31*, 7440–7449. [CrossRef] [PubMed]
26. Wang, F.; Tan, R.; Feng, K.; Hu, J.; Zhuang, Z.; Wang, C.; Hou, J.; Liu, X. Magnetic Resonance Imaging-Based Radiomics Features Associated with Depth of Invasion Predicted Lymph Node Metastasis and Prognosis in Tongue Cancer. *J. Magn. Reson. Imaging* **2022**, *56*, 196–209. [CrossRef] [PubMed]
27. Kubo, K.; Kawahara, D.; Murakami, Y.; Takeuchi, Y.; Katsuta, T.; Imano, N.; Nishibuchi, I.; Saito, A.; Konishi, M.; Kakimoto, N.; et al. Development of a radiomics and machine learning model for predicting occult cervical lymph node metastasis in patients with tongue cancer. *Oral Surg. Oral Med. Oral Pathol. Oral Radiol.* **2022**, *134*, 93–101. [CrossRef] [PubMed]
28. Zhong, Y.-W.; Jiang, Y.; Dong, S.; Wu, W.-J.; Wang, L.-X.; Zhang, J.; Huang, M.-W. Tumor radiomics signature for artificial neural network-assisted detection of neck metastasis in patient with tongue cancer. *J. Neuroradiol.* **2022**, *49*, 213–218. [CrossRef]
29. Committeri, U.; Fusco, R.; Di Bernardo, E.; Abbate, V.; Salzano, G.; Maglitto, F.; Orabona, G.D.; Piombino, P.; Bonavolontà, P.; Arena, A.; et al. Radiomics Metrics Combined with Clinical Data in the Surgical Management of Early-Stage (cT1–T2 N0) Tongue Squamous Cell Carcinomas: A Preliminary Study. *Biology* **2022**, *11*, 468. [CrossRef]
30. Kudoh, T.; Haga, A.; Kudoh, K.; Takahashi, A.; Sasaki, M.; Kudo, Y.; Ikushima, H.; Miyamoto, Y. Radiomics analysis of [18F]-fluoro-2-deoxyglucose positron emission tomography for the prediction of cervical lymph node metastasis in tongue squamous cell carcinoma. *Oral. Radiol.* **2023**, *39*, 41–50, Erratum in: *Oral. Radiol.* **2022**, *39*, 51–52. [CrossRef]
31. Traverso, A.; Abdalaty, A.H.; Hasan, M.; Tadic, T.; Patel, T.; Giuliani, M.; Kim, J.; Ringash, J.; Cho, J.; Bratman, S.; et al. PO-1549: Non-invasive prediction of lymph node risk in oral cavity cancer patients. *Radiother. Oncol.* **2020**, *152*, S838. [CrossRef]
32. Traverso, A.; Hosni-Abdalaty, A.; Hasan, M.; Kim, J.; Ringash, J.; Cho, J.; Hope, A. Investigating Radiomics to Predict Positive Lymph Nodes in Oral Cavity Squamous Cell Carcinoma (OSCC). Scientific Abstracts and Sessions. *Med. Phys.* **2019**, *46*, e94–e670. [CrossRef]
33. Ren, J.; Yuan, Y.; Tao, X. Histogram analysis of diffusion-weighted imaging and dynamic contrast-enhanced MRI for predicting occult lymph node metastasis in early-stage oral tongue squamous cell carcinoma. *Eur. Radiol.* **2022**, *32*, 2739–2747. [CrossRef] [PubMed]
34. Zhang, Y.-M.; Gong, G.-Z.; Qiu, Q.-T.; Han, Y.-W.; Lu, H.-M.; Yin, Y. Radiomics for Diagnosis and Radiotherapy of Nasopharyngeal Carcinoma. *Front. Oncol.* **2022**, *11*, 767134. [CrossRef] [PubMed]
35. Rajgor, A.D.; Patel, S.; McCulloch, D.; Obara, B.; Bacardit, J.; McQueen, A.; Aboagye, E.; Ali, T.; O'hara, J.; Hamilton, D.W. The application of radiomics in laryngeal cancer. *Br. J. Radiol.* **2021**, *94*, 20210499. [CrossRef] [PubMed]
36. Gul, M.; Bonjoc, K.-J.C.; Gorlin, D.; Wong, C.W.; Salem, A.; La, V.; Filippov, A.; Chaudhry, A.; Imam, M.H.; Chaudhry, A.A. Diagnostic Utility of Radiomics in Thyroid and Head and Neck Cancers. *Front. Oncol.* **2021**, *11*, 639326. [CrossRef] [PubMed]
37. Aringhieri, G.; Fanni, S.C.; Febi, M.; Colligiani, L.; Cioni, D.; Neri, E. The Role of Radiomics in Salivary Gland Imaging: A Systematic Review and Radiomics Quality Assessment. *Diagnostics* **2022**, *12*, 3002. [CrossRef]
38. Giannitto, C.; Mercante, G.; Ammirabile, A.; Cerri, L.; De Giorgi, T.; Lofino, L.; Vatteroni, G.; Casiraghi, E.; Marra, S.; Esposito, A.A.; et al. Radiomics-based machine learning for the diagnosis of lymph node metastases in patients with head and neck cancer: Systematic review. *Head Neck* **2023**, *45*, 482–491. [CrossRef]
39. Romeo, V.; Cuocolo, R.; Ricciardi, C.; Ugga, L.; Cocozza, S.; Verde, F.; Stanzione, A.; Napolitano, V.; Russo, D.; Improta, G.; et al. Prediction of Tumor Grade and Nodal Status in Oropharyngeal and Oral Cavity Squamous-cell Carcinoma Using a Radiomic Approach. *Anticancer. Res.* **2020**, *40*, 271–280. [CrossRef]
40. Van den Brekel, M.W.; Castelijns, J.A.; Stel, H.V.; Golding, R.P.; Meyer, C.J.; Snow, G.B. Modern imaging techniques and ultrasound-guided aspiration cytology for the assessment of neck node metastases: A prospective comparative study. *Eur. Arch. Otorhinolaryngol.* **1993**, *250*, 11–17. [CrossRef]
41. Sun, R.; Tang, X.; Yang, Y.; Zhang, C. 18FDG-PET/CT for the detection of regional nodal metastasis in patients with head and neck cancer: A meta-analysis. *Oral Oncol.* **2015**, *51*, 314–320. [CrossRef]
42. De Bree, R.; Takes, R.P.; Castelijns, J.A.; Medina, J.E.; Stoeckli, S.J.; Mancuso, A.A.; Hunt, J.L.; Rodrigo, J.P.; Triantafyllou, A.; Teymoortash, A.; et al. Advances in diagnostic modalities to detect occult lymph node metastases in head and neck squamous cell carcinoma. *Head Neck* **2015**, *37*, 1829–1839. [CrossRef] [PubMed]
43. Hosny, A.; Parmar, C.; Quackenbush, J.; Schwartz, L.H.; Aerts, H.J.W.L. Artificial intelligence in radiology. *Nat. Rev. Cancer* **2018**, *18*, 500–510. [CrossRef] [PubMed]
44. Reel, P.S.; Reel, S.; Pearson, E.; Trucco, E.; Jefferson, E. Using machine learning approaches for multi-omics data analysis: A review. *Biotechnol. Adv.* **2021**, *49*, 107739. [CrossRef]

45. Quinn, T.P.; Senadeera, M.; Jacobs, S.; Coghlan, S.; Le, V. Trust and medical AI: The challenges we face and the expertise needed to overcome them. *J. Am. Med. Inform. Assoc.* **2021**, *28*, 890–894. [CrossRef]
46. Babushkina, D. Are we justified attributing a mistake in diagnosis to an AI diagnostic system? *AI Ethics* **2023**, *3*, 567–584. [CrossRef]

Disclaimer/Publisher's Note: The statements, opinions and data contained in all publications are solely those of the individual author(s) and contributor(s) and not of MDPI and/or the editor(s). MDPI and/or the editor(s) disclaim responsibility for any injury to people or property resulting from any ideas, methods, instructions or products referred to in the content.

MDPI
St. Alban-Anlage 66
4052 Basel
Switzerland
www.mdpi.com

Journal of Clinical Medicine Editorial Office
E-mail: jcm@mdpi.com
www.mdpi.com/journal/jcm

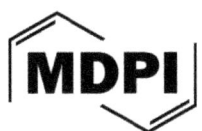

Disclaimer/Publisher's Note: The statements, opinions and data contained in all publications are solely those of the individual author(s) and contributor(s) and not of MDPI and/or the editor(s). MDPI and/or the editor(s) disclaim responsibility for any injury to people or property resulting from any ideas, methods, instructions or products referred to in the content.

www.ingramcontent.com/pod-product-compliance
Lightning Source LLC
LaVergne TN
LVHW070626100526
838202LV00012B/736